THE OCULAR FUNDUS IN SYSTEMIC DISEASE

THE OCULAR FUNDUS IN SYSTEMIC DISEASE

A CLINICAL PATHOLOGICAL CORRELATION

EDWARD M. CHESTER, M.D.
ASSOCIATE PROFESSOR OF MEDICINE
ASSOCIATE IN THE DIVISION OF RESEARCH IN MEDICAL EDUCATION
CASE WESTERN RESERVE UNIVERSITY
DIRECTOR, AMBULATORY TEACHING CLINIC
CLEVELAND METROPOLITAN GENERAL HOSPITAL

FOREWORD BY
THOMAS HALE HAM, M.D.
Director, The Division of Research in Medical Education
Hanna Payne Professor of Medicine
Case Western Reserve University

ILLUSTRATED BY
MARITA BITANS
Medical Illustrator
Cleveland Metropolitan General Hospital

PHOTOMICROGRAPHS BY
ROLLA B. McCASHEN
Supervisor, Division of Photography
Cleveland Metropolitan General Hospital

Retinal photographs by the author

THE PRESS OF CASE WESTERN RESERVE UNIVERSITY 1973

Distributed by Year Book Medical Publishers, Inc.
35 East Wacker Drive, Chicago 60601

Publication of this book was generously supported to assist in medical education and health care, by gifts from

The Carnegie Corporation of New York
The Division of Ophthalmology, Professor Charles I. Thomas, M.D., Director
The Department of Surgery, William D. Holden, M.D., Oliver H. Payne Professor and Director of Surgery, University Hospitals, Case Western Reserve University
The University Hospitals of Cleveland
Eli Lilly and Company, Indianapolis, Indiana
The Webster-Underhill Foundation, Mrs. Harold T. White, Chairman—Board of Trustees

Division of Research in Medical Education
School of Medicine
Case Western Reserve University
This publication was supported in part by NIH grant LM 00673 from the National Library of Medicine.

Library of Congress Catalog Card Number: 72-77961
International Standard Book Number: 0-8151-1657-8

To my wife, Mary

Contents

CHAPTER II. ARTERIAL AND ARTERIOLAR DISEASE

CHAPTER III. EXTRAVASCULAR LESIONS OF THE RETINA

CHAPTER IV. RETINAL VENOUS DISEASE

CHAPTER V. THE MICROANEURYSM

CHAPTER VI. NEOVASCULARIZATION AND PROLIFERATIVE RETINOPATHY

CHAPTER VII. DISEASE OF THE OPTIC NERVE

LISTS OF ILLUSTRATIONS

All the retinal photographs and photomicrographs have been enlarged two to four times in an attempt to accentuate the normal and abnormal findings. Scales indicated are those of the original photomicrographs.

CODE:

(D) Plate accompanied by drawing
(C) Color composite painting
(C) (D) Color composite painting and drawing
(FI) Fluorescein angiogram
Fig. Figure number . . .

THE NORMAL OCULAR FUNDUS

COMMON VARIANTS FROM NORMAL

Anomalies

LESIONS, ACCORDING TO DISEASE

Diabetic Retinopathy

ARTERIOLAR DISEASE

VENOUS DISEASE

LESIONS, ACCORDING TO DISEASE (cont.)

Diabetic Retinopathy (cont.)

MICROANEURYSM

RETINAL PHOTOGRAPHS

Illus. No.	Page No.
B8	110
135	127
136	127
137 (FI)	127
138	128
139	128
140	129
141	129
160 (D)	140
161 (D)	141
C2	158
C8	166
C9	167
C10	167
C11	167
C13	170
D5	206
228 (C)	217
229 (C)	218
230 (C)	219
231 (C)	220

PHOTOMICROGRAPHS

Illus. No.	Page No.
68	63
142	130
143	130
144	131
145	131
146	131
147	132
148	132
151	133
152	133
153	133

NEOVASCULARIZATION

RETINAL PHOTOGRAPHS

Illus. No.	Page No.
93	82
96 (D)	83
128	122
154	138
155	138
156	138
157	138
158	139
159 (D)	140
160 (D)	140
161 (D)	141
166 (D)	145
167 (D)	145
168	146
169 (D)	146
170 (D)	147

PHOTOMICROGRAPHS

Illus. No.	Page No.
162 (D)	142
163 (D)	142
164 (D)	142
165 (D)	142

PROLIFERATIVE RETINOPATHY

PHOTOGRAPHS OF OTHER ABNORMALITIES IN THE EYE IN THE DIABETIC PATIENT

Diabetic Retinopathy (cont.)

EXTRAVASCULAR LESIONS

Cotton Wool Patch

Hypertensive Retinopathy (cont.)

Hypertensive Retinopathy (cont.)

EXTRAVASCULAR LESIONS (con't.)

Hemorrhage

Occlusion of Central Retinal Artery

Retinopathy in Some Hematologic and Metabolic Disorders (cont.)

Optic Nerve (cont.)

PAPILLEDEMA

LESIONS, ACCORDING TO DISEASE (cont.)

Optic Nerve (cont.)

OPTIC NEURITIS (OPTIC NEUROPATHY)

OPTIC ATROPHY

ILLUSTRATIONS, IN ORDER OF PRESENTATION

CHAPTER I

CHAPTER II

CHAPTER III (cont.)

CHAPTER IV

CHAPTER V

CHAPTER VI

CHAPTER VIII

FOREWORD

It is a gratifying experience to study the retina with Edward M. Chester, M.D., in this remarkable result of life–long research, a book designed especially for the learner. The inquiry is exciting because we find that the eye becomes a unique window for observing the retina as part of the brain with its dynamic nerve tissues, vascular bed, and supporting structures. The pathophysiology of changes in the retina leads us to observe processes local to the eye and local to the brain, general to the body, and general to the brain.

For example, the sequential retinal photographs in one patient with accelerated hypertension are worth their weight in gold because they tell us something that most of us do not know, namely, that amazing resolution can occur in the vascular changes that were extremely severe initially. Here, then, is the place to observe regression from disease in the same patient over time. As learners, it is a joy to have each unit begin with clinical examples, stimulating us to observe carefully and to ask why, then to have Dr. Chester discuss the pathogenesis and histology, with concise statements of the significance and limits of present knowledge. The classifications of disease processes and mechanisms are related to the pathologic changes which are handsomely shown.

The introduction of "unknowns," in the form of unlabeled illustrations, challenges learners to ask a whole series of questions as they try to be definitive about the range of the normal and of the kind of abnormality that is before us; participation is built into the approach. The answers are appropriately available and carefully written to state the limitations in diagnosis and mechanism.

The normal structures are vividly presented in Chapter I so that we can review them as necessary and become oriented to landmarks. In the same chapter, classic abnormalities are presented, and we learn how to record the data on these. Each of the subsequent chapters forms a distinct unit; we learn about diseases of the vascular units, hypertensive changes, diabetic retinopathy, microaneurysms, exudates, optic nerve changes, changes from diseases of the eye, and systemic, congenital, and hereditary abnormalities.

We can go back again and again to review these units, to test our visual perception, interpretation, and limitations. Because this book has been designed for and pretested with students of all levels, we feel the warmth and insight of Dr. Chester as physician–teacher as though he were with us. Our experience with this book brings new knowledge, new skill that we can apply immediately at the bedside to the benefit of the patient, and satisfaction to us as the observers. This book is a model for self–instruction and self–evaluation based on excellence in clinical investigation.

Thomas Hale Ham, M.D.
Director, The Division of Research
in Medical Education
Hanna Payne Professor of Medicine
School of Medicine
Case Western Reserve University

PREFACE

This book correlates funduscopic changes in systemic disease with the corresponding pathology. Although such information is available to ophthalmologists and pathologists, it is not widely disseminated to most other physicians. Since the ophthalmoscopic examination provides a reliable bedside method for visualization of small blood vessels and the optic nerve, it is important that all physicians understand the pathology, pathogenesis, and significance of the abnormalities which can be detected by this technique.

My interest in this approach developed during my training in internal medicine, which emphasized cardiovascular disease. Later as a clinician and teacher, I was able to utilize funduscopic changes frequently as reliable diagnostic clues and indicators of either progression or regression of certain local and systemic diseases. The need for a better understanding of the clinical pathological correlation became more intense fifteen years ago, when I attempted to develop a better understanding of diabetes mellitus and its associated vascular lesions. Ten years ago, in an attempt to understand the pathology and pathogenesis of ophthalmoscopic abnormalities, I developed a histology laboratory for the study of retinal tissue. I was fortunate, at that time, to learn the basic neuropathology of the retina and optic nerve by working with Betty Q. Banker, M.D., Professor of Pathology at Case Western Reserve University. My understanding of retinal abnormalities was increased when I spent part of one summer in the Howe Laboratories at the Massachusetts Eye and Ear Infirmary. There, through the kindness of David G. Cogan, M.D., Professor of Ophthalmology at Harvard Medical School and Director of the Howe Laboratories, and Toichiro Kuwabara, M.D., Associate Professor of Pathology in the Department of Ophthalmology of Harvard Medical School, I learned some of their advanced histologic techniques and was permitted to study many of their retinal preparations.

These experiences, in addition to the previously developed interest and laboratory experience in retinal and optic nerve changes in systemic disease, provided sufficient material to develop a syllabus which was used to teach medical students and house officers. It was Thomas Hale Ham, M.D., Hanna Payne Professor of Medicine and Director of the Division of Research in Medical Education at Case Western Reserve University, who urged me to develop the accumulated information into a book. With a great deal of help, criticism, and encouragement from him, other colleagues, medical students, house officers at Cleveland Metropolitan General Hospital, and members of the Case Western Reserve University Press, the format and contents of this book were tested and moulded into their present form.

The material presented in this book is based upon clinical observations of patients and histologic studies performed by me. A large portion of the histologic studies were performed in conjunction with Betty Q. Banker, M.D. The narrative, which is derived from a review of literature and personal observation, is reinforced through the use of appropriate photographs and drawings of the ophthalmologic abnormalities and their corresponding histologic changes. Self–testing of the reader is introduced through the use of unlabeled retinal photographs and unlabeled photomicrographs (test plates), and by the presentation of the clinical findings. In this exercise, the reader is questioned about the funduscopic findings, their pathologic equivalent, and when appropriate, their relationship to systemic and local disease.

The book was designed primarily for medical students and house officers. Hopefully, it may also be of value to physicians in many specialities. Through use of this book, it is hoped that the reader will develop a greater incentive to do a careful funduscopic examination and become more efficient in the use of the ophthalmoscope. A better understanding of the pathologic basis of the lesions of the retina and optic nerve and the ability to correlate such lesions with local and systemic disease will also result.

I am indebted to many of my colleagues and friends for helpful suggestions and reviews. They include Betty Q. Banker, M.D. (Professor of Pathology, Case Western Reserve University), C. Susan Chester, M.D., David G. Cogan, M.D. (Henry Willard Williams Professor of Ophthalmology, Harvard Medical School, and Director of the Howe Laboratories), Thomas Hale Ham, M.D. (Director, The Division of Research in Medical Education, Hanna Payne Professor of Medicine, Case Western Reserve University), John W. Harris, M.D. (Professor of Medicine, Case Western Reserve University), Richard Honard, M.D., Irwin Jacobs, M.D., Everett Madson, M.D., Louis Rakita, M.D. (Professor of Medicine, Case Western Reserve University), Charles I. Thomas, M.D. (Professor of Ophthalmology, Director of the Division of Ophthalmology, Case Western Reserve University), Martin Wand, M.D., Maurice Victor, M.D. (Professor of Neurology, Case Western

Reserve University), many medical students of Case Western Reserve University, and house officers at Cleveland Metropolitan General Hospital.

All the drawings except Figure VI, by Miss Mary Dawson, were done by Miss Marita Bitans, Medical Illustrator, Cleveland Metropolitan General Hospital. Most of the photomicrographs were made by Rolla B. McCashen, Chief Photographer, Cleveland Metropolitan General Hospital. Several retinal photographs were taken by Everett Madson, M.D., Malcolm Tarkanian, M.D., and Martin Wand, M.D., while they were working with me. Except for a few others taken by Lee R. Wolin, Ph.D., Director of the Laboratory of Neuropsychology, Cleveland Psychiatric Institute, the retinal photography was done by me.

A deep sense of gratitude goes to my wife, Mary H. Chester, for her skillful preparation of the eye tissue in the laboratory, for helpful advice in the development of the book, and for bearing with me during its preparation. The enormous amount of time, deep interest, and effort exerted by my secretary, Miss Frances Apltauer, who typed an endless number of drafts and performed many other essential duties in its preparation, deserves my deepest appreciation. To Miss Betty Stein, Medical Librarian, Cleveland Metropolitan General Hospital, and Miss Betty Joy, Assistant Medical Librarian, Cleveland Metropolitan General Hospital, who obtained the many books and journals used for reference and for their careful and helpful bibliography search, I am also indebted. The personal satisfaction of developing the book resulted to a great extent from the warmth engendered by my association with members of the Case Western Reserve University Press. I am most grateful to them for their expert advice, intense interest, and understanding.

This work was supported by the Division of Research in Medical Education of Case Western Reserve University through a grant from the National Library of Medicine. Its initial development as a syllabus for medical students was supported by the Webster–Underhill Foundation. Many of the clinical and histological observations, which serve as the basis for the book, were the result of clinical investigations supported, in part, by the Health Fund of Greater Cleveland and the Cleveland Diabetes Fund.

E.M.C.

THE OCULAR FUNDUS IN SYSTEMIC DISEASE

Chapter I
THE RETINA AND OPTIC NERVE

EMBRYOLOGY

The initial recognizable event in the development of the eye is the formation of two lateral depressions (optic sulci) in the cephalic portion of the neural plate (Fig. I). By the fourth week of embryonic development, these concavities deepen and form the single–walled, primary optic vesicles which extend from the lateral walls of the forebrain and lie beneath the ectoderm which later forms the lens (Fig. II). Shortly thereafter the vesicles invaginate to form double–walled optic cups (Fig. III). Differentiation of the two layers of the optic cups then begins (Fig. IV). The outer layer becomes thinner and ultimately is converted into a single row of melanin–containing hexagonal cells, the pigment cell layer of the retina. The inner layer develops into highly organized nervous tissue, the sensory retina. Cells from the inner layer of the optic cup grow through its attachment to the diencephalon (optic stalk) and form a fiber tract of the brain, the optic nerve (Fig. V). The space that exists in the embryo between the two layers of the optic cup (Fig. IV) is the potential site of the separation of the sensory retina from the pigment cell layer, known as retinal detachment.

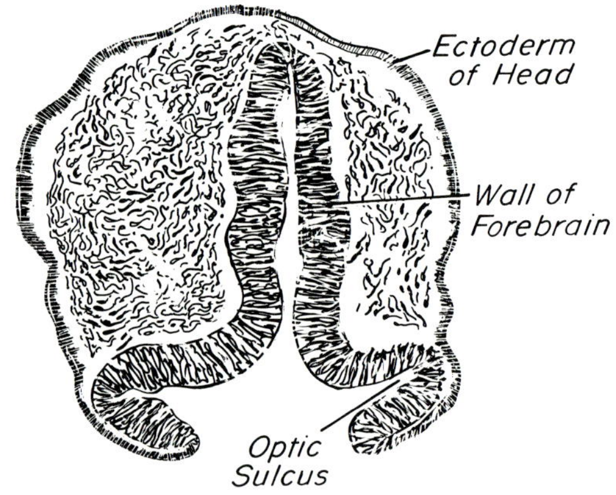

(I) 14 Somites

Figure I. The development of the lateral depressions (optic sulci) in the cephalic portion of the neural plate (from Patten).

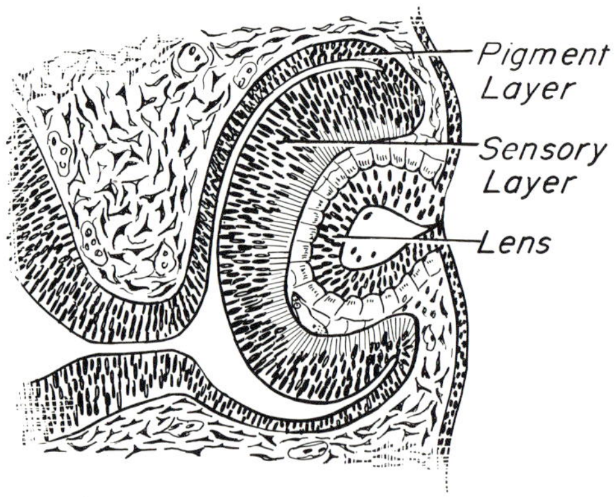

(IV) 7mm.

Figure IV. Differentiation of the two layers of the optic cup (from Patten).

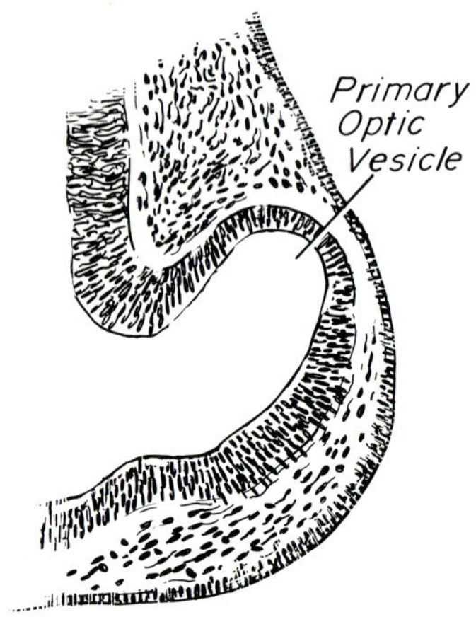

(II) 4mm.

Figure II. The formation of the primary optic vesicle in the lateral walls of the forebrain (from Patten).

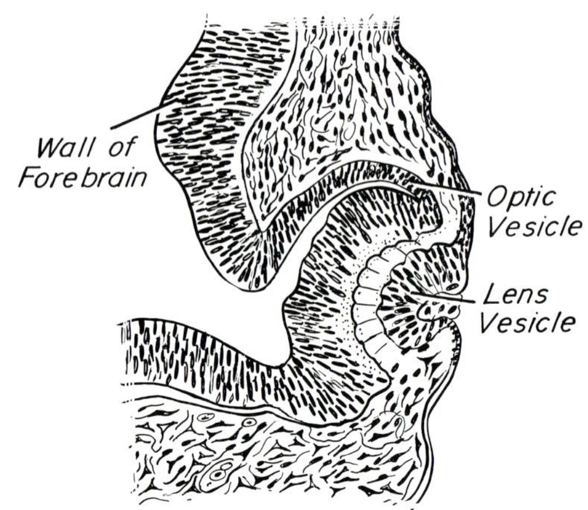

(III) 5mm.

Figure III. Invagination of the optic vesicle to form the double-walled optic cup (from Patten).

The invagination of the optic cup produces a gap in the continuity of its inferior wall—the choroid or hyaloid fissure—which continues along the optic stalk as a groove for the hyaloid artery (Fig. V). Eventually the fissure fuses and encloses the hyaloid artery within the optic stalk and cup. Failure of the hyaloid fissure to fuse results in a congenital defect known as a coloboma. This anomaly may appear as either a crater around the optic disc or as a cleft below the disc which extends through the choroid and retina. In the fetus, the hyaloid artery, a continuation of the central retinal artery, extends through the vitreous to the posterior part of the lens and supplies the anterior segment of the developing eye. This vessel normally disappears before birth. It may, however, persist as a blood–filled vessel or as a stringlike structure extending into the vitreous from either the optic disc or the lens (see pp. 24–25).

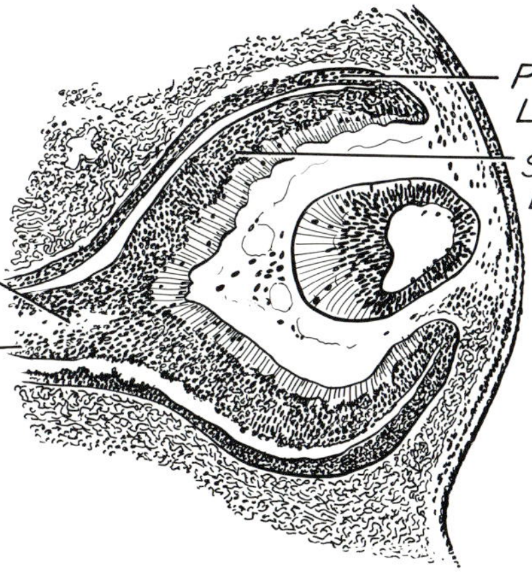

(V) 10 mm.

Figure V. Further differentiation of the layers of the optic cup to form the pigment cell layer of the retina and the sensory retina. The formation of the optic nerve (from Patten).

THE ANATOMY OF THE EYE

The eye includes the eyeball and its connection to the brain, the optic nerve. The eyeball is a sphere (Fig. VI). Its wall consists of three layers. They are (1) an outer fibrous tissue which forms the sclera posteriorly and the cornea anteriorly; (2) a middle, pigmented vascular tissue, the uvea, which consists of choroid posteriorly and the ciliary body and iris anteriorly; and (3) an inner layer of nervous tissue, the retina, which is continuous with the optic nerve. The cavity within the eyeball contains the following structures: (1) the vitreous body, which contains a transparent jellylike substance and lies anterior to the retina; (2) the crystalline lens; and (3) the anterior chamber which contains the aqueous humor.

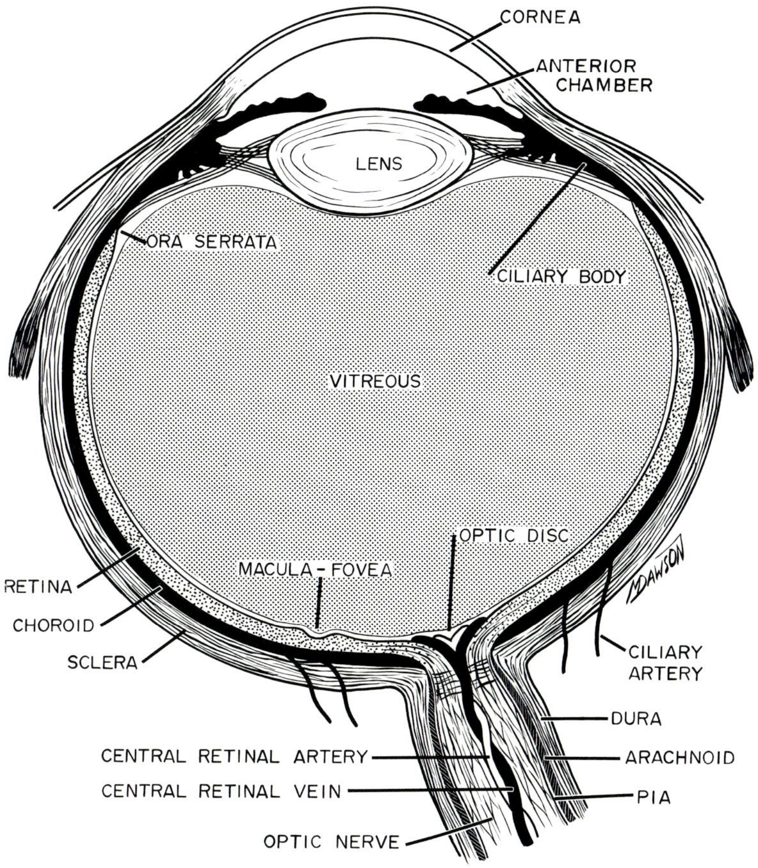

Figure VI. A horizontal section of the eye.

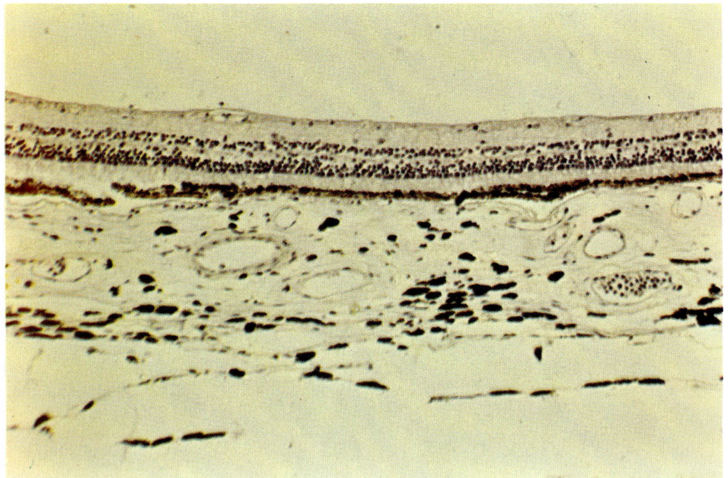

Plate 1. Vertical section of normal retina and choroid (hematoxylin and eosin, H&E, × 80).

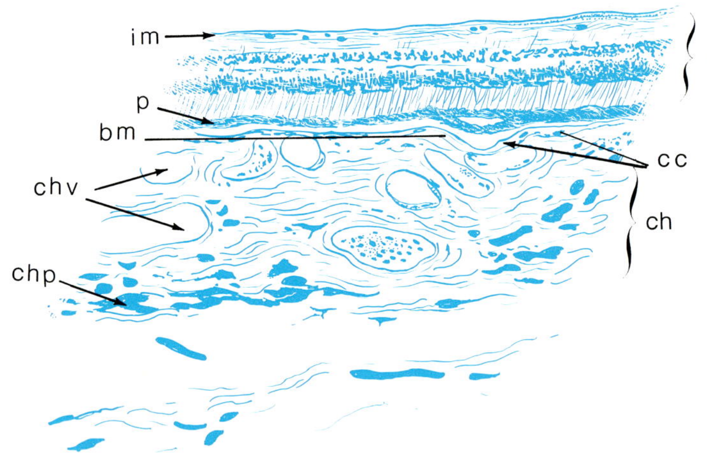

Drawing 1. Plate 1 (r, retina; ch, choroid; im, internal limiting membrane; p, pigment cells; bm, Bruch's membrane; cc, choriocapillaris; chv, choroidal blood vessels; chp, choroidal pigment).

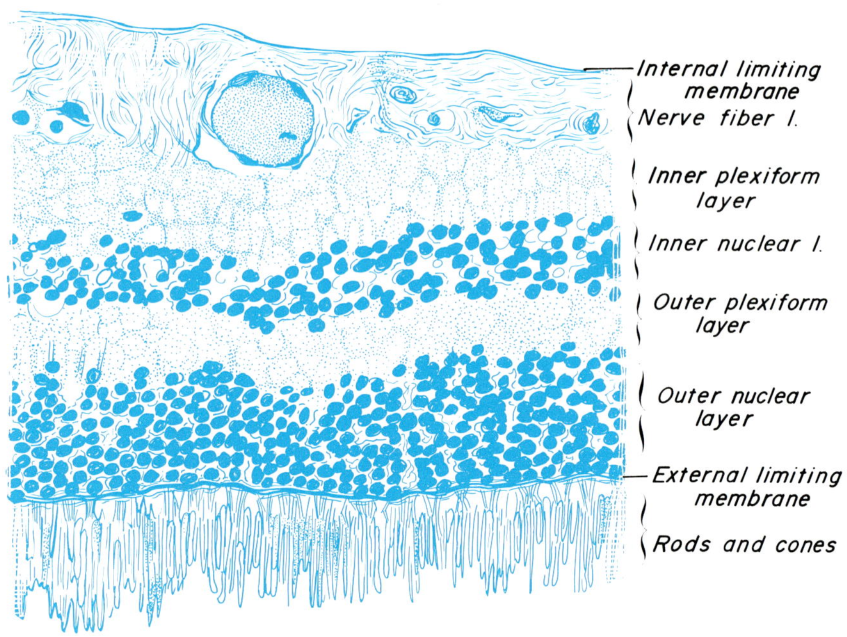

Figure VII. A vertical section of the retina.

The Retina, Anatomy and Histology

The *retina* is a thin, transparent membrane which varies in thickness from 90 to 350 micra.[1 (p. 91)] Although loosely attached to the pigment cells, it is firmly anchored to the optic disc posteriorly and to the *ora serrata* anteriorly[2 (p. 469)] (Fig. VI). The vitreous body is immediately anterior to the retina. The pigment cell layer of the retina is attached posteriorly to the choroid.

The retina is composed of ten layers (Fig. VII, Plate 1 and Drawing 1). From within outward these are:

1. Internal limiting membrane
2. Nerve fiber layer
3. Ganglion cell layer
4. Inner plexiform layer
5. Inner nuclear layer
6. Outer plexiform layer
7. Outer nuclear layer
8. External limiting membrane
9. Layer of rods and cones
10. Pigment cell layer

1. The *internal limiting membrane* is a thin, acellular, basement membrane. Anteriorly it is loosely attached to coalesced vitreous fibers known as the hyaloid membrane. The internal limiting membrane extends over the entire retina with the exception of the optic nerve.[3 (p. 16)]

2. The *nerve fiber layer* consists of the axons of the ganglion cells. Most of the axonal fibers of the ganglion cells are directed horizontally.* In the periphery they form an open network so that the spaces between bundles are round or polygonal.[4 (p. 128)] Fibers of the

*The internal limiting membrane will be used as a point of reference. Horizontal direction refers to fibers which are parallel to it; fibers perpendicular to the membrane are designated as vertical.

Müller cells of the inner nuclear layer extend vertically through the nerve fiber layer and are attached to the internal limiting membrane. Lemmocytes, bipolar cells with elongated nuclei, are present in the nerve fiber layer.[5]

3. The *ganglion cell layer* is composed of nerve cells which vary in size, number, and arrangement of their processes.[6 (pp. 9-18)] The ganglion cells have abundant cytoplasm and large nuclei with prominent Nissl granules. The cells increase in number as they approach the macular area and become sparse in the periphery of the retina. Astrocytes found among the ganglion cells attach their processes to blood vessels in that layer.[5]

4. The *inner plexiform layer* is a fine network of nerve fibers formed by the synapses of the axons of the bipolar and amacrine cells of the inner nuclear layer with the dendrites of the ganglion cells. Numerous astrocytes are also present.[5]

5. The *inner nuclear layer* contains the following four cell types (Fig. VIII): the *bipolar cells,* whose dendrites synapse with the axons of the cells of the rods and cones; the *horizontal cells,* which provide fibers that synapse with the axons of the rod and cone cells as well as with adjacent bipolar cells; the *amacrine cells,* which extend processes that synapse with the dendrites of the ganglion cells in the inner plexiform layer; the *Müller cells,* whose fibers provide the supporting framework of the retina; these fibers extend anteriorly to the inner limiting membrane and posteriorly to form part of the external limiting membrane.

6. The *outer plexiform layer* is composed of axons of the rod and cone nuclei and the dendrites of the bipolar and horizontal cells of the inner nuclear layer. These fibers generally are arranged in vertical rows.

7. The *outer nuclear layer* consists of eight or nine layers of cells. Two types of cells are described. The rods arise from the cells which contain small and densely stained nuclei. Cells with larger and more weakly stained nuclei give rise to the cones.

8. The *external limiting membrane* is perforated, thus permitting passage for the fibers of the rods and cones.

9. The *rods and cones* are the photoreceptors. The rods are slender and cylindrical. The cones are flask–shaped and shorter than the rods.

10. External to the rods and cones and adjacent to Bruch's membrane of the choroid is the *pigment cell layer* of the retina. It is composed of a single layer of hexagonal cells which contain granules of melanin. It is loosely attached to the rods and cones.

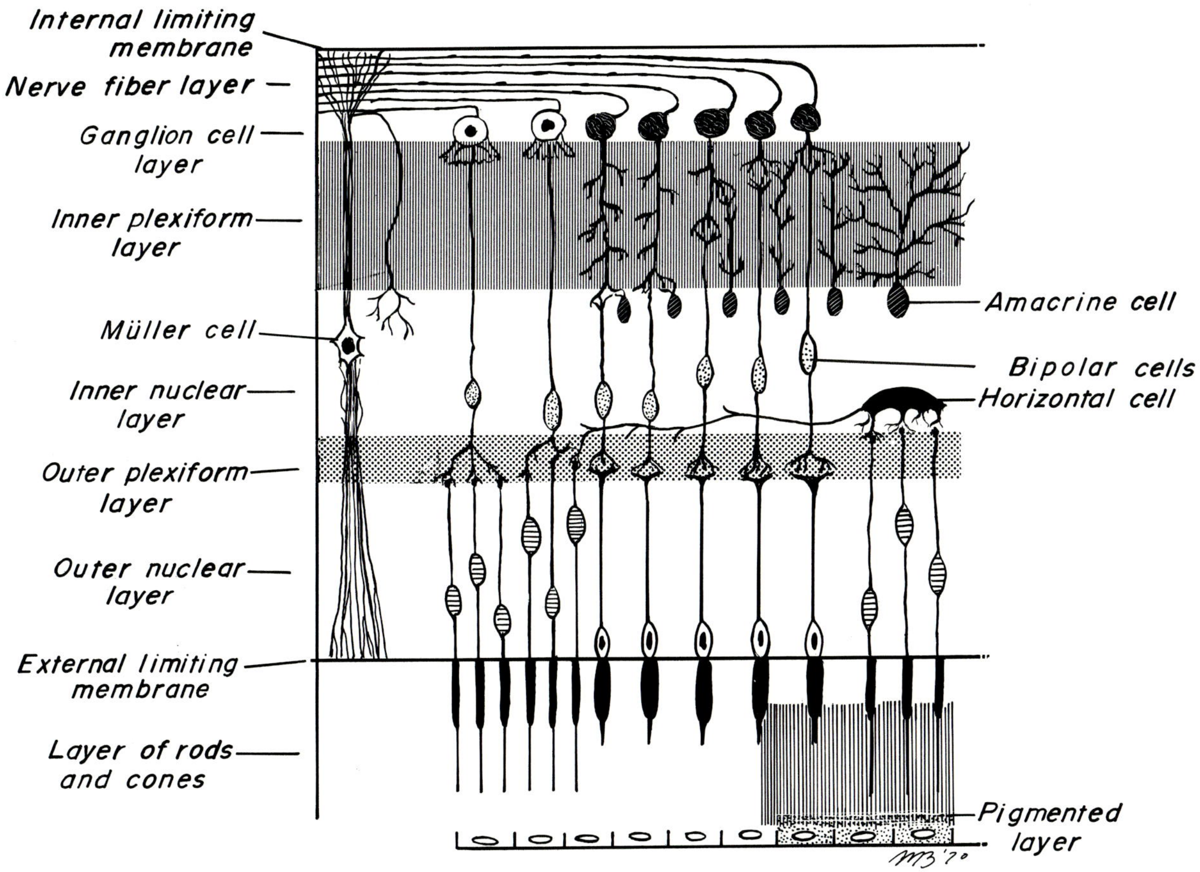

Figure VIII. Cell types and glia within the retina (from Cogan and Kuwabara).

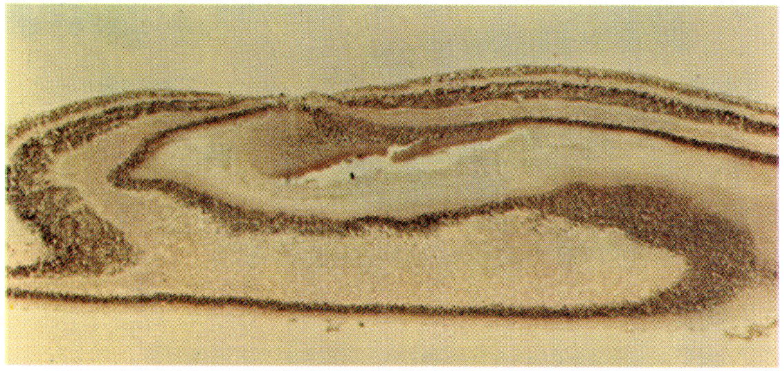

Plate 2. Section of retina through the macula. Note the depression at the fovea and the broad outer plexiform layer which radiates toward the fovea (H&E, × 11).

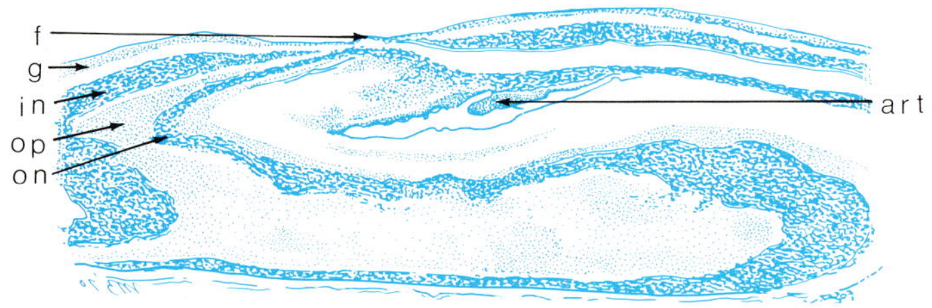

Drawing 2. Plate 2 (f, fovea; g, ganglion cells; in, inner nuclear layer; op, outer plexiform layer; on, outer nuclear layer; art, artefact).

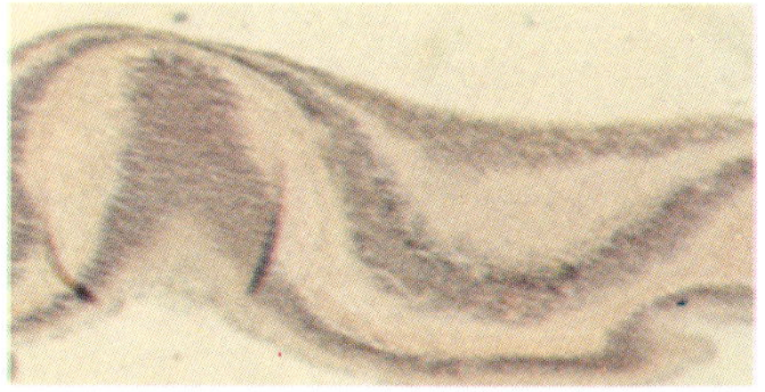

Plate 3. Section of normal macula approaching the fovea. Note the following in the region of the fovea: (1) the absence of blood vessels; (2) the extremely thin nerve fiber layer; (3) the absence of ganglion cells; (4) the narrow inner nuclear layer; (5) the broad outer plexiform layer, whose fibers are directed toward the fovea (H&E, approx. × 20).

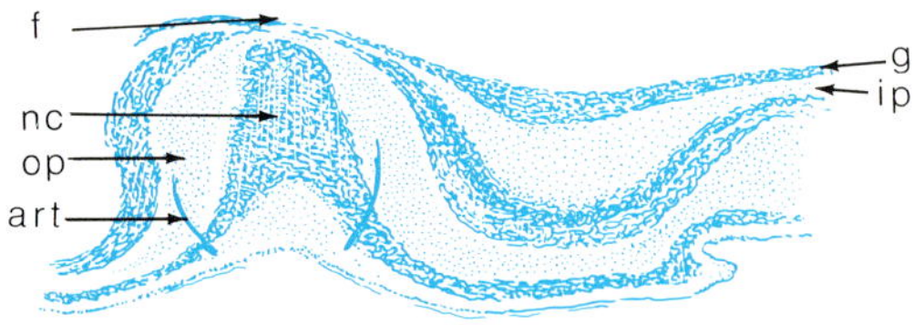

Drawing 3. Plate 3 (f, fovea; g, ganglion cells; ip, inner plexiform layer; op, outer plexiform layer; nc, nuclei of cones; art, artefact).

The *macula* is a circular pigmented area approximately the same size as the optic disc. It is located approximately 1½ disc diameters temporal to the disc. The small central depression of the macula is called the *fovea.* Near the fovea, structural changes occur (Plates 2 and 3 and Drawings 2 and 3). The changes include a decrease in the number of ganglion cells and attenuation of the nerve fiber layer. Blood vessels disappear, the inner nuclear layer narrows, and the outer plexiform layer increases in size. At the fovea, there are only cones and a thin nerve fiber layer. In the macular region the synaptic arrangement is on a one–to–one relationship, unlike the remainder of the retina. Because of the absence of ganglion cells and an inner nuclear layer in the fovea, the axons of the cones in the outer plexiform layer radiate outward to reach the dendrites of the bipolar and amacrine cells of the adjacent inner nuclear layer. The fibers of the outer plexiform layer of the macula radiate from the central foveal hub like the spokes of a wheel. Because of this anatomic arrangement, outer plexiform lesions of the macula assume a starlike pattern.

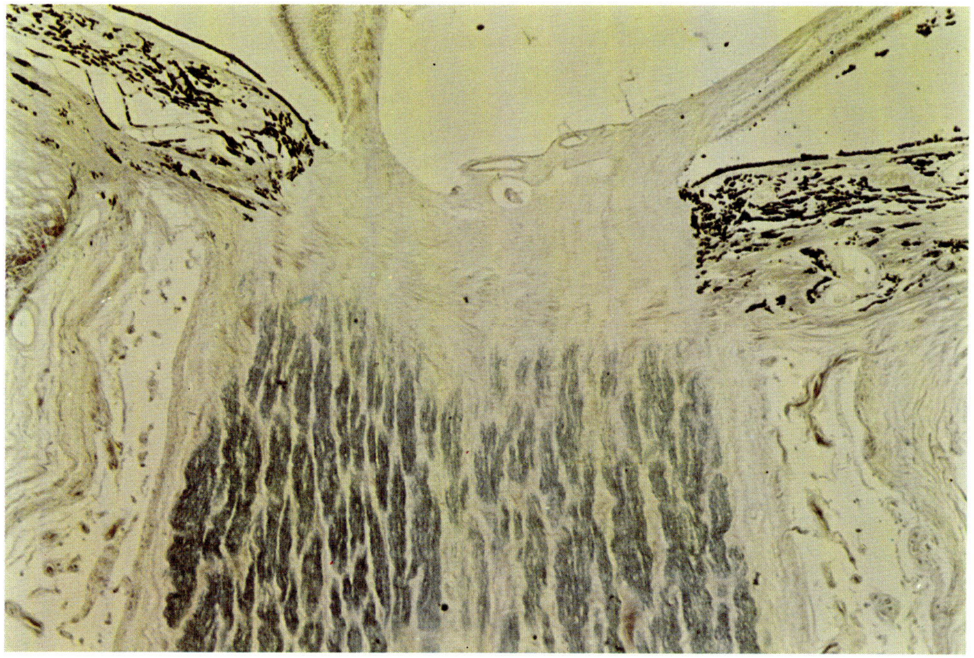

Plate 4.* Section of the retina, choroid, sclera, and optic nerve. Note that nerve fibers of the retina enter the optic nerve and acquire myelin sheaths (stained blue) after they pass through the lamina cribrosa (myelin sheath stain, × 20).

*Separation of retina and choroid is an artefact. It often occurs when the tissue is processed for histologic study.

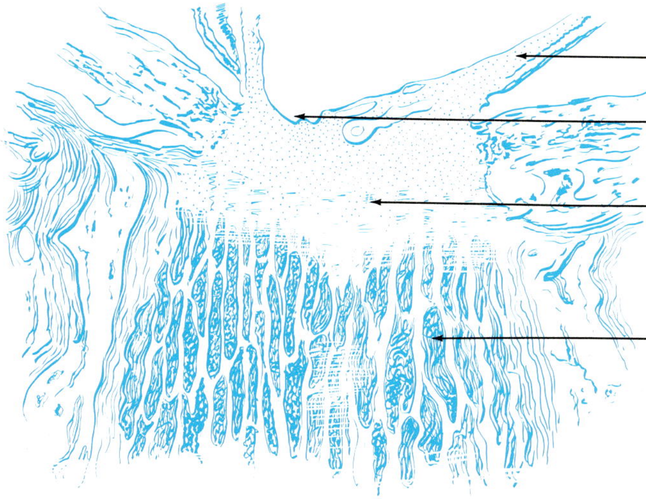

Drawing 4. Plate 4 (nf, nerve fiber layer; pc, physiologic cup; lc, lamina cribrosa; mnf, myelinated nerve fibers).

The Optic Nerve, Anatomy and Histology

The optic nerve, which consists of white matter, is a fiber tract of the central nervous system and is formed by the axons of the retinal ganglion cells. These nerve fibers acquire myelin sheaths after they leave the globe and penetrate the lamina cribrosa, a sievelike structure, which is formed chiefly by the sclera (Plate 4 and Drawing 4).

From the globe to the optic chiasm, the nerve measures approximately 5 cm in length. Anatomically, it is divided into four segments

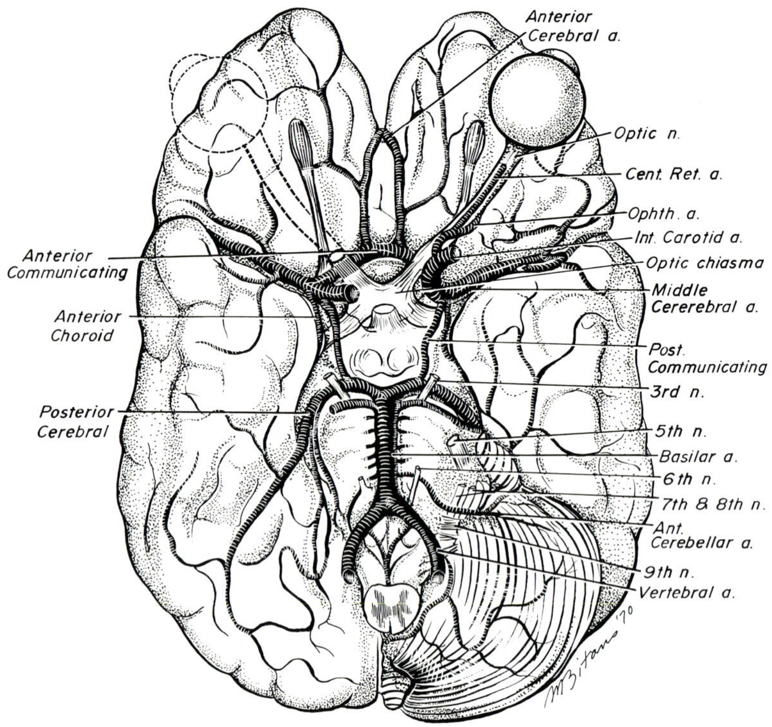

Figure IX. The inferior surface of the brain illustrating the course of the optic nerve and its relationship to other structures.

—intraocular, intraorbital, intracanalicular, and intracranial. The short intraocular portion, the central retinal artery, and the vein emerge through the nasal side of the globe. The intraorbital portion extends to the optic foramen and is surrounded by the dural, arachnoid, and pial membranes of the brain. The dura merges with sclera. The arachnoid and subarachnoid space are continuous with the arachnoid and subarachnoid space of the brain. The pia is tightly bound to the optic nerve and is the most vascular layer of the three membranes. Its fibrous extensions envelop capillaries as they enter and subdivide the nerve into longitudinally arranged fiber compartments. The interstitial cells of the nerve include oligodendroglia, astrocytes, and microglia. The nerve fibers first acquire myelin sheaths in the intraorbital segment.*

The intracanalicular portion of the nerve extends from the optic foramen along the lesser wing of the sphenoid bone for a short distance. The next segment of the nerve, the intracranial portion, passes backward and fuses with the other optic nerve to form the optic chiasm in the region of the sella turcica (Fig. IX).

The Visual Pathway (Fig. X)

The visual impulse is initiated by light stimulation of the photosensitive pigment of the rods and cones of the retina. A neural discharge follows and is transmitted by way of the bipolar cells to the ganglion cells of the retina. The fibers of the medial portions of the optic nerve which arise from the nasal segment of the retina (defined by a line through the center of the fovea) cross to the opposite side at the optic chiasm and terminate in the contralateral geniculate body. The axons that arise from the lateral half of the retina are situated in the lateral part of the optic nerve. They do not cross and terminate in the homolateral geniculate body. The pathway then continues through the geniculocalcarine radiation to the striate area of the occipital cortex.

*The nerve fibers of the retina may acquire myelin sheaths before they leave the globe via the lamina cribrosa. Clinically this anomaly most commonly appears as a white patch which extends from the optic disc. The white patch has striated edges, and it often extends along the nerve fibers of the retina (see pp. 21, 104).

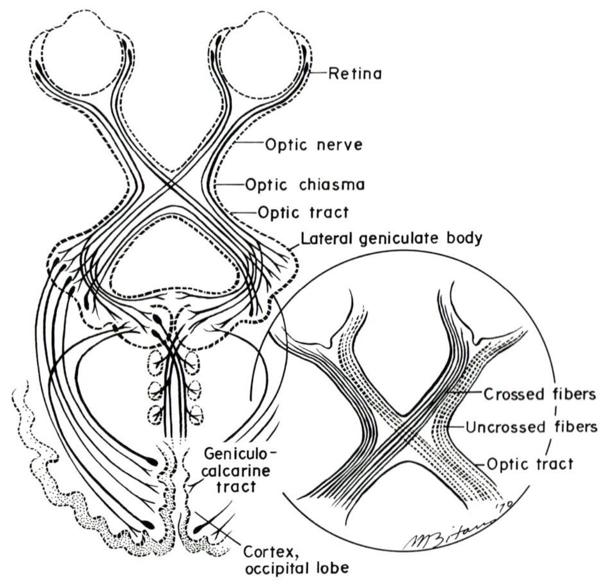

Figure X. The visual pathway.

BLOOD SUPPLY OF THE EYE

Blood Supply of the Optic Nerve (Fig. XI)

The blood supply of the optic nerve is highly variable. The main capillary networks are the periaxial and axial systems. The contribution of the central retinal artery is made by way of its pial branches which anastomose with the circle of Zinn–Haller.[7] The latter, found in the region of the lamina cribrosa and optic nerve, originates from the short posterior ciliary branches of the ophthalmic artery.*

The periaxial capillary network is formed by anastomoses of vessels which originate from the ophthalmic, short posterior ciliaries, anterior cerebral, internal, and external carotid, lacrimal, and middle meningeal arteries.[8] The resulting capillary network supplies the pia and sends branches along the pial septa which enter the optic nerve.

The axial capillary network supplies the central portion of the optic nerve. This system is highly variable. Frequently, a branch of the ophthalmic artery called the central optic nerve artery arises proximal to the origin of the central retinal artery and passes through the center of the optic nerve.[9] The central optic nerve artery supplies the macular fibers, serves as vasavasorum for the central retinal artery, and anastomoses with capillaries arising from the arterial circle of Zinn–Haller.[9]

*In approximately 20% of the population, an aberrant vessel—the cilioretinal artery—arises from the circle of Zinn–Haller. It passes forward with the optic nerve without entering it or joining the central retinal artery. The cilioretinal artery is observed at the edge of the disc, usually the temporal side, and forms part of the blood supply of the retina (see pp. 24–25).

The central retinal artery passes directly through the subarachnoid space and enters the optic nerve. In contrast, the corresponding vein crosses directly in less than one half of the nerves studied; in the remainder the intravaginal course is prolonged.[10] Venous return may be impeded in that unprotected portion of the vein whether by an accumulation of blood, exudate, tumor, or by an increased subarachnoid fluid pressure around the optic nerve. The resulting increase in central retinal vein pressure is considered to be one of the mechanisms involved in the production of papilledema (see p. 180).

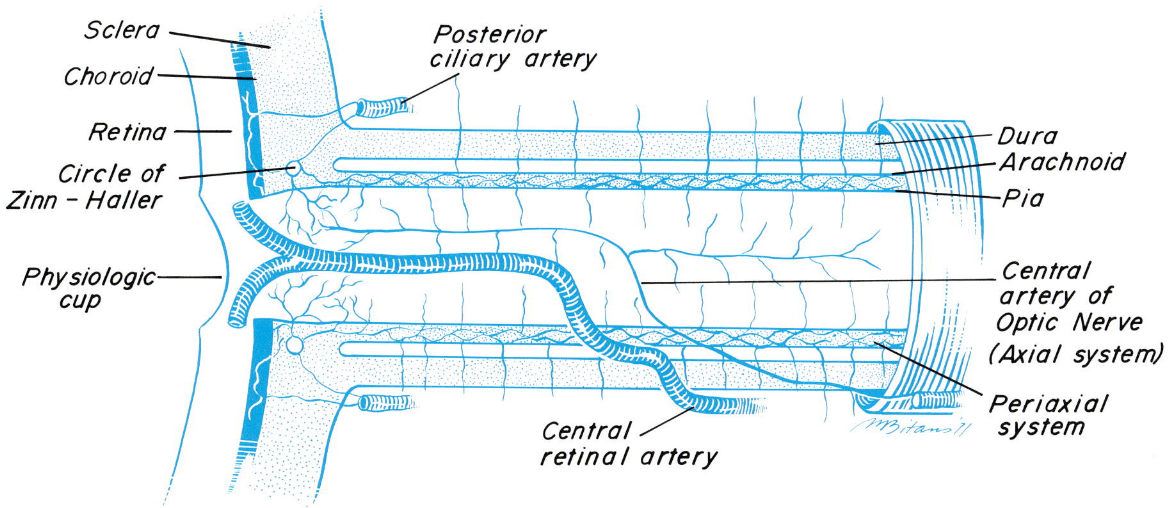

Figure XI. The arterial supply of the optic nerve (from Francois and Neetens).

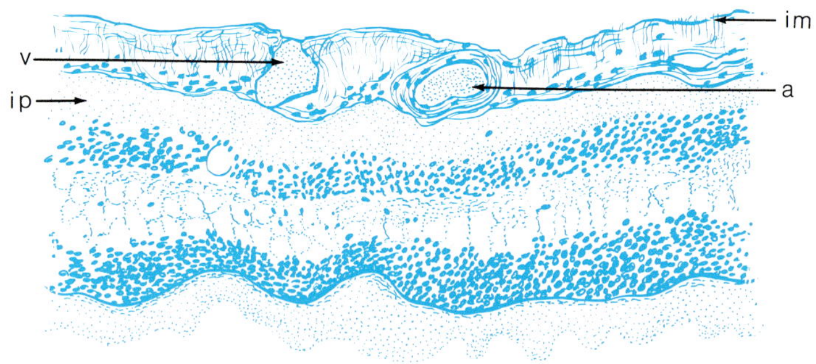

Drawing 5. Plate 5 (im, internal limiting membrane; a, arteriole; v, vein; ip, inner plexiform layer).

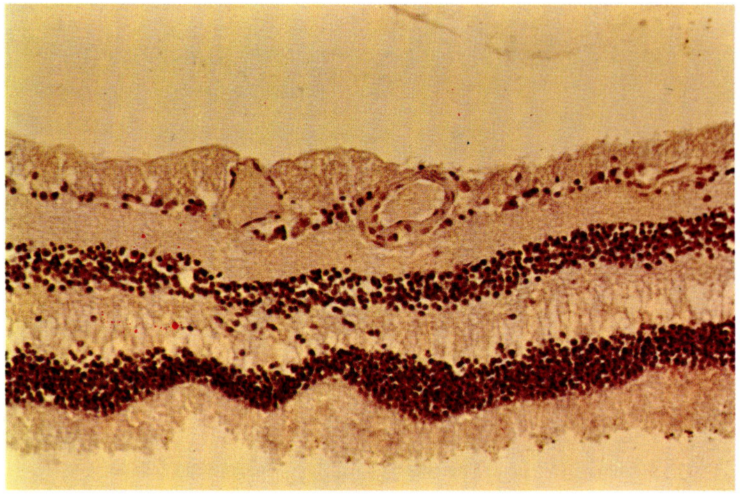

Plate 5. Section of retina. Normal arteriole and venule in the nerve fiber layer. The arteriolar wall is thicker than that of the venule. The lumen of the latter is the larger of the two (H&E, × 120).

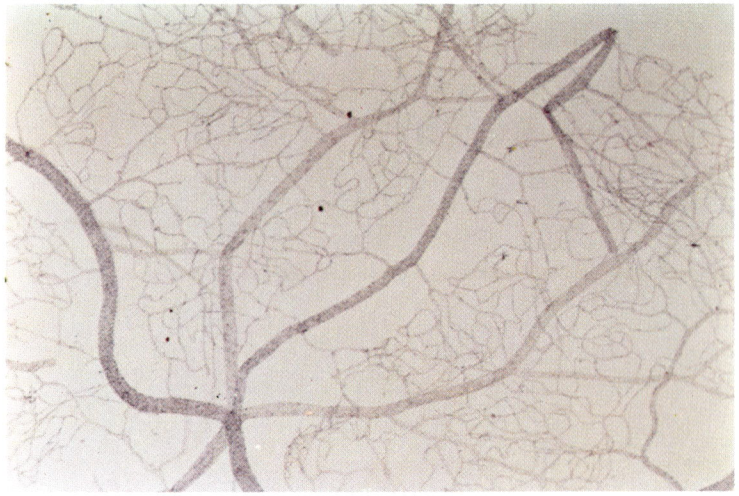

Plate 6. Trypsin–digest; flat mount; normal arteriole, venule, and capillary anastomosis (H&E, × 20).

Blood Supply of the Retina

The retina is nourished through two routes. The posterior third of the retina, which includes the outer plexiform and outer nuclear layers, the rods and cones, and the pigment cells, has no intrinsic blood supply and receives its nourishment by diffusion through the semipermeable Bruch's membrane via the choriocapillaries. The anterior two–thirds (nerve fiber layer to the most anterior part of the outer plexiform layer) of the retina is supplied by the central retinal artery and its branches.

The central retinal artery originates from the ophthalmic branch of the internal carotid artery. Before the central retinal artery enters the eye, it has a structure typical of an artery. After it passes through the lamina cribrosa, the vessel wall undergoes a number of changes. These changes include a reduction in size; the internal elastic lamella becomes thinner and disappears entirely after the first or second bifurcation; although the muscular layer becomes thinner, it remains continuous until it reaches a distance of one disc diameter from the optic disc or at the second bifurcation. Distal to those sites the arterial branches have only widely separated and isolated muscle fibers. As a result of these changes, the branches of the central retinal artery can be classified as arterioles (Plate 5 and Drawing 5).

The four branches are distributed throughout the temporal and nasal portions of the retina in the superior and inferior quadrants. Venous branches, in general, are distributed in the same manner, emptying into the central retinal vein which returns to the optic nerve through the lamina cribrosa. According to Wolff,[1 (p. 128)] the superior and inferior retinal veins join at the lamina cribrosa and form the vena centralis. The latter, after receiving a branch from the superior ophthalmic vein, generally continues to the cavernous sinus.

The major branches of the central retinal artery extend peripherally from the optic nerve within the nerve fiber layer of the retina. According to Michaelson,[11] divisions of these vessels remain in that layer until precapillaries are formed. He defines two groups of capillaries, one arising superficially, the other, designated as the deep group, extending to the junction of the inner nuclear and outer plexiform layers. Anastomotic capillaries join these two capillary networks. In the region of the macula and optic disc, the capillary layers increase to three and four respectively. Toussaint, Kuwabara, and Cogan's[12] studies provide reason to question the concept of the laminar distribution of capillaries in the retina. These studies demonstrate that capillaries exist at all levels of the anterior two–thirds of the retina without evidence of layering.

The trypsin digestion technique devised by Kuwabara and Cogan[13] has provided a method for the study of the vasculature of the retina after the nervous tissue has been removed. With this technique the vascular topography remains intact so that the relationship between arterioles, capillaries, and venules can be studied satisfactorily. In addition, histologic characteristics of such vessels can be detected.

Arterioles and Venules

Flat mounts of trypsin–digested retina disclose that retinal venules differ from arterioles in size, staining characteristics, and nuclear structure. Retinal venules have a wider diameter, stain lightly, and have fewer nuclear structures. In contrast the arterioles are narrower, stain deeply, and have numerous nuclear structures directed along both the longitudinal and horizontal axis of the vessel (Plate 6).

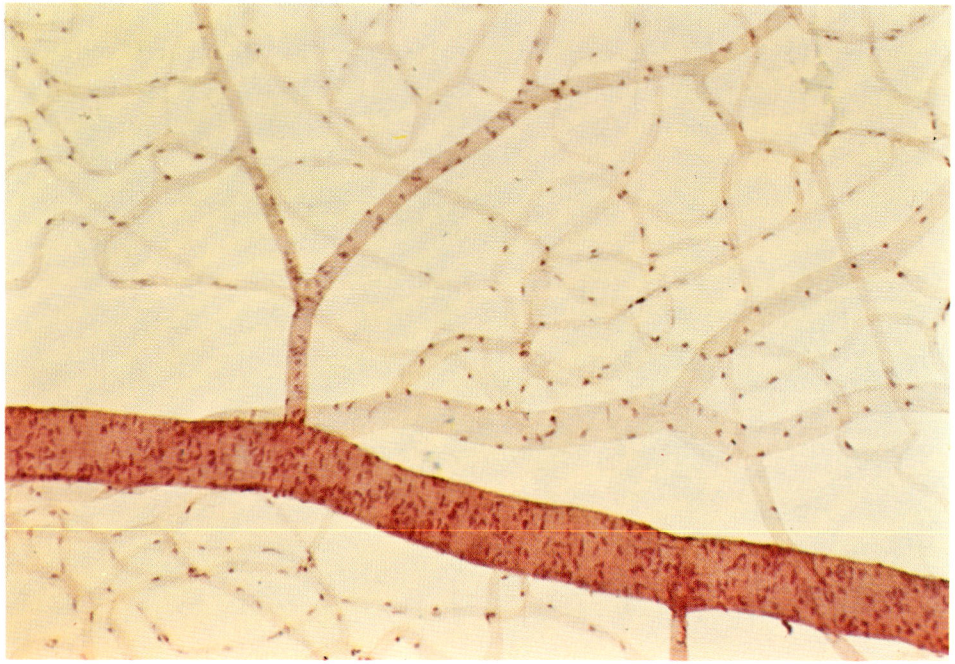

Plate 7. Trypsin–digest; flat mount. Normal capillaries. Note the uniformly distributed nuclei of endothelial and mural cells (phosphotungstic acid hematoxylin stain—PTAH, approx. × 80).

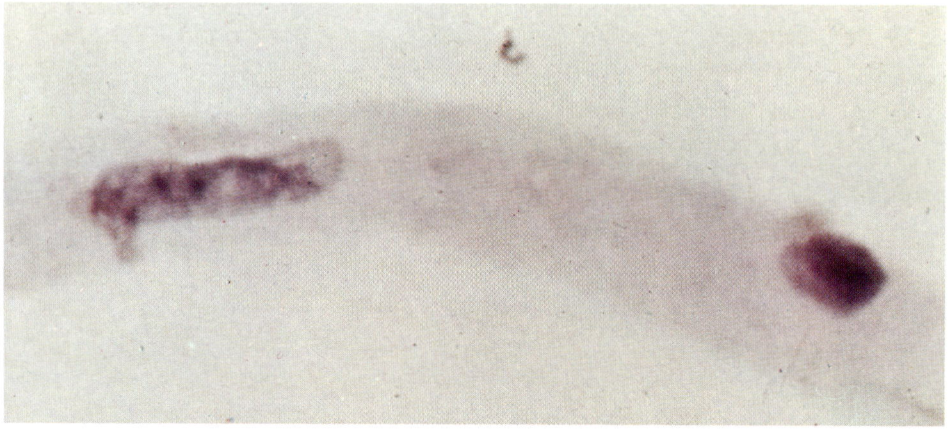

Plate 8. Trypsin–digest; flat mount. Single capillary endothelial and mural cell nuclei (PTAH, approx. × 300).

Capillaries

The capillaries appear as light–staining tubular structures (Plates 7 and 8). The elongated nuclei of their endothelial cells are directed along the long axis of the vessel.[13] The nucleus of another cell, the pericyte, is spherical and stains deeply.[14] It is located on the outer portion of the vessel wall and electron microscopy discloses it to be enclosed within a split in the basement membrane.[14-17] Kuwabara and Cogan[13, 17] refer to it as the mural cell. The pericytes (mural cells) and endothelial cells are roughly equal in number and are randomly distributed.

EXAMINATION OF THE EYE

Although our attention will be focused on the method and value of the examination of the optic fundus, it is understood that the physician will recognize the importance of other aspects of the ophthalmologic examination.* The physician should be capable of detecting the common abnormalities of the visual system. Visual acuity can be tested with the Snellen chart and visual fields by confrontation. Exophthalmos, nystagmus, and extraocular muscle disorders are detected readily. Direct inspection of the cornea, conjunctiva, and sclera can be made with adequate light. Pupillary abnormalities such as inequality, failure to respond to light, and failure of response in accommodation are easily detected. Tonometry can be performed with safety.

*The reader is referred to textbooks of ophthialmology for more comprehensive presentation of the examination of the eye.

Technique of Funduscopy

The ophthalmoscopic examination should proceed in the following manner. Every effort should be made to provide a comfortable position for the patient during the procedure. If possible he should be seated on the edge of a bed or examining table with you standing. If the patient is in a chair, the examination can be performed well with you seated on either side. The examination is best performed in a darkened room. If no contraindications exist, the pupils should be dilated (see p. 17).

The patient should be asked to fix one eye on an object in front of him while you examine the other eye. Use your right eye to examine the patient's corresponding eye and your left eye to examine his left. Begin the examination with a +20 lens (black), moving your ophthalmoscope 6–12 inches away from the patient until you can see the red reflex. Then bring the instrument as close to him as possible. Try to avoid obstruction of the vision of the other eye. Examine the media (cornea, anterior chamber, lens, and vitreous). Lenticular and vitreous opacities are often apparent with a +20 lens; however, vitreous lesions are observed more clearly within +10 to +2.

The retina is usually clearly focused within the range of +1 to −1 (red). An imaginary vertical line drawn through the center of the optic disc anatomically divides the fundus into temporal and nasal segments (Fig. XII). The optic disc then becomes the central reference point. The temporal and nasal portions of the retina can be divided into superior and inferior quadrants.

Examine the margins of the optic disc and the number of small vessels that cross its edges. Note the color and shape of the disc and the depth and size of the physiologic cup. Does the central retinal vein pulsate? Follow the four branches of the central retinal artery and vein through the four quadrants of the fundus. Examine their caliber, contour, color, and relationship at the crossings. Look for abnormalities of the retina such as hemorrhage, degeneration (exudates), and pigmentation after you have examined the blood vessels. If such extravascular lesions are observed, describe their location, color, configuration, and relationship to the retinal blood vessels. To obtain a better view of the temporal part of the fundus and macula, have the patient look directly into the light of the ophthalmoscope with the eye under examination. Note the oval, pigmented macula. Is the normal orderly pigment pattern intact? Can you see the foveal reflex? The nasal portion of the fundus is seen best when the patient directs the eye under examination toward the nose. Then have him look up, then down, and examine the superior and inferior segments of the retina.

The order of the examination of the fundus becomes an individual choice; an orderly and thorough examination, however, is essential. The purpose of funduscopy is rarely understood by the patient. He generally associates

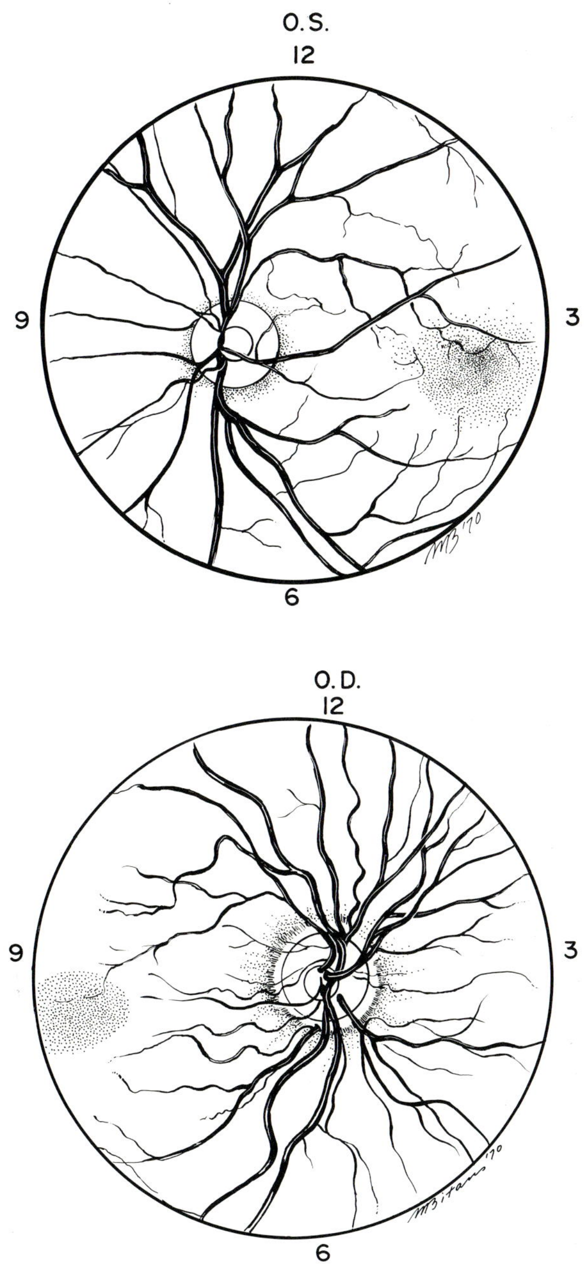

Figure XII. The optic fundi.

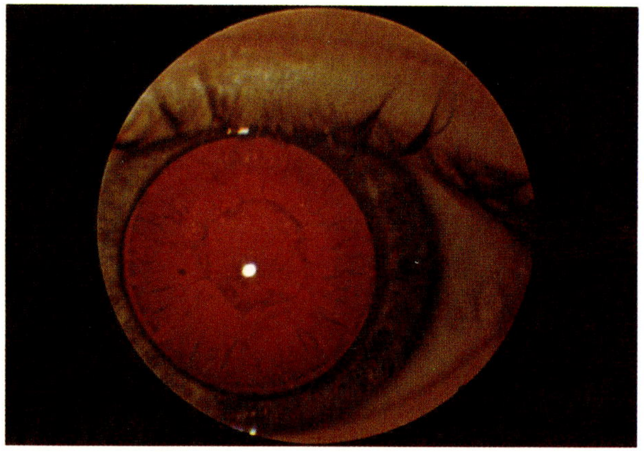

Plate 9. Photograph of lens taken with a +20 lens. Note striate, linear, dark areas radiating toward a central ring–shaped opacity.

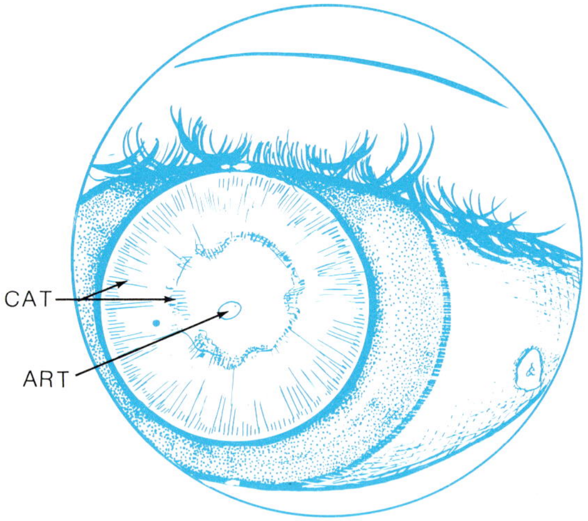

Drawing 9. Plate 9 (CAT, cataract; ART, artefact).

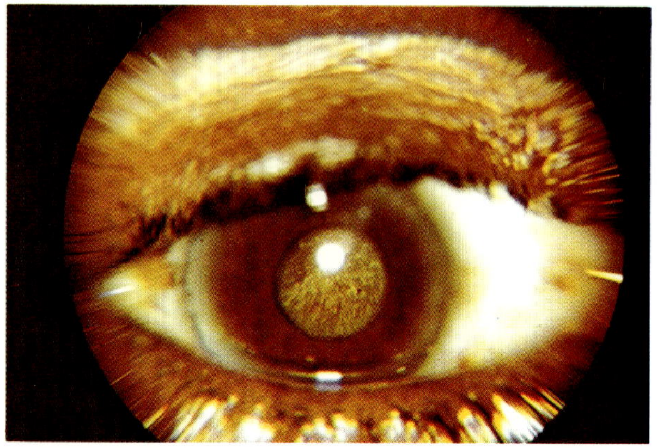

Plate 10. Many white opacities were observed within the red reflex with a +20 lens. They were clearly outlined at +8, becoming less clear with a 0 lens, at which level the retina came into sharp focus.

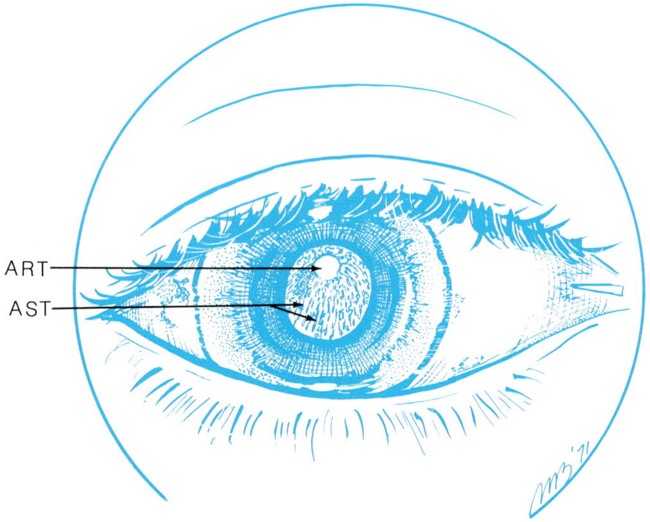

Drawing 10. Plate 10 (AST, asteroid bodies; ART, artefact).

it with visual acuity and often expresses concern. If the purpose of the examination is explained, namely, a statement is made of the importance of direct observation of the optic nerve, blood vessels, and structure of the retina, the patient may be relieved of his anxiety. A statement that no abnormalities are present is reassuring. When there are changes present, they may be tactfully stated.

The transparency of the normal cornea, aqueous humor, lens, and vitreous provides no barrier to the light of the ophthalmoscope and permits the examiner to see the optic fundus clearly (Fig. VI). Opacifications of the cornea and lens, depending upon their extent, can interfere with funduscopic examination. Disturbances of the anterior chamber and the vitreous such as hemorrhage, inflammation, and floating bodies may obscure the underlying retina. Examination of the cornea, anterior chamber, lens, and vitreous can be performed best with the slit lamp. However, disorders of the media (cornea, anterior chamber, lens, and vitreous) may be detected with the ophthalmoscope. Examination of the media is started with a strongly positive lens (+20). If the media are clear the pupil appears to be a red circular structure (red reflex). The oxyhemoglobin of the blood in the choriocapillaries provides the red color. Ordinarily lenticular opacities (cataracts) are seen clearly within the range of +20 to +12 lenses of the ophthalmoscope. The opacities appear black against the red background and assume a variety of forms. They may appear as spokes radiating from the lens periphery toward a central ring (Plate 9 and Drawing 9), circular–central, or wedge–shaped densities. They may opacify the entire lens.[2 (pp. 655-678), 18, 19] As the examiner reduces the positivity of the lens of the ophthalmoscope to +10, he reaches the region of the vitreous. Lesions of the vitreous, although visible at +20, come into focus sharply between +10 and +2 (Plate 10 and Drawing 10). It may, at times, be difficult to distinguish between lenticular and vitreous lesions. Generally they can be distinguished by the examiner slowly moving his head while funduscopy is being performed. The lenticular lesion will remain fixed while the examiner performs this maneuver. In contrast, vitreous lesions will move in the opposite direction. The opacities noted in Plate 9 were fixed. The lesion in Plate 9 is a cataract.[2 (pp. 655-678), 18, 19] In contrast, the opacities noted in Plate 10 floated in the vitreous and moved in the opposite direction when the examiner moved his head.

The lesions noted in Plates 10 and 11 and Drawings 10 and 11 are called *asteroid hyalitis*[2 (pp. 641-654), 20-22] Asteroid hyalitis is usually unilateral. It is commoner in the male and is generally found in older patients. Diabetes mellitus and primary amyloidosis may be related diseases.

After the media have been examined, the physician sees the retina clearly with a slightly positive or negative lens. The examination must be done systematically in order to avoid errors of omission. Examination of the retina is best performed through a dilated pupil. A mydriatic may be used in patients with glaucoma when the clinical findings absolutely demand observation of the optic fundus, but must be used with great caution. If one locates the optic disc first, this can be used as the central point. The term *optic disc* is applied to the ophthalmoscopic view of the intraocular portion of the optic nerve as it enters the globe. The retinal nerve fibers which enter and overlie the optic nerve fibers form the papilla.

METHOD OF EXAMINATION OF THE OPTIC FUNDUS

The structures of the normal optic fundus and some of its variations will be presented as though the author were performing the ophthalmoscopic examination. Figure XII presents a view of the fundus of each eye. The numerals at the rim of the circles are arranged as the face of a clock with the optic disc as the center. This enables the examiner to identify the location of abnormalities. (A description of methods of recording ophthalmoscopic abnormalities follows this section.)

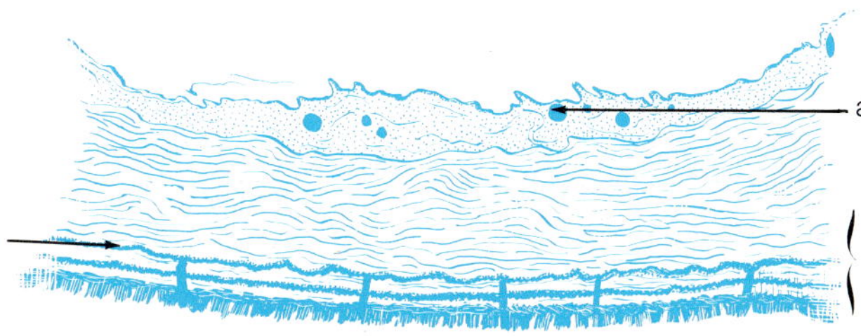

Drawing 11. Plate 11 (ast, asteroid bodies; v, vitreous fibers; r, retina; im, internal limiting membrane).

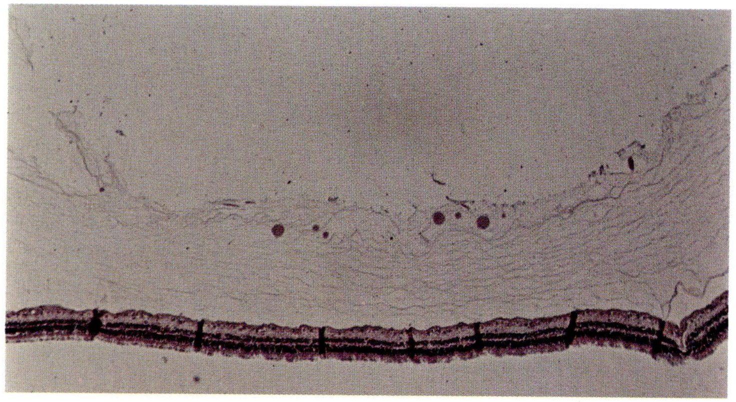

Plate 11. Note the small oval bodies lying within the fibers which are in front of the retina. The fibers are the condensations of precipitated vitreous. The oval bodies are the lesions noted in Plate 10 (H&E, × 27).

Plate 12. Normal disc. Note color, margins, and vessels. Do you notice the fine sunburst effect around the optic disc?

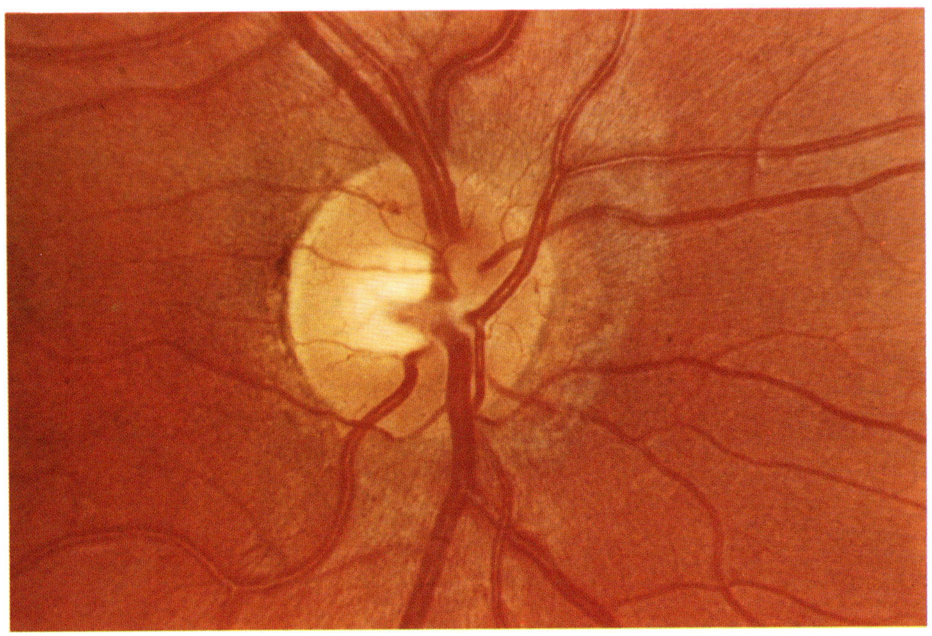

The Normal Optic Fundus

THE OPTIC DISC

The optic disc is either round or oval, and measures approximately 1.5 mm in diameter (Plate 12). It appears to have a pale, red blush superimposed upon a faint yellow color. The numerous peripapillary capillaries produce the red blush. The temporal margin of the disc is generally more distinct than the nasal one. The converging axons of the nerve fiber layer may produce a sunburst effect as they enter the optic disc (Plate 12). A white circle (scleral ring) may either envelop the disc or produce a pale temporal crescent (Plate 13). This variant occurs when the choroid does not make intimate contact with the optic nerve. As a result, sclera is visible in the gap. In severe myopia the scleral ring may

Plate 13. O.S. (left eye). A white scleral ring surrounds the temporal margin of the optic disc.

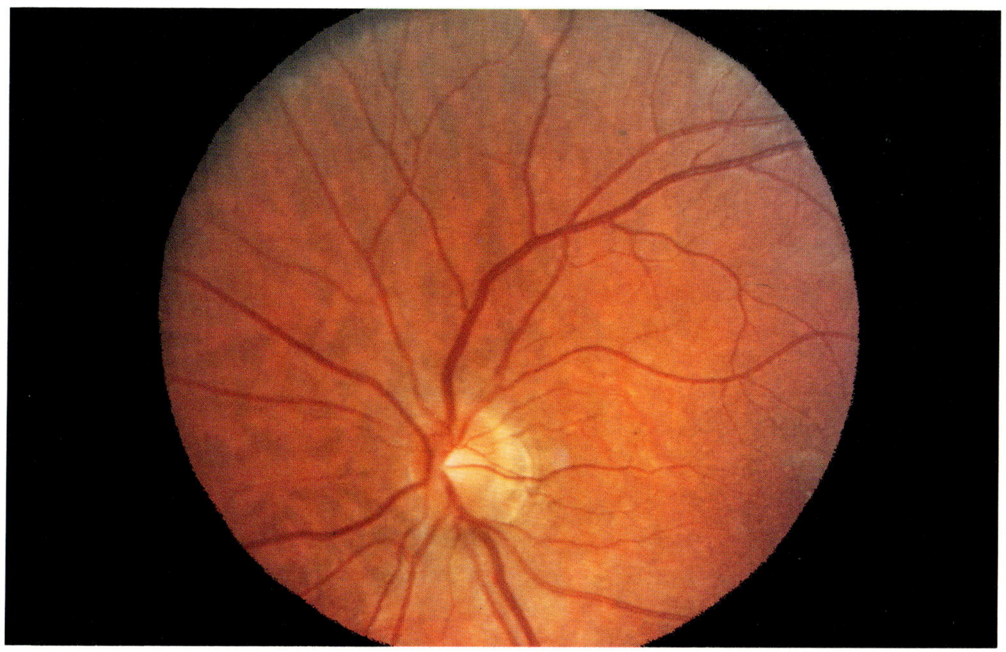

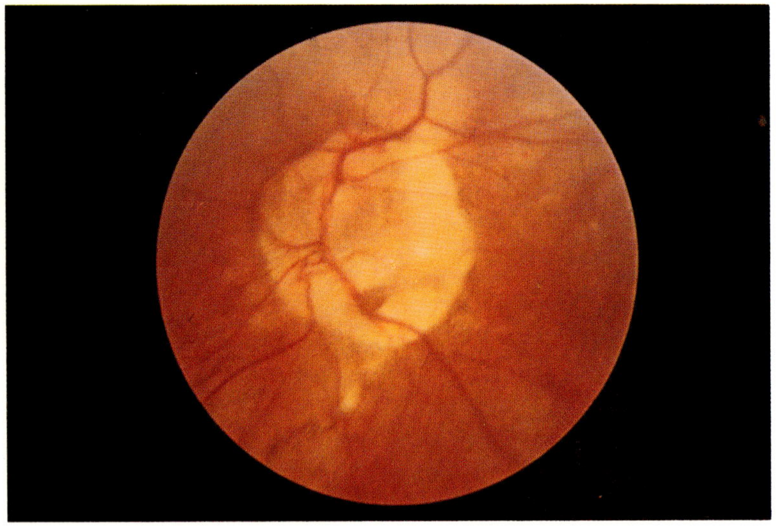

Plate 14. A broad, temporal, scleral crescent outlines a normal disc in a patient with severe myopia. A choroidal vessel, visible as a broad orange band, lies behind the inferior temporal vein.

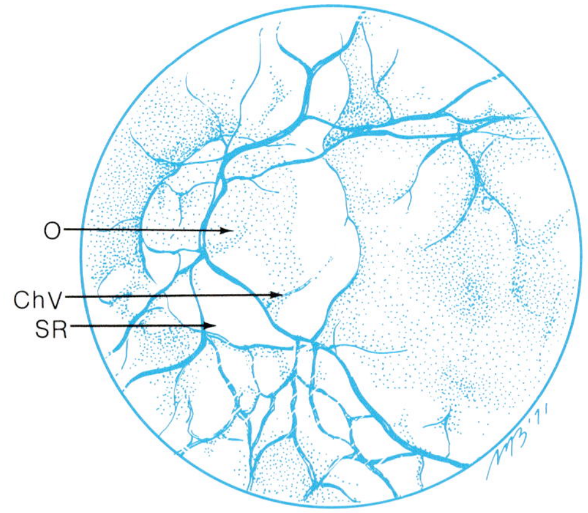

Drawing 14. Plate 14 (O, optic disc; SR, scleral ring; CHV, choroidal blood vessel).

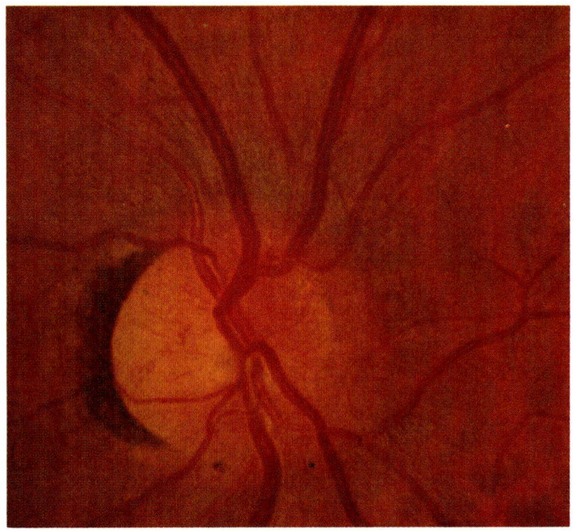

Plate 15. O.D. (right eye). Pigmented crescent at temporal margin of disc.

Figure XIII. The lamina cribrosa of the optic disc.

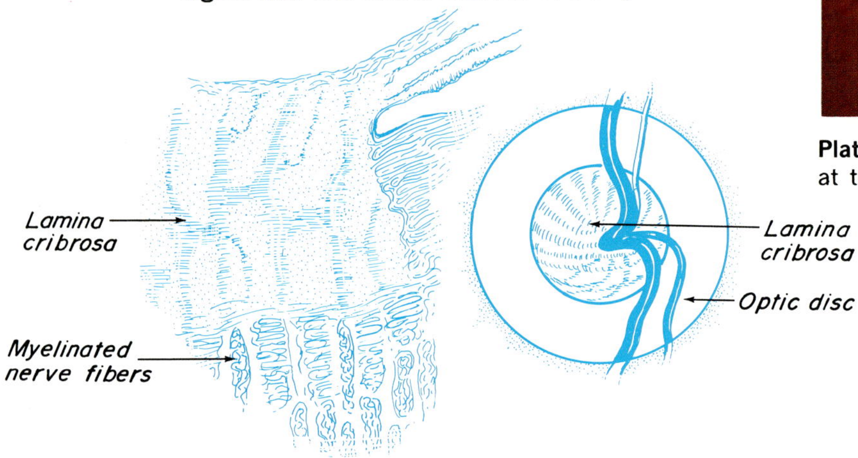

be broad and completely surround the disc (Plate 14 and Drawing 14). Choroidal vessels may be visible in the scleral ring (Plate 14 and Drawing 14; see p. 187 for a discussion of the effects of myopia). Thickening of the retinal pigment layer before it reaches the optic nerve frequently produces a pigmented ring temporal to the disc (pigmented crescent, Plate 15). The scleral ring and pigmented crescent may be present in the same eye.

In the center or slightly nasally, a small depression, the physiologic cup, is visible in the disc (Plate 12); through it the retinal vessels emerge. Within this depression, a sieve-like membrane, the lamina cribrosa, may be visible (Fig. XIII). This structure is formed by the fibers of the sclera, the pia mater, and perivascular sheaths of the central retinal vessels. Normally the axons of the ganglion cells of the retina do not acquire myelin sheaths until they penetrate the lamina cribrosa (see p. 9). A striking abnormality, known as myelinated or medullated nerve fibers (Plate 16), occurs when anomalous myelination exists in retinal and optic nerve fibers before they enter the lamina cribrosa.[23 (pp. 646-652)] Plate 17 and Drawing 17 demonstrate a group of myelinated nerve fibers situated above the lamina cribrosa.

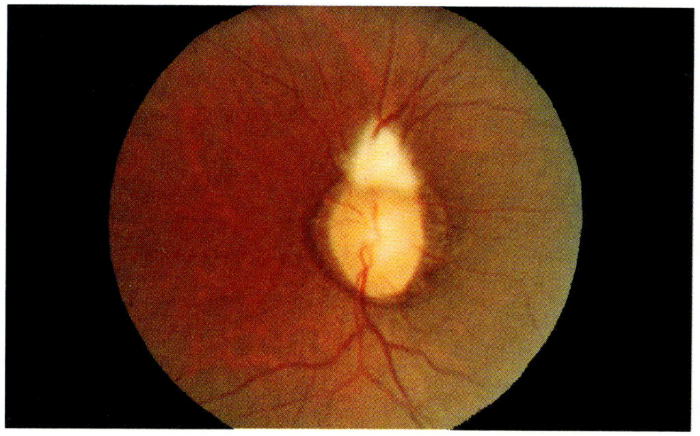

Plate 16. O.S. Myelinated nerve fibers. A white, irregular patch arises from the superior aspect of the disc. It overlies the superior retinal vessels.

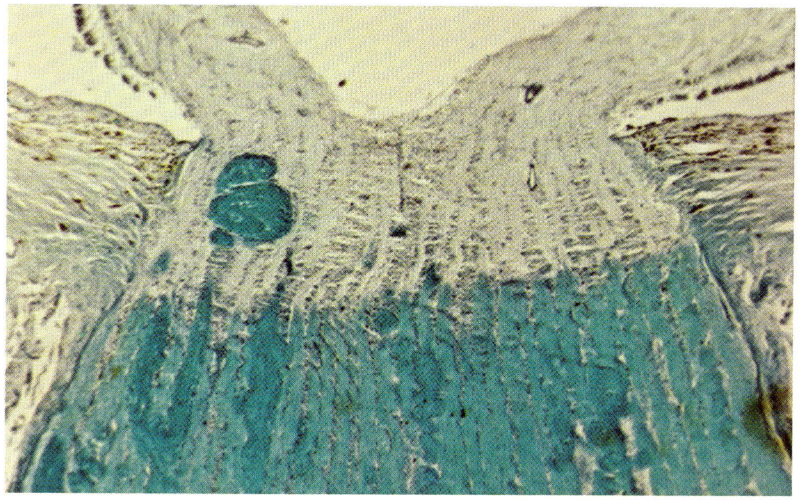

Plate 17. (Luxol fast blue, × 11½).

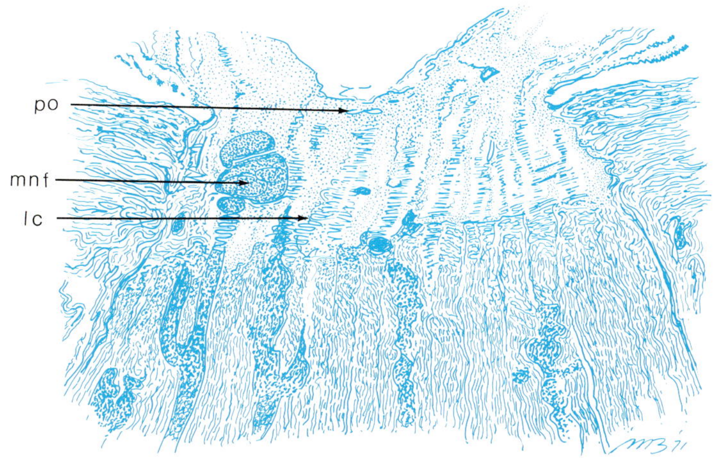

Drawing 17. Plate 17 (po, optic papilla; lc, lamina cribrosa; mnf, myelinated nerve fibers).

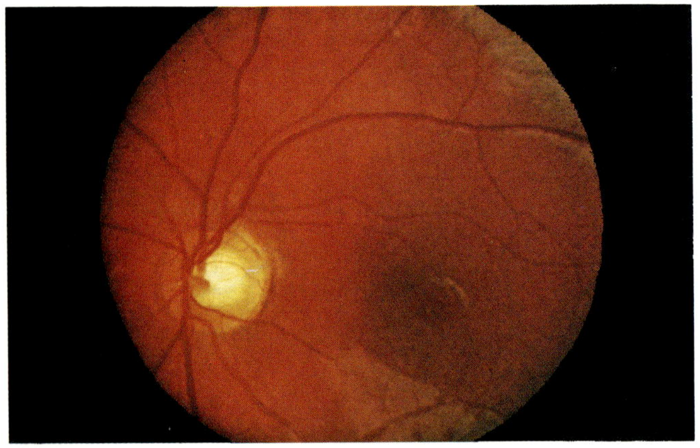

Plate 18. O.D. The fundus color is orange–red. The patient has fair skin and light brown hair. Note the macula, a dark brown, oval area, inferior and temporal to the disc.

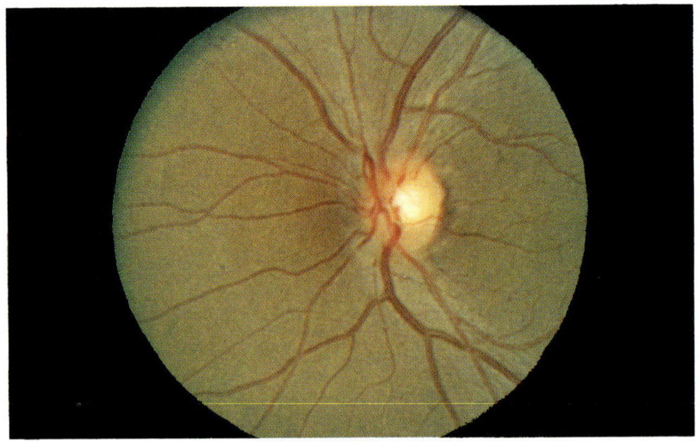

Plate 19. O.S. The fundus of a negro is a mixture of red, brown, and black.

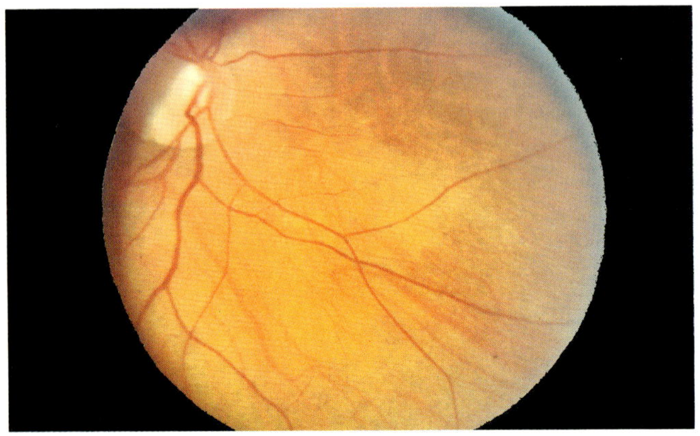

Plate 20. O.D. Fundus of a blond. Note the absence of pigment below the disc. The choroidal blood vessels are visible behind those of the retina. Pigment is present in the portion of the fundus adjacent to the nerve head.

Plate 21. O.S. Note brown–black islands of color that are separated by the orange–red choroidal blood vessels.

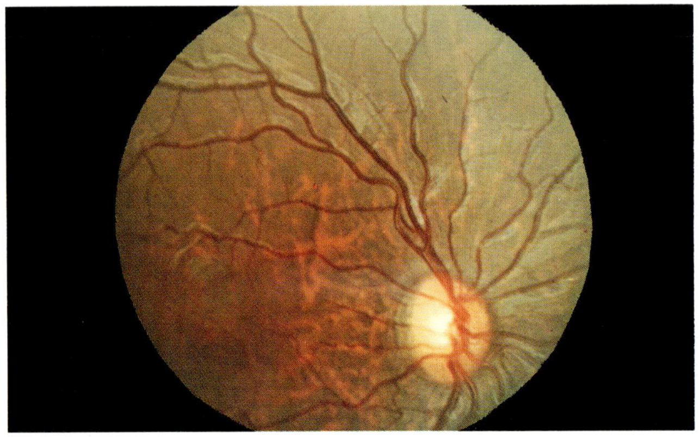

THE RETINA

With the light supplied by the ophthalmoscope, the color of the fundus is orange–red (Plate 18). Although the color is determined by the amount of oxyhemoglobin in the choroidal vessels, it is modified by the amount of melanin in the choroid and the pigment cell layer of the retina. As a result, the fundal reflex of the dark brunette and negro is a mixture of red, brown, and black (Plate 19). In contrast, the fundus color of the blond is red. In very light blonds or albinos, the decreased amount or absence of melanin in the choroid and pigment cell layers of the retina allows the choroidal vessels to be seen as broad orange bands behind the retinal vessels (Plate 20). The tigroid or tessellated fundus (Plate 21) provides a mosaic of islands of pigmentation which are separated by the visible choroidal vessels. This normal variant appears most commonly after middle age. It is the result of patchy melanin depletion in the pigment cell layer of the retina. The fundus appears pale in those with severe anemia and blue–red in patients who are cyanotic.

A cellophane–like glaze or "water–silk" appearance is frequently visible in the fundus of the young patient (Plate 22). It is believed to be the result of the reflection of the light of the ophthalmoscope as it strikes the internal limiting membrane and it is called retinal sheen. It is most prominent temporal, superior, and inferior to the disc, and along the retinal vessels. A change in the angle of the head of the ophthalmoscope will generally eliminate the perivascular sheen. These reflections of light are normal phenomena in the young and generally disappear after age forty. At times, the sheen may assume linear, dotted, or circular forms. The latter may appear as a ring about the macula or as a semicircle close to the disc.

THE MACULA

The macula is an ovoid pigmented area temporal and slightly inferior to the disc (Plates 23 and 24). It is generally the same size as the disc and approximately 1½ disc diameters from the temporal margin. Fine twiglike branches of the superior and inferior temporal vessels terminate at its border (Plate 25). The fovea, which is located in the center of the macula, is avascular (see p. 8 for a review of the histology of the macula). This avascular area appears as a small, orange–red reflex (foveal reflex). It is observed best when the patient looks directly into the light of the ophthalmoscope. Since the fovea contains a thin nerve fiber layer with neither ganglion cells nor inner nuclear layer, the oxyhemoglobin of the blood in the choriocapillaries is readily visible and accounts for this normal reflex.

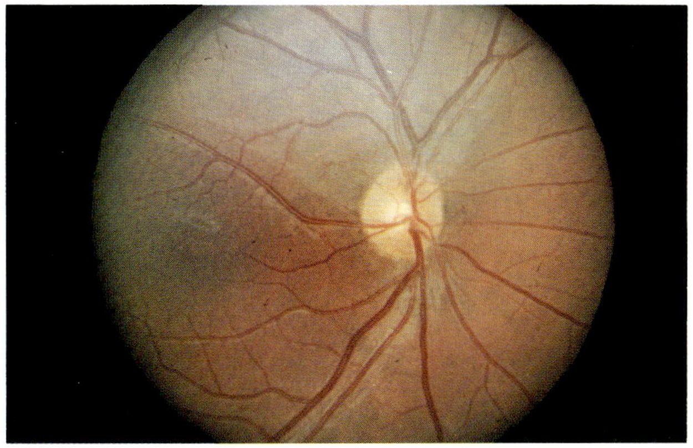

Plate 22. O.D. Normal fundus. Note white reflection of light extending over the upper portion of the retina and along the inferior central vessels.

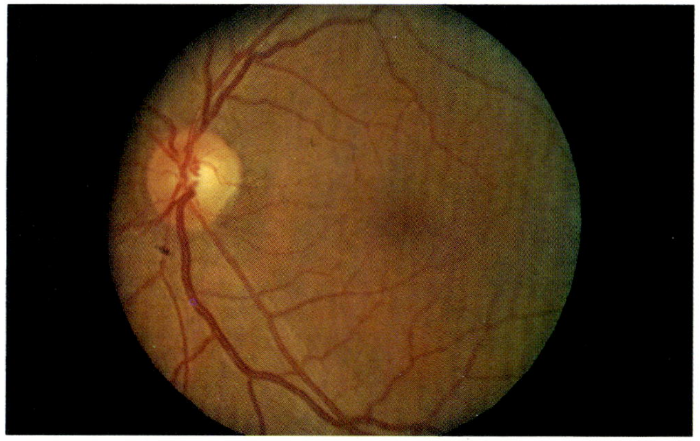

Plate 23. O.S. The macula is a darkly pigmented, circular area, located approximately 1½ disc diameters temporal to the optic disc.

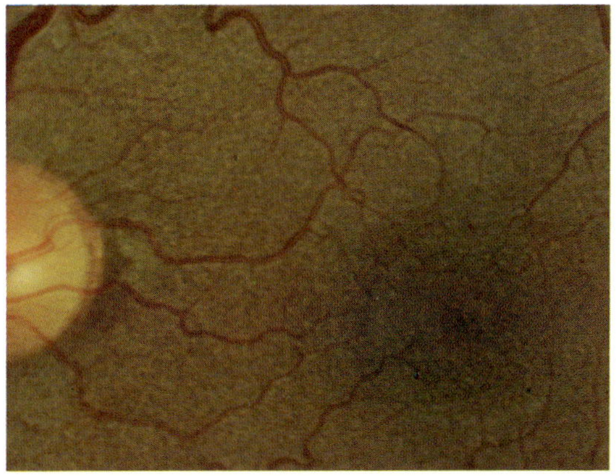

Plate 24. O.S. A magnified view of the macula. Note the central light area, the fovea.

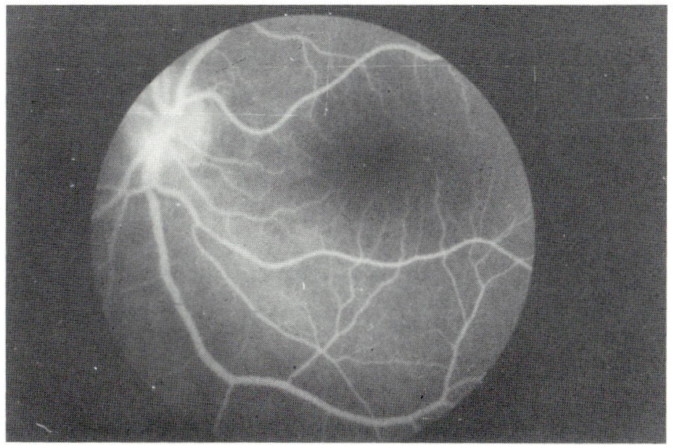

Plate 25. O.S. Fluorescein angiogram of the retina which demonstrates the arrangement of the dye–filled blood vessels in the macular region during the arteriovenous phase. (See Refs. 24–26 for a description of fluorescein angiography.)

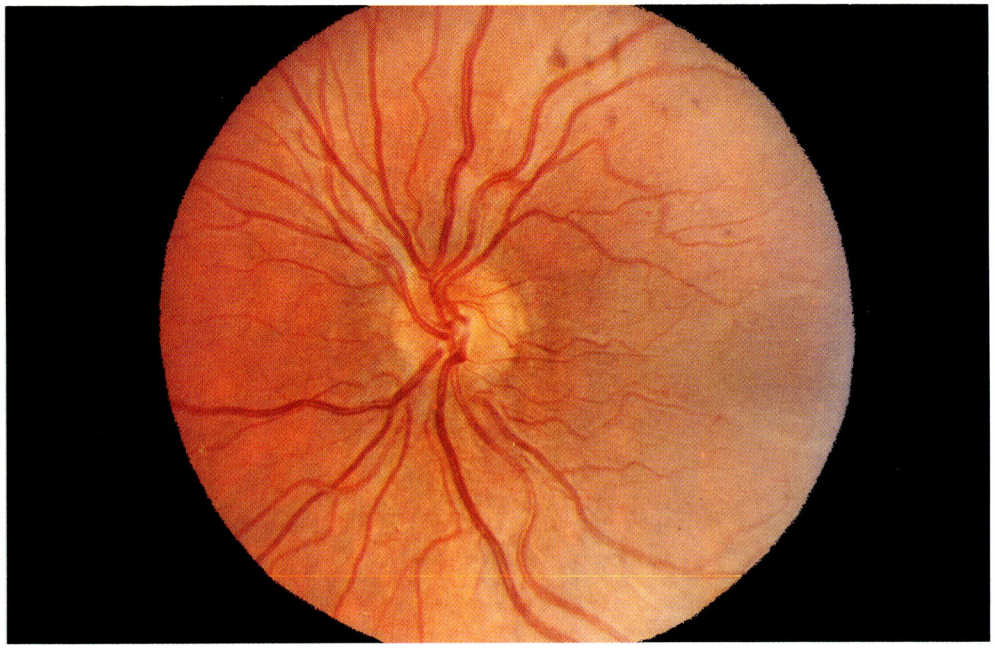

Plate 26. O.S. Normal fundus. The retinal blood vessels emerge from the physiologic cup of a normal optic disc. Superior and inferior arteriolar and venular branches extend into the nasal and temporal portions of the retina. The venules are darker and broader than the arterioles. Normal arteriovenous crossings are observed in the superior and inferior nasal quadrants. Note the white reflex (sheen) which surrounds the macula.

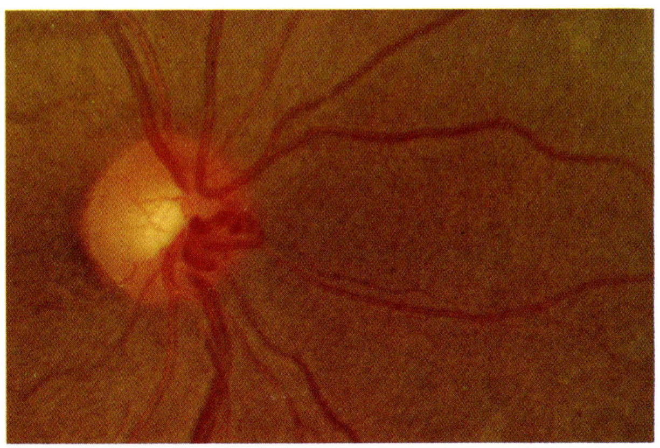

Plate 27. O.S. Persistent hyaloid vessels. A coil of blood vessels extends forward from the nasal portion of the disc. These anomalous vessels are in sharp focus with a +8 lens.

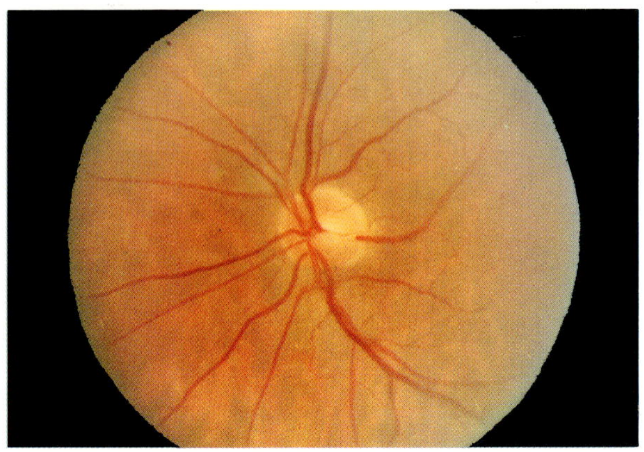

Plate 28. O.S. Cilioretinal artery. A small blood vessel, unattached to the central retinal vessels, extends from the temporal edge of the disc.

THE RETINAL VESSELS

Pulsation of the central retinal vein is a normal phenomenon. If absent, it can often be elicited in the normal patient with gentle eyeball pressure.* The central retinal artery normally does not pulsate. The four branches of the central retinal artery and vein traverse the four quadrants of the retina (Plate 26). Particularly in the young, the blood vessels curve in broad sweeps. They are even in caliber, tapering gradually as they extend toward the periphery. As previously indicated, the arterial branches have the histologic characteristics of arterioles. Secondary branches generally occur at approximately right angles. The temporal vessels distribute fine arteriolar branches which end in the macular region. The arterioles are lighter in color and narrower than the venules, roughly in the ratio of 2 to 3. These vessels cross each other at several points; generally the arteriole crosses the venule. The outline of the underlying venule remains intact at the crossing. A central light reflection is often visible in the normal arteriole; it tends to be patchy in the venular wall. Two concepts are offered to explain the so–called central light streak. The more frequently quoted explanation states that the phenomenon results from the reflection of the light of the ophthalmoscope as it strikes the interface of the column of blood and the concave vascular wall. Reflection of light from the internal limiting membrane is offered as the explanation of this sign by others.

Common congenital anomalies of the retinal circulation include persistent hyaloid vessels and the cilioretinal artery. Persistent hyaloid vessels remain visible as either blood–filled vessels (Plate 27) or as a cordlike structure which extends anteriorly from the optic disc.[23 (pp. 764-793)] As indicated previously (see

*As a solitary finding, absence of pulsation of the central retinal vein is not significant.

p. 4) the hyaloid artery is a continuation of the central retinal artery in the fetus. The former extends anteriorly through the vitreous to the posterior aspect of the lens and supplies the anterior segment of the eye. Normally the hyaloid vessels are obliterated before birth and leave no visible remnants. When they persist as anomalous structures, they produce no ill effects.

The cilioretinal artery, the other anomaly, is observed at the edge of the optic disc, usually on the temporal aspect (Plate 28). It extends laterally and may be the major source of nourishment of the macula. It arises from the circle of Zinn–Haller (see p. 11). It travels forward with the optic nerve without entering it and is not joined to the central retinal artery.[23 (pp. 764-793)] The vascular anomaly is present in approximately 20% of the population. Since it often provides the major blood supply of the macula, it may spare that vital part of the retina in patients with central retinal artery occlusion (see p. 31). Persistent hyaloid vessels and the cilioretinal artery may be present in the same patient (Plate 29).

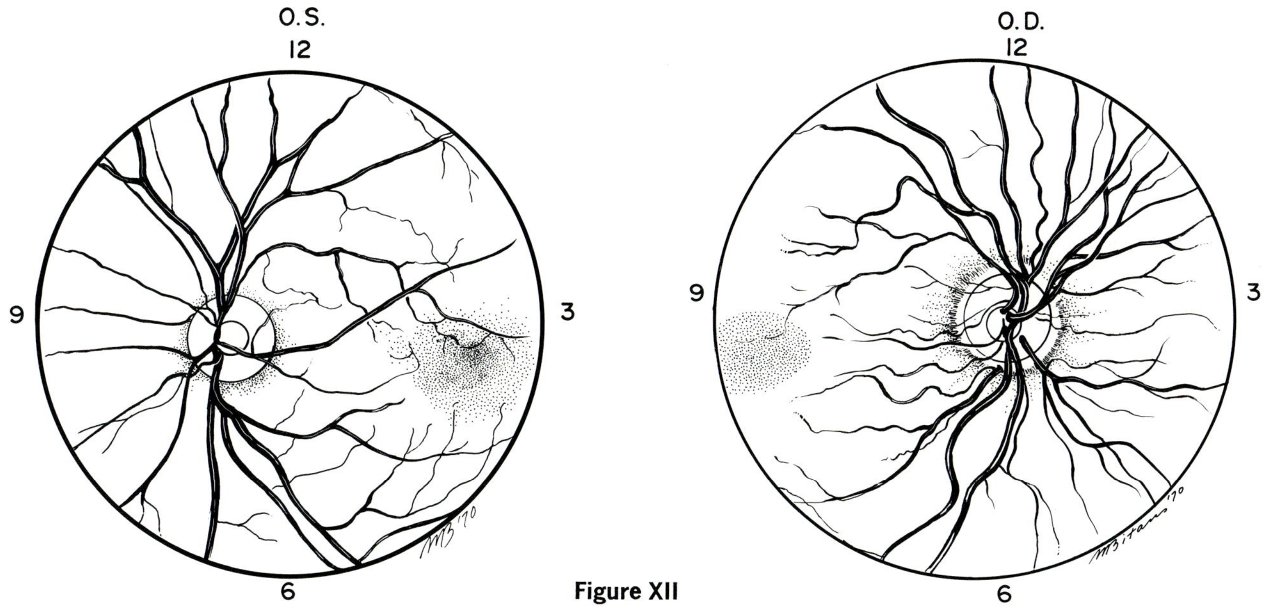

Figure XII

METHODS OF RECORDING RESULTS OF FUNDUSCOPIC EXAMINATION

The results of the examination can be recorded by either narrative description or a sketch. Either method of recording is simplified if one accepts the fundus as the face of a clock with the disc in the center and the numerals at the periphery (Fig. XII). Lesions of the retina can then be described or drawn according to their location on the clock, measuring so many disc diameters from the optic nerve. The symbol O.U. (oculi unitas) represents both eyes; O.D. (oculus dexter) and O.S. (oculus sinister) are used to represent the right and left eye respectively. The de-

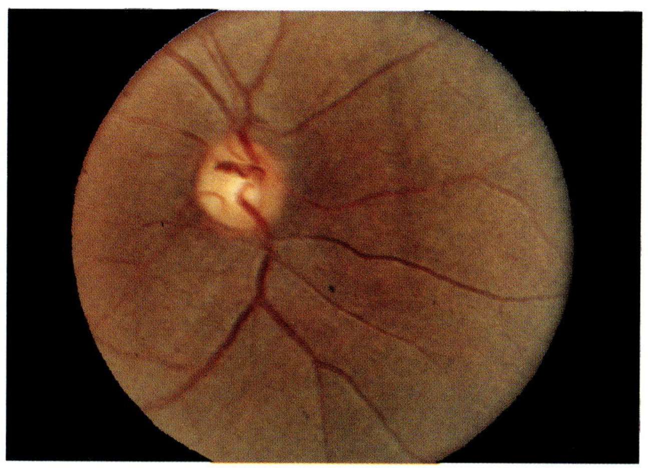

Plate 29. O.D. Persistent hyaloid vessel and cilioretinal artery. The cilioretinal artery arises from the temporal part of the disc. It is not connected to the central retinal artery. The hyaloid vessel arises from the central retinal vessels.

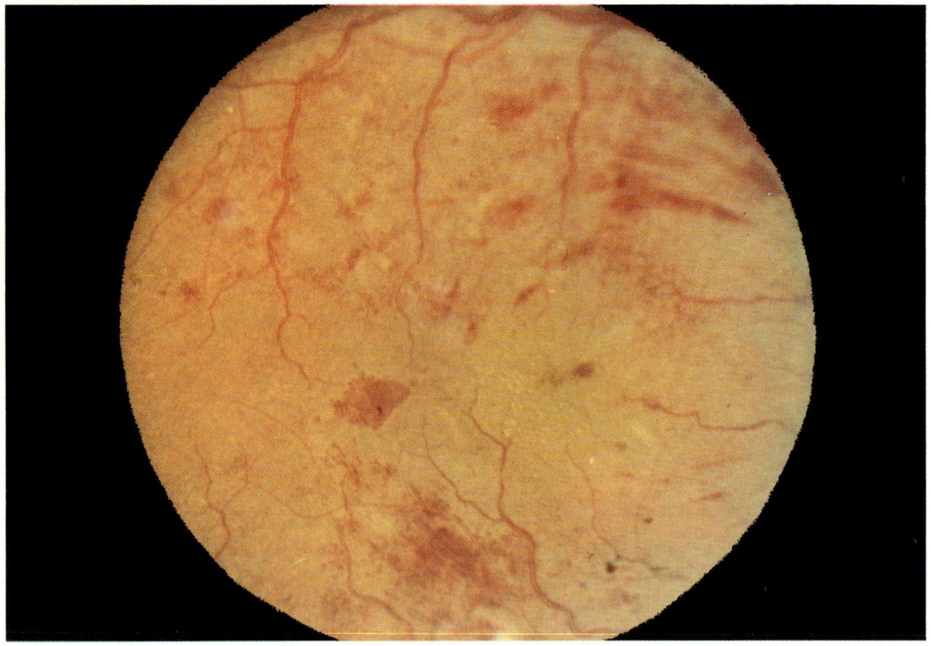

Plate 30. O.D. Temporal. There are numerous flame–shaped and linear hemorrhages; many of them overlie blood vessels. In addition, several round (dot and blot) hemorrhages are behind retinal vessels. Several small, discrete, white lesions are crossed by blood vessels (hard exudates).

scription of each eye may be listed separately. However, the author prefers to list the findings common to both eyes, followed by any differences in each eye. For example:

O.U.—The media are clear. Both optic discs are flat and their margins are distinct. The central retinal veins pulsate spontaneously. The arterioles are normal. Marked venular tortuosity and segmentation are observed. The maculae are normal with good foveal reflexes. There are no retinal abnormalities except as described below.

O.D.—There is a large flame–shaped hemorrhage at 3 o'clock, one disc diameter from the optic nerve. Several microaneurysms are present at 9 o'clock medial to the macula.

O.S.—There are several small, sharply defined, yellow areas of degeneration (exudates) at 6 o'clock, two disc diameters below the optic nerve. Several small blood vessels cross over the lesions.

The accuracy of the record is increased when the narrative description is combined with either a line drawing or retinal photographs.

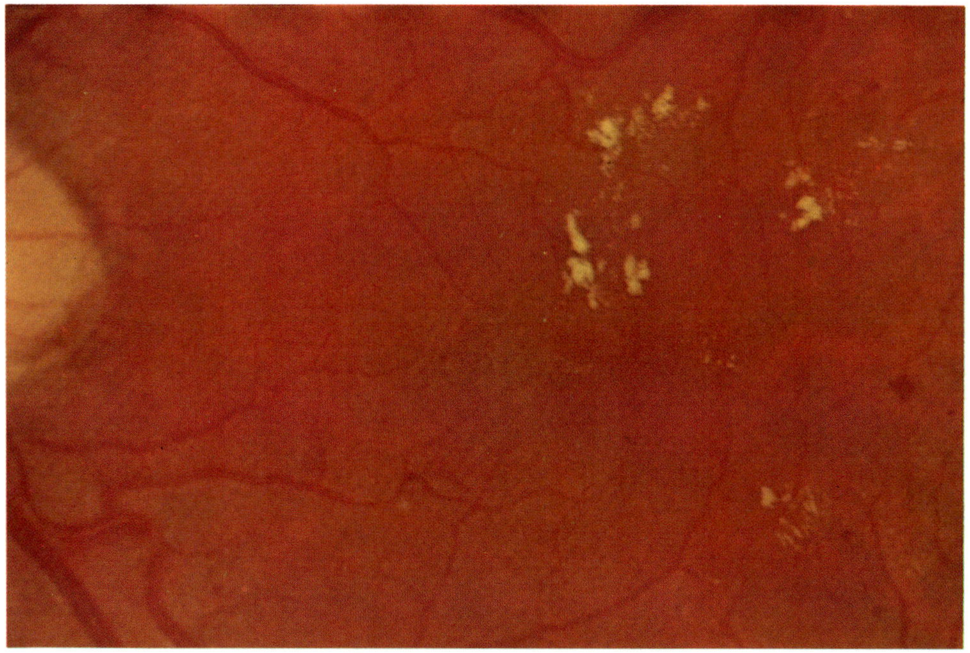

Plate 31. O.S. Temporal; hard exudates. The darkly pigmented area, the macula, is $1\frac{1}{2}$ disc diameters from the temporal margin of the nerve head. There are several small, discrete, white areas of degeneration in the macular region. Similar areas of degenération are noted at 5 o'clock, inferior to the macula and 3 disc diameters from the optic nerve. Blood vessels cross over several of those lesions. A flame–shaped hemorrhage is present below and temporal to the macula. Several small red dots (probably microaneurysms) are visible between the disc and the macula.

RECOGNITION OF THE CHARACTER AND LOCATION OF RETINAL ABNORMALITIES

The understanding of the normal histology and blood supply of the retina can help the examiner determine the location and character of various abnormalities of the retina. As examples we shall discuss hemorrhage, cotton wool patches, and hard exudates.* (Review histology and blood supply of the retina, pp. 6–8 and 12–14.) For example, hemorrhage in the nerve fiber layer of the retina is confined by the horizontal nerve fibers in that area. As a result, hemorrhages in the nerve fiber are linear and flame–shaped (Plate 30). In addition, such hemorrhages generally overlie the blood vessels in that layer. The round hemorrhages (Plate 30) are in the outer plexiform layer. Their shape is determined by the pressure exerted by the vertical fibers of that layer. Blood in that area spreads the fibers and accumulates in the form of a cylinder. It appears round when viewed end–on with the ophthalmoscope. In addition, the round or oval (dot and blot) hemorrhages lie behind the retinal blood vessels (Plate 30). The hard exudate is also found in the outer plexiform layer. It appears as a discrete lesion located behind the retinal blood vessels (Plate 31).

When outer plexiform lesions are present in the macula, they assume a starlike form (Plate 32).

The cotton wool patch (soft exudate) develops in the nerve fiber layer. Characteristically, it has irregular or striate borders and usually obscures the underlying blood vessels (Plate 33).

*The abnormalities are discussed in Chapter III, the extravascular lesions, pages 58 through 69.

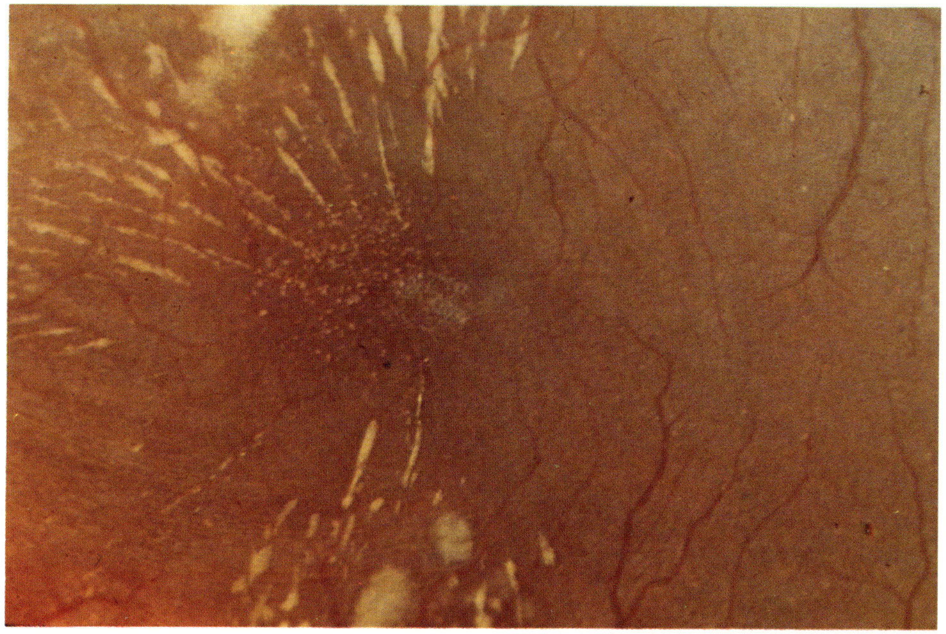

Plate 32. O.S. Macula; macular star. The macula, a dark, pigmented area, is in the center. There are linear white lesions radiating from its superior and inferior aspects. Note that blood vessels cross over several of the linear lesions. In addition there are three white lesions, with irregular borders (cotton wool patches) above and below the macula.

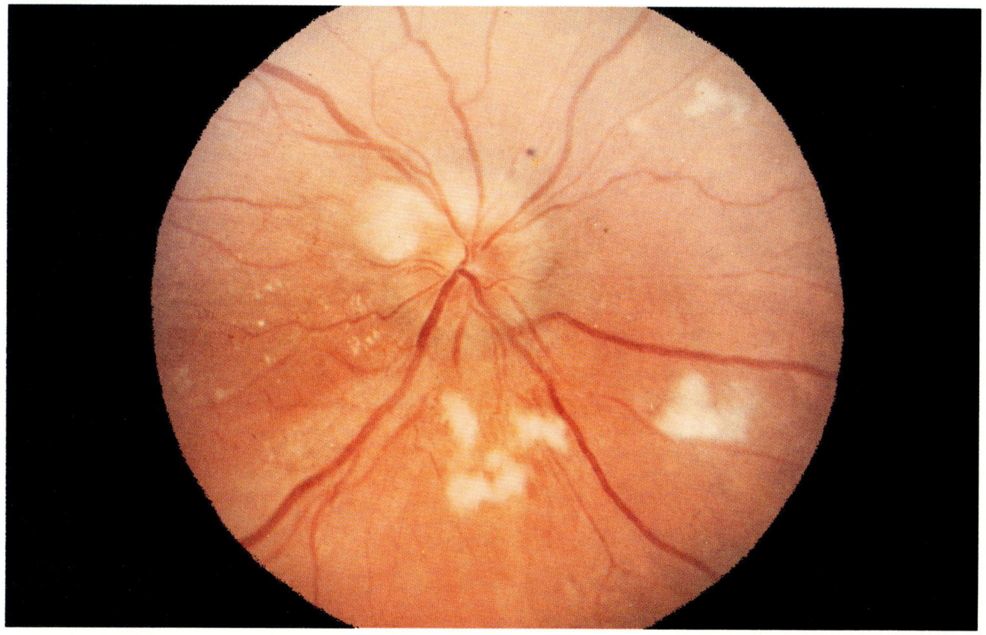

Plate 33. O.D. Central; cotton wool patches. The optic disc is hyperemic and its margins are indistinct (papilledema). There are irregular white lesions at 1, 5, and 6 o'clock (cotton wool patches). Several of these lesions overlie blood vessels. One cotton wool lesion, at 11 o'clock, encroaches upon the swollen optic disc. A linear hemorrhage is present above the cotton wool patch at 5 o'clock. There are several hard exudates between 7 and 11 o'clock, within one disc diameter of the nerve head.

ANNOTATED BIBLIOGRAPHY

Embryology

Allan, F. D.: *Essentials of Human Embryology,* pp. 166–171, Oxford University Press, New York, 1960. A clear and concise outline of the embryology of the eye.

Patten, B. M.: *Human Embryology,* 2nd ed., pp. 396–411, Blakiston Co., New York, 1952. A detailed discussion of the embryology of the eye.

Anatomy of the Retina and Optic Nerve

Duke–Elder, W. S. and Wybar, K. C.: *The Anatomy of the Visual System,* in Duke–Elder, W. S. (ed): *System of Ophthalmology,* Vol. II, Mosby, St. Louis, 1961; retina, pp. 220–273; optic nerve, pp. 273–293. An excellent description of the anatomy of the retina and optic nerve.

Hogan, M. J. and Zimmerman, L. E. (eds.): *Ophthalmic Pathology. An Atlas and Textbook,* 2nd ed., Saunders, Philadelphia, 1962; retina, pp. 469–475; optic nerve, pp. 571–577. A clear and concise presentation of anatomy of the retina and optic nerve.

Wolff, E.: *Anatomy of the Eye and Orbit, Including the Central Connections, Development, and Comparative Anatomy of the Visual Apparatus,* 5th ed., revised by R. J. Last, Saunders, Philadelphia, 1961; retina, pp. 88–114; optic nerve, pp. 295–317. A detailed presentation of the anatomy of the retina and optic nerve.

Blood Supply of the Retina

Kuwabara, T. and Cogan, D. G.: *Studies of Retinal Vascular Patterns, Part I. Normal Architecture,* Arch. Ophthalmol., **64:** 904, 1960. An excellent presentation of a superb method for the study of the small retinal vessels.

Michaelson, I. C.: *Retinal Circulation in Man and Animals,* Charles C Thomas, Springfield, Ill., 1954. An interesting presentation of the retinal circulation.

Blood Supply of the Optic Nerve

Francois, J. and Neetens, A.: *Vascularization of the Optic Pathway. I. Lamina Cribrosa and Optic Nerve,* Brit. J. Ophthalmol., **38:** 472, 1954.

Singh, S. and Dass, R.: *The Central Artery of the Retina. II. A Study of Its Distribution and Anastomoses,* Brit. J. Ophthalmol., **44:** 280, 1960.

The two articles complement each other, presenting a good review of the blood supply of the optic nerve.

General Examination of the Eye

Berens, C.: *The Eye and Its Diseases; By Ninety–Two International Authorities,* 2nd ed., pp. 149–161, Saunders, Philadelphia, 1949. A presentation of the importance of the ophthalmologic history, the scope of the general examination of the eye, and methods of testing visual acuity.

Examination of the Fundus

Ballantyne, A. J. and Michaelson, I. C.: *Textbook of the Fundus of the Eye,* 2nd ed., Williams & Wilkins, Baltimore, 1970; methods of examination, pp. 1–49; the normal fundus, pp. 53–86. This text has excellent discussions.

Congenital Anomalies

Duke–Elder, W. S.: *Normal and Abnormal Development. Part 2, Congenital Deformities,* in Duke–Elder, W. S. (ed.): *System of Ophthalmology,* Vol. III, Mosby, St. Louis, 1963; vascular anomalies, pp. 764–793; optic disc anomalies, pp. 668–688, colobomata, pp. 456–481; medullated (myelinated) nerve fibers, pp. 646–652. Clear presentations of some of the more common anomalies.

Chapter II

ARTERIAL AND ARTERIOLAR DISEASE

ARTERIAL AND ARTERIOLAR DISEASE OF THE RETINA

The term arteriosclerotic retinopathy has been applied to the vascular lesions which affect the retinal circulation. Since arteriosclerosis includes three major types of pathologic change—intimal atherosclerosis, arteriolarsclerosis, and medial calcification—the term arteriosclerotic retinopathy is ambiguous and misleading. Of the three forms of arteriosclerosis, only intimal atherosclerosis and arteriolarsclerosis affect the retinal vessels.

Atherosclerosis affects large and small arteries with the main pathologic change in the intima. Lipid–containing cells accumulate between the internal elastic lamella and endothelium. The atheroma increases in size and may occlude the lumen of medium size and small arteries with or without thrombosis. The internal elastic lamella may become fragmented and the atheromata may be replaced by fibrous tissue. Medial fibrosis and sclerosis may occur as well. The central retinal artery and its branches close to the disc are true arteries and may be the site of atherosclerosis and subsequent occlusion.

Arteriolarsclerosis involves arterioles throughout the body. Its histologic changes consist of endothelial hyperplasia, intimal hyalinization, and medial hypertrophy. Arteriolarsclerosis is commonly associated with hypertension and generally produces clinical alterations of the retinal blood vessels (see pp. 36–47). In malignant or accelerated hypertension, the morphologic changes in the arterioles include fibrinoid degeneration of their walls, often called fibrinoid necrosis or necrotizing arteriolitis.

RETINAL ARTERIAL DISEASE

Occlusion of the Central Retinal Artery

Occlusive disease of the central retinal artery or its branches may be the result of the following pathological states:

1. Atherosclerosis
2. Embolism
   a. occlusive disease of the internal carotid arteries
   b. following arteriography
   c. associated with thromboendarterectomy
   d. aortic and mitral valve disease
   e. following valvulotomy
   f. auricular fibrillation and mural thrombosis of the left atrium
   g. subacute bacterial endocarditis
   h. myocardial infarction and mural thrombosis of the left ventricle
   i. endocardial myxoma
   j. fat embolism
3. Vascular inflammatory disease
   a. temporal arteritis
   b. polyarteritis nodosa
   c. pulseless disease
4. Sickle cell disease
5. Angiospasm
   a. migraine
   b. pregnancy
   c. tobacco
6. Drugs
   a. oral contraceptives
   b. quinine

Plate 34. O.S. Central retinal artery occlusion in the presence of a cilioretinal artery in a black patient. The arterioles are narrow. The retina is pale with the exception of the triangular, normal segment immediately temporal to the disc. Did you notice the cilioretinal artery emerging from the temporal side of the disc? It apparently nourishes the normal segment. Note the brown–red fovea (cherry–red spot) temporal to the segment of normal retina. There is a flame–shaped hemorrhage overlying the disc at 7 o'clock.

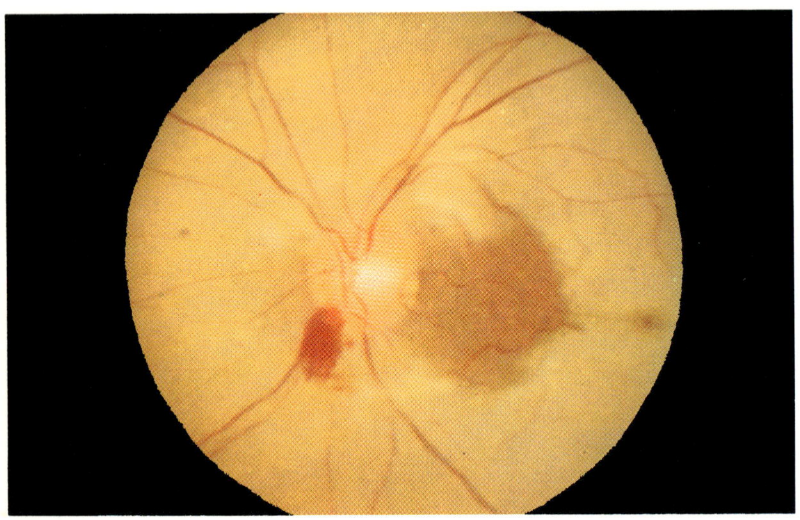

Drawing 34. Plate 34 (O, optic disc; HEM, hemorrhage; CRA, cilioretinal artery; R, normal retina; FO, fovea).

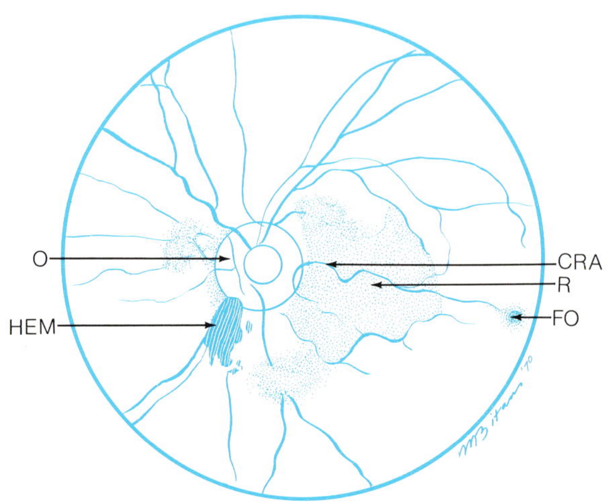

Clinical Findings

Characteristically there is a sudden, painless loss of vision in the affected eye. The pupil is dilated and does not react with direct stimulation of light. The arterioles are narrow and the retina is opaque and white. In sharp contrast, the oxyhemoglobin in the uninvolved underlying choroidal blood vessels appears as a red or brown spot at the fovea (cherry–red spot) (Plate 34 and Drawing 34). Clumping of red blood cells in the venules produces the "boxcar" effect. Fluorescein angiography discloses a similar change in the arterioles as well.[27] Retinal hemorrhage may occur, although it is unusual. If a cilioretinal artery is present, the segment of the retina which it supplies may be preserved and retain its normal appearance (Plate 34 and Drawing 34).

Within several weeks the retina regains its transparency and the normal fundus color returns (Plate 35 and Drawing 35). Optic atrophy, characterized by a sharply marginated, pale disc, develops frequently (Plate 35). (See pp. 185 and 193 for a detailed presentation of optic atrophy.) Months later, the arterioles may appear as white threads ("silver wire" change, see pp. 40 – 41). Secondary glaucoma is a rare complication.[28] If a single branch of the retinal artery is occluded, the retinal changes are limited to the area supplied by that vessel.

Drawing 35. Plate 35 (O, sharply outlined optic disc with few blood vessels crossing its margins; D, areas of degeneration; M, macula; CRA, ciliretinal artery).

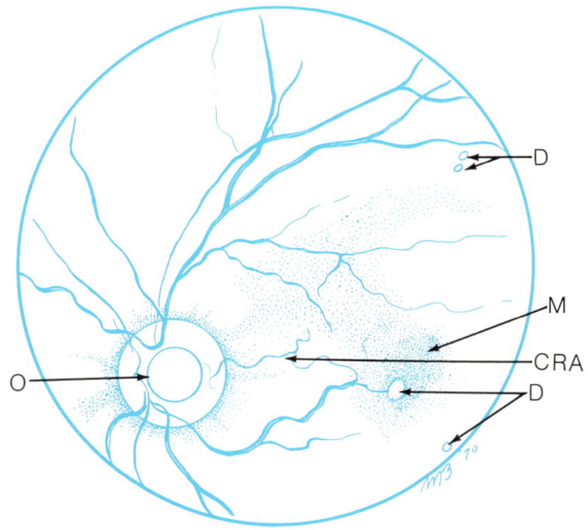

Plate 35. O.S. Temporal. Same patient as Plate 34, 7 months later. The normal fundus color has returned; the disc is pale, contains few vessels, and has sharp borders. The arterioles are narrow. Note circular yellow lesions which represent areas of degeneration in the macula and in the peripheral retina inferior and temporal to the macula. In this instance, the cilioretinal artery (arising along the temporal part of the disc) did not protect the macula.

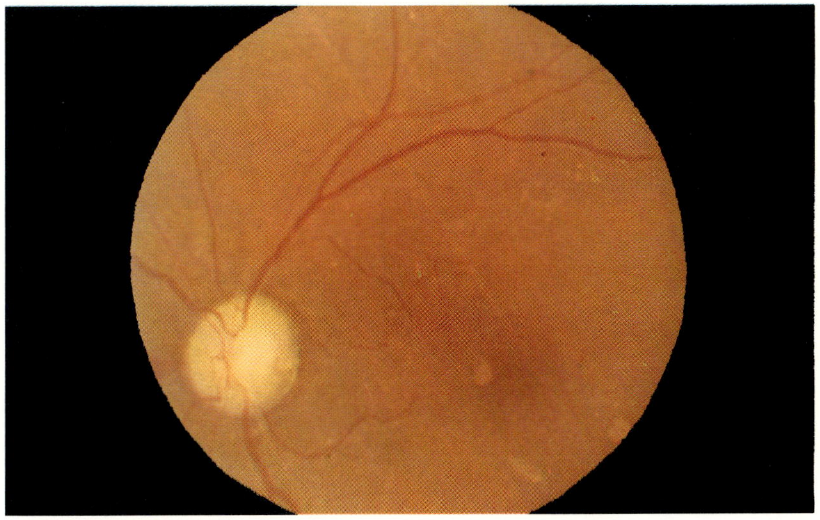

Plate 36. Atheromatous embolus of a branch of the central retinal artery. A glistening orange plaque (cholesterol embolus) is visible at the bifurcation of an arteriole.

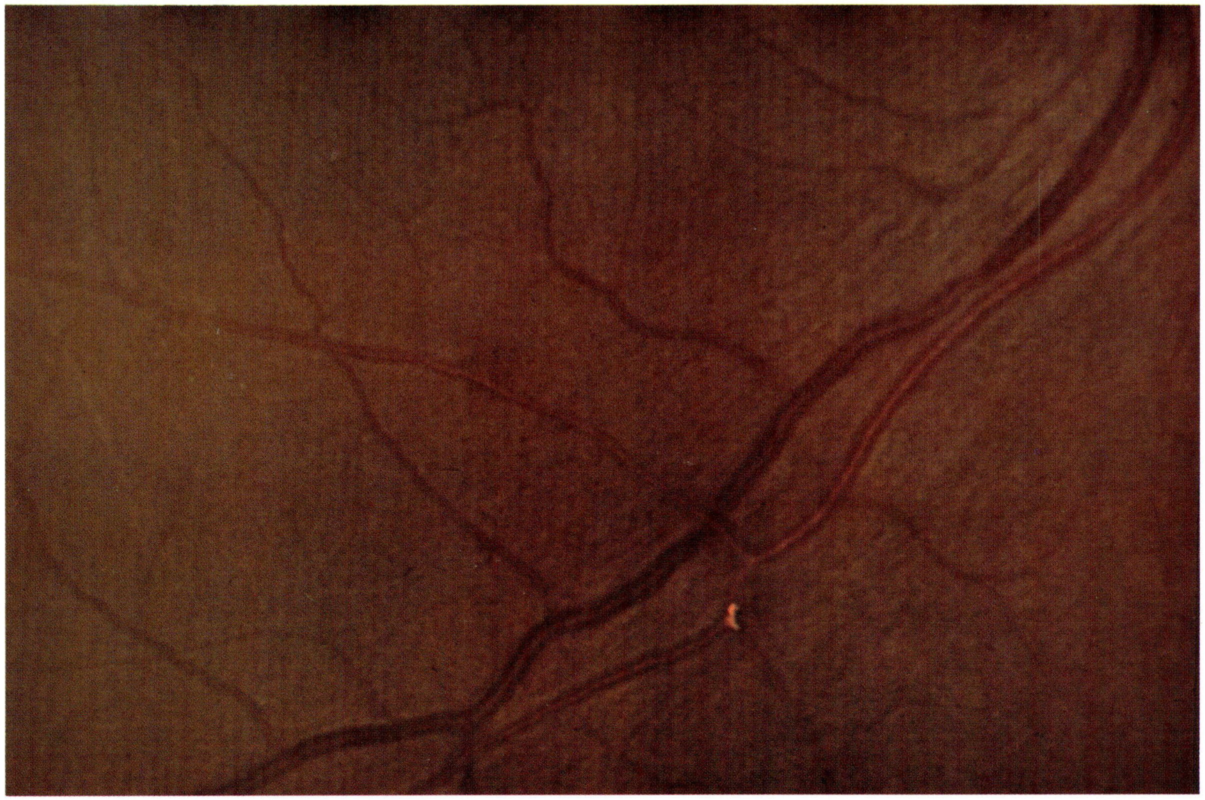

A transient, unilateral blindness, amaurosis fugax, at times accompanied by a temporary contralateral hemiparesis, has been observed in patients with occlusive disease of the interior carotid artery.[29, 30, 31, 32, 33] The visual loss occurs suddenly, and generally lasts less than one minute, leaving no scotomata. During the acute episode, the pupil of the affected eye does not constrict with direct stimulation of light. Funduscopy often discloses the presence of white or glistening orange plaques in the arterioles[29, 30, 32] (Plate 36). Peripheral movement of these intravascular inclusions and their ultimate disappearance have been observed.[29, 30, 32] In a recent review of fifty-four patients with rheumatic heart disease, eighteen (33%) gave a history of transient loss of vision.[34] Auricular fibrillation and sinus rhythm were observed with equal frequency. The majority of the patients had clinical evidence of mitral valve disease; the remainder had involvement of both the mitral and aortic valves or only aortic valve disease.

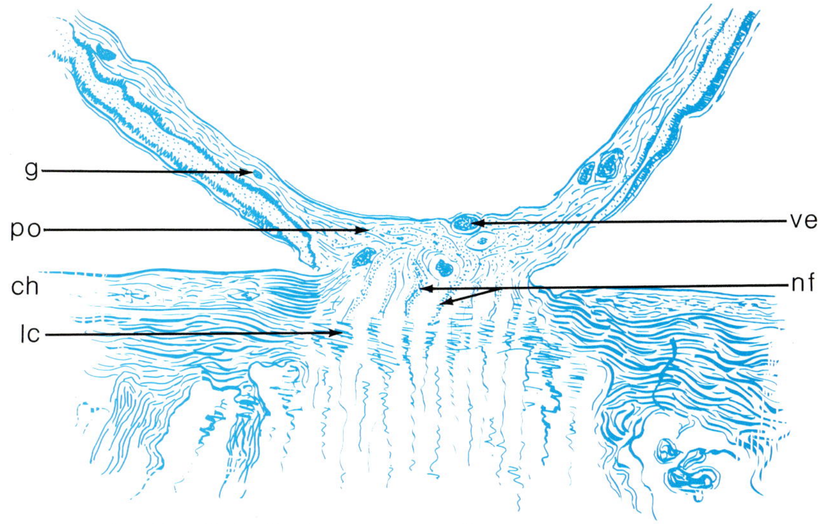

Drawing 37. Plate 37 (po, optic papilla; r, retina; ch, choroid; nf, swollen nerve fibers; ve, vascular engorgement; g, ganglion cells; lc, lamina cribrosa).

Plate 37. Central retinal artery occlusion. Many of the nerve fibers anterior to the lamina cribrosa are necrotic and swollen; others accept the stain poorly. Ganglion cells are decreased in number. Vascular engorgement and a perivascular inflammatory response are present. The outer plexiform and nuclear layers are normal (PTAH, × 20).

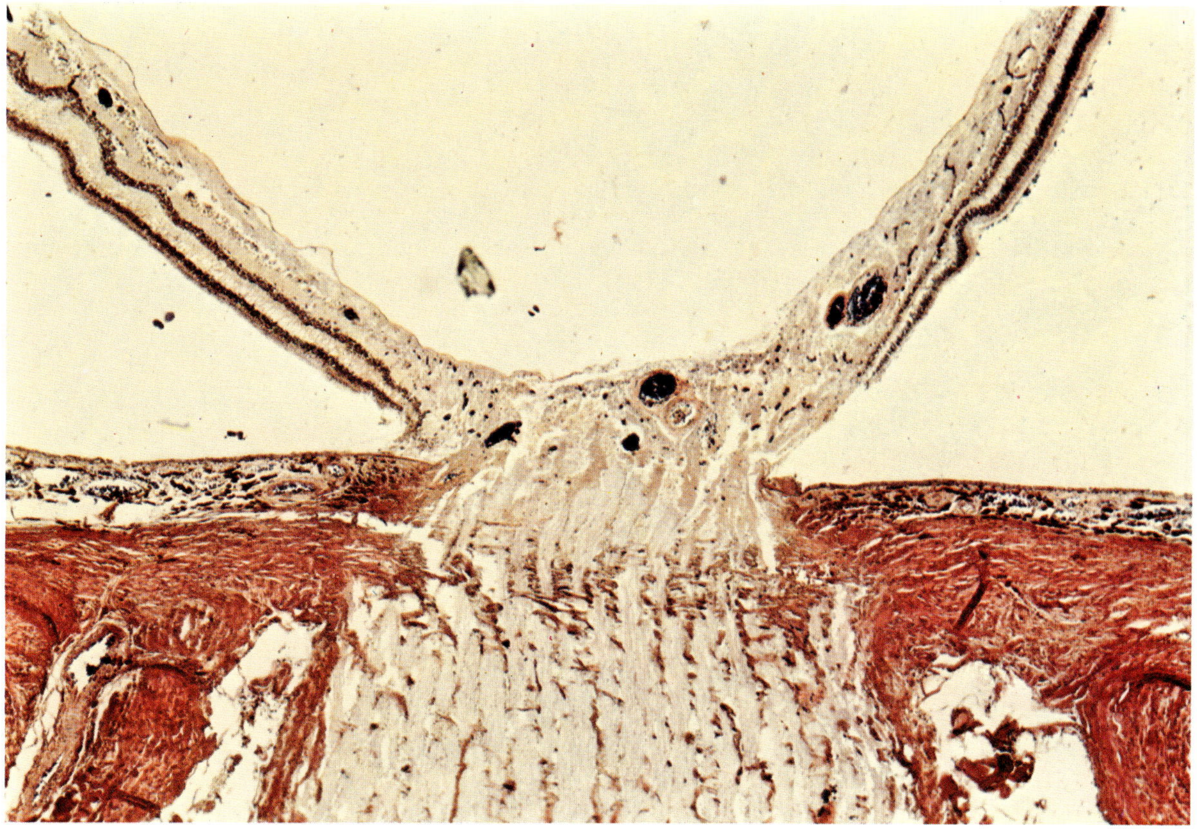

Pathology

Obstruction of the central retinal artery is followed by edema of the inner retinal layers.[35] (Review blood supply of the retina, pp. 12–14.) Necrosis of nerve cells, particularly ganglion cells and nerve fibers, occurs (Plate 37 and Drawing 37). The resulting cellular debris is removed by macrophages. Marked shrinkage of the involved layers and loss of nuclear structures are the end results.[2 (p. 495)] Retinal gliosis is usually absent.[2 (p. 495)] The loss of ganglion cells is followed by ascending degeneration of the fibers of the optic nerve with subsequent optic atrophy (see ischemic neuropathy of the optic nerve, p. 193). The outer plexiform layer, the rods and cones, and their nuclei remain intact when the central retinal artery is occluded, since the integrity of these structures is not dependent upon that artery.

Utilizing the squirrel monkey, a primate with an optic disc, blood vessels, and macula similar to man, Kroll[36] studied the clinical and histologic changes that followed experimental occlusion of the central retinal artery. Serial fundus photographs and fluorescein angiography demonstrated changes similar to those observed in the spontaneously developed disease in man. In the monkey, within 15 minutes after ligation of the central retinal artery, electron microscopy disclosed mitochondrial swelling in the neurons of the inner retinal layers. Progressive changes included swelling of the endoplasmic reticulum and cell cytoplasm. After 3½ hours, clumping of nuclear chromatin and rupture of cytoplasmic membranes were observed. Destruction of all cells anterior to the outer nuclear layer was noted after 16 hours. The photoreceptor cells were spared. In the same study, when tissue was studied by phase microscopy, changes were observed 40 minutes after the central retinal artery was ligated. Edema of the inner retinal layers was accompanied by vacuolization of the axons of the nerve fiber layer and the ganglion cells After 3½ hours, there was massive edema of the inner layers and marked vacuolization of the ganglion cells and their axons. Vacuoles were also observed in the inner plexiform layer and the nuclei of the cells in the inner nuclear layer were pyknotic. The outer plexiform fibers and the rods and cones and their nuclei were unaffected.

Such evidence strongly suggests that a comparable sequence of events occurs in man after sudden and complete occlusion of the central retinal artery.

Pathogenesis

The abnormalities responsible for occlusion of the central retinal artery include atherosclerosis, embolism, vascular inflammatory disease, and angiospasm.

1. Atherosclerosis of the central retinal artery is most prominent at the site where that vessel penetrates the dural sheath of the optic nerve and at the lamina cribrosa.[2 (p. 66)] Obliterative endarteritis or local thrombosis superimposed upon atheromata provide the actual occlusion.

2. Embolism. An embolus may completely obstruct the central retinal artery in the region of the lamina cribrosa. Smaller emboli lodge in the arteriolar branches. Occlusive disease of the internal carotid arteries is the most frequent source of the emboli.[37] Small segments of atheromatous plaques or of the thrombus which overlie these lesions may become dislodged spontaneously,[30] after either arteriography[38] or thromboendarterectomy.[39] The emboli consist of cholesterol esters,[40] neutral fat,[41] masses of platelets,[39] segments of mural thrombi,[42] bacterial vegetations from infected heart valves, portions of an endocardial myxoma,[43] and calcium.[44-46] The emboli composed of calcium either arise spontaneously from diseased aortic valves[44,46] or they follow valvulotomy.[45]

3. Vascular inflammatory disease. The vascular inflammatory diseases that are associated with clinical evidence of central retinal artery occlusion include temporal arteritis, polyarteritis nodosa, and pulseless disease. Pathologic confirmation of involvement and occlusion of the central retinal artery has been demonstrated in temporal arteritis.[47, 48] Only clinical observations have been made in polyarteritis nodosa.[49] In pulseless disease, the ischemic changes in the retina are the result of occlusion of common carotid arteries.[50]

a. Temporal arteritis is a generalized panangitis which characteristically involves the temporal arteries. Other cranial arteries, particularly the carotid system and the aortic arch and its branches, may also be affected. The involved arteries may develop nodules and often become solid cords. Histologic findings include intimal proliferation with varying degrees of luminal obstruction. A granulomatous inflammation of the media is the characteristic change. The inflammatory process spreads to the adventitia as well. The etiology of temporal arteritis is not known.

b. Polyarteritis nodosa is a progressive, systemic, necrotizing inflammation of small arteries and arterioles. The initial inflammatory changes, which occur primarily in the media and spread to the intima and adventitia, consist of polymorphonuclear cells and eosinophils. They are eventually replaced by mononuclear cells, including lymphocytes, plasma cells, and macrophages. Aneurysms may form at the sites of necrosis of the vessel wall. Fibrous and thrombotic occlusions of the involved vessels are common. Although the etiology of this disease is not clear, it is generally considered a manifestation of hypersensitivity and it is classified as one of the vascular connective tissue disorders.

c. Pulseless disease (Takayasu's disease or the aortic arch syndrome) is a giant cell arteritis of the major arteries that arise from the aortic arch. Microscopic changes include an inflammatory response in the entire vessel wall. The lymphocytic and giant cell response is accompanied by subintimal fibrosis, which results in narrowing and often obliteration of the vascular lumen. Since the disease involves the common carotid arteries, manifestations of retinal ischemia are common.

The etiology of pulseless disease is not known.

4. Sickle cell disease. Clinical manifestations of central retinal artery occlusion are described in sickle cell disease.[4 (p. 290)] Although vascular occlusion is known to be a manifestation of sickle cell disease, histologic evidence of involvement of the central retinal artery is lacking.

5. Angiospasm. The concept that transient visual loss may result from spasm of the retinal artery and its branches is well established in ophthalmoscopic literature.[4 (pp. 195-196)] Such visual loss has been reported by patients with migraine, by pregnant women, and by users of tobacco.[4 (p. 196)] The validity of vasospasm as a mechanism for the production of transient visual loss is seriously threatened by the previously cited relationship between retinal arterial and arteriolar embolism in amaurosis fugax.

6. Drugs.

a. Oral contraceptives. Clinical evidence of central retinal artery occlusion which results from the use of oral contraceptives is well documented.[51] Although histologic evidence of alterations of the vasculature of the retina is not available, there is ample evidence of systemic arterial disease following ingestion of such drugs.[52] The arterial changes include thrombosis, intimal thickening and fibrosis, and disruption of the media.[52] Less common changes are endothelial and intimal proliferation, and local nodular fibrosis of intima, media, and adventitia. These are observed in the absence of thrombosis.[52]

b. Quinine is included in the list of drugs allegedly associated with retinal artery occlusion, presumably on the basis of vasospasm.[4 (p. 196)]

Occlusion of the Central Retinal Artery and Clinical States

Obstruction of the central retinal artery occurs most commonly after age fifty in patients who have hypertension and diabetes mellitus.[53] The reported high frequency of embolic occlusion of the cerebral and retinal arterial systems associated with atherosclerosis and mural thrombosis of the internal carotid arteries is striking.[30, 33, 37] It should be emphasized that both arteriography and thromboendarterectomy of the carotid arterial system may be further sources of such embolic phenomena.[38, 41] Calcific aortic valve disease, particularly after valvulotomy, may produce the same complications.[44-46, 54] Mitral valve disease,[34, 53] subacute bacterial endocarditis, myocardial infarction with mural thrombosis,[42] and left atrial myxoma[48] provide other sources of such embolic phenomena. Fat embolism may follow severe trauma with multiple fracture of bones.[55, 56] Thrombotic occlusion has been reported in association with skull fracture.[57]

Temporal arteritis usually occurs in elderly patients and may affect one or both central retinal arteries. In this disorder, the symptoms and signs of central retinal artery occlusion are accompanied by severe headache, nodular, tender, and thrombosed temporal arteries, fever, and leukocytosis.[47, 58-68] Temporal artery biopsy often discloses the presence of the characteristic arteritis. Since steroid therapy halts the progression of the disease, early diagnosis and treatment, particularly in unilateral central retinal artery occlusion, may prevent the development of ischemic optic neuropathy and optic atrophy in the other eye[69] (see p. 193).

Documented central retinal artery occlusion is rare in polyarteritis nodosa.[49] Since steroid therapy may be effective, early diagnosis is important. Multisystem involvement, often associated with fever, weight loss, hypertension, peripheral neuropathy, arthralgia, and leukocytosis with eosinophilia should suggest this diagnosis. Muscle, skin, and renal biopsy often provide histologic evidence of its presence.

The retinal ischemia in pulseless disease results from occlusion of the carotid arteries as they arise from the aortic arch.[50, 70] The ocular abnormalities include cataract, optic atrophy, microaneurysms, cotton wool patches, and hemorrhage.[70-73] The systemic manifestations include symptoms of cerebral ischemia, such as vertigo, seizures, syncope, transient hemiparesis, and aphasia.[72] These findings are accompanied by the absence or diminution of arterial pulsations and blood pressure in the upper extremities. Hypertension in the legs is often present. Fever, leukocytosis, and elevated sedimentation rate may accompany the other findings. Reversibility of the manifestations of cerebral and retinal ischemia has been reported after thromboendarterectomy[75] and the placement of bypass grafts between the aorta and internal carotid arteries.[75]

Central retinal artery occlusion is a rare complication of sickle cell disease.[4 (p. 290), 76] It has been reported in heterozygous, SA[77] as well as in the homozygous, SS form.[76] In SA disease the central retinal artery occlusion was bilateral and the patient also had documented lupus erythematosus.[77] Although central retinal artery occlusion has not been reported in lupus erythematosus, one cannot be certain that the sickle cell trait was the sole offender.[77]

Cryoglobulinemia is an extremely rare cause of occlusion of the central retinal artery.[78]

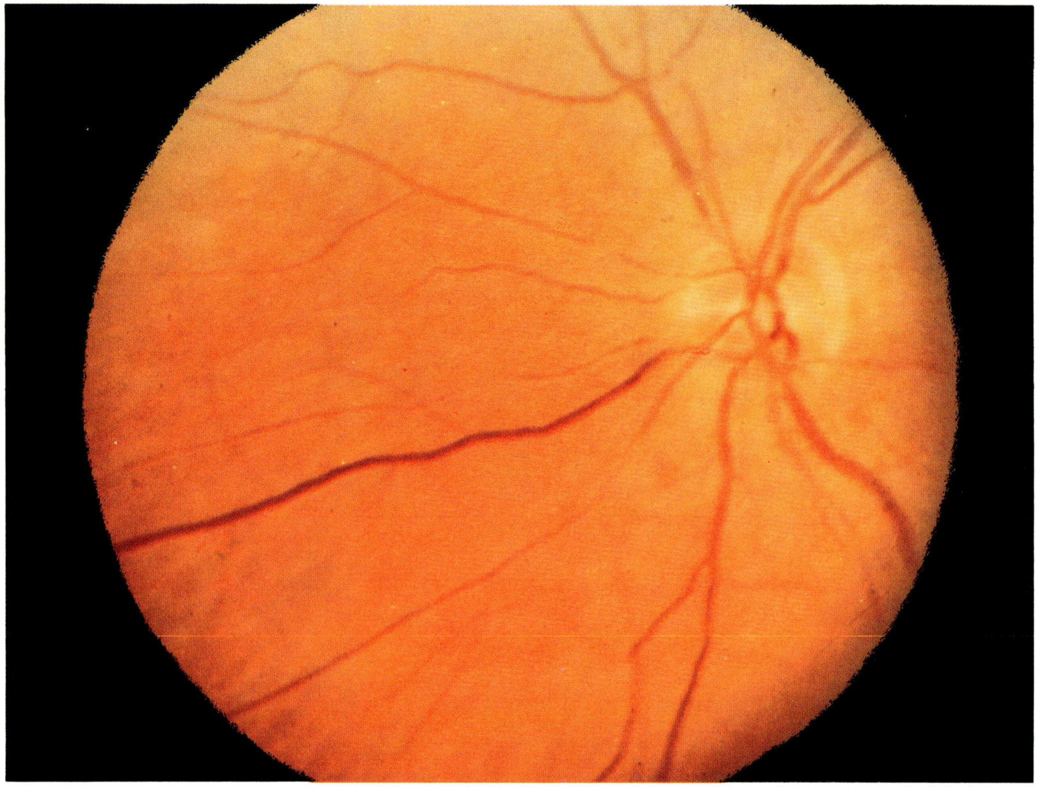

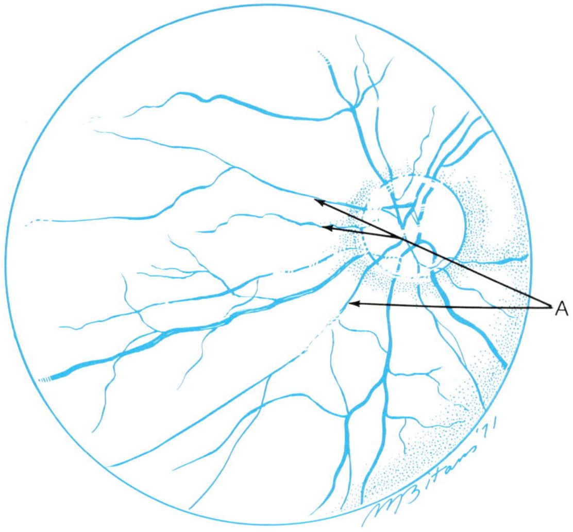

Drawing 38. Plate 38 (A, arteriolar narrowing).

Plate 38. O.S. Diffuse arteriolar narrowing and straightening.

The alarming, recently described neuro–ophthalmologic complications associated with the widespread use of oral contraceptives is a major source of concern.[51, 52, 79, 80] The manifestations include: migraine, chiefly in patients with a previous history of vascular headache; transient cerebral ischemia and cerebral thrombosis in previously healthy young women; and occlusion of the central retinal artery and vein.

RETINAL ARTERIOLARSCLEROSIS

As previously stated, the branches of the central retinal artery acquire the characteristics of arterioles distal to their first or second bifurcations. In hypertension, which serves as an excellent model, arteriolarsclerosis is the basic pathologic change. It is characterized by the presence of endothelial hyperplasia, intimal and medial hyalinization, and medial hypertrophy. In the retina, the clinical manifestations of that pathologic state are not only readily recognized but they also offer the possibility of estimating generalized arteriolar change.

ARTERIOLAR DISEASE

The clinical manifestations of arteriolar disease consist of the following:

I. Alteration of caliber
   A. Narrowing
      1. Diffuse
      2. Segmental
      3. Alterations of arteriolar–venular ratio (A–V ratio)
      4. Straightening
   B. Widening
      1. Diffuse
      2. Segmental
   C. Tortuosity
II. Alteration of central light streak
   A. Broadening of light streak
   B. "Copper wire" change
   C. "Silver wire" change
III. Sheathing
   A. Parallel
   B. Pipe–stem
IV. Arteriolar–venular compression (arteriovenous compression)
   A. A–V displacement
   B. A–V nicking or compression

Alteration of Caliber

Narrowing of retinal arteroles may be diffuse (Plate 38 and Drawing 38) or segmental

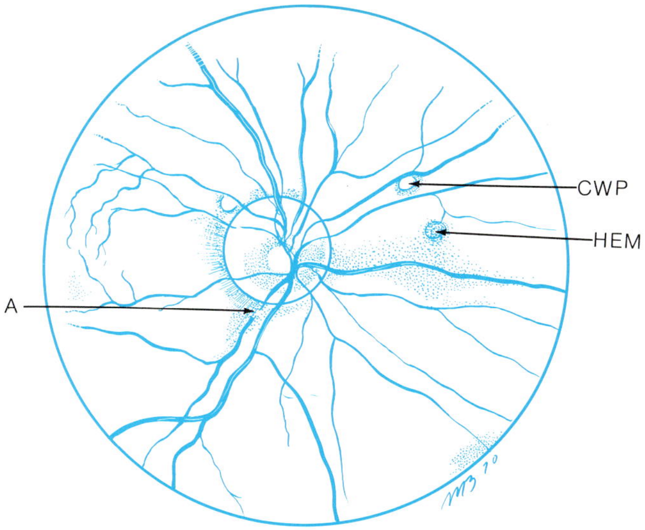

Drawing 39. Plate 39 (CWP, cotton wool patch; A, segmental arteriolar narrowing; HEM, hemorrhage).

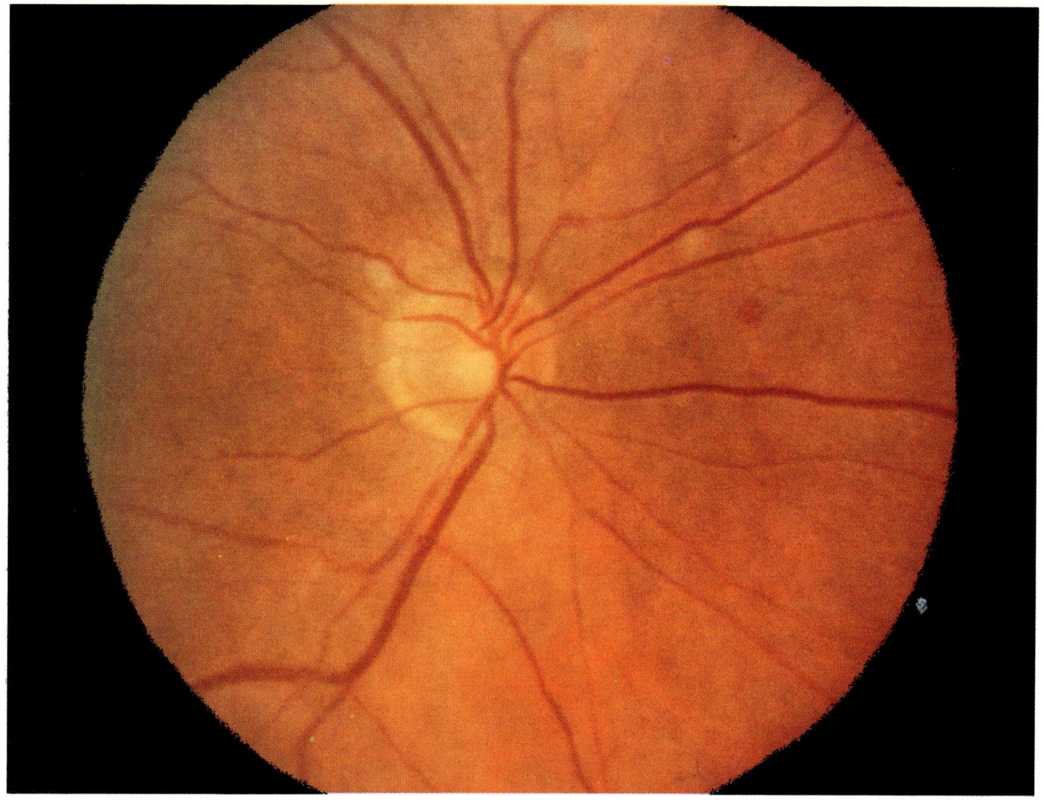

Plate 39. O.D. Focal (segmental) arteriolar narrowing at 6 o'clock close to the disc. Note the hemorrhage at 2 o'clock and the cotton wool patch at 1 o'clock, one disc diameter from the disc.

(Plate 39 and Drawing 39). Although such changes are generally found in young patients with hypertension or toxemia of pregnancy, Leishman[81] describes similar changes in older patients without hypertension and refers to such alterations as the "senile retinal arteriole." Occlusion of the central retinal artery is known to cause arteriolar narrowing as well (Plate 34 and Drawing 34).

In toxemia of pregnancy[82] and early in the course of hypertensive disease the diminished caliber of retinal arterioles is believed to be the result of vasospasm associated with elevated blood pressure.[83, 84] The reversibility of arteriolar narrowing after therapeutic reduction of diastolic blood pressure in those diseases justifies the concept of vasoconstriction and suggests that fixed arteriolar changes may be absent during some stage of hypertensive disease.[82, 84, 85] Although Sieker and Hickam[86] demonstrated that retinal arterioles of normal individuals constrict after inhalation of a high concentration of oxygen, they were unable to reproduce this change in a group of patients with hypertension. It has been well documented that focal and diffuse retinal arteriolar narrowing may become irreversible in patients with hypertension despite adequate blood pressure response to sympathectomy[82, 84] or drug therapy.[87, 88] In a study of 33 patients with chronic renal disease and hypertension prior to renal transplantation, retinal arteriolar narrowing was observed in 26.[89] Post–operatively that abnormality persisted in 23 of the group even though papilledema and such extravascular lesions as cotton wool patches and hemorrhage disappeared. These observations indicate that retinal arteriolar narrowing becomes fixed as the hypertensive state progresses.

Plate 34. O.S. Central retinal artery occlusion in the presence of a cilioretinal artery in a black patient. The arterioles are narrow. The retina is pale with the exception of the triangular, normal segment immediately temporal to the disc.

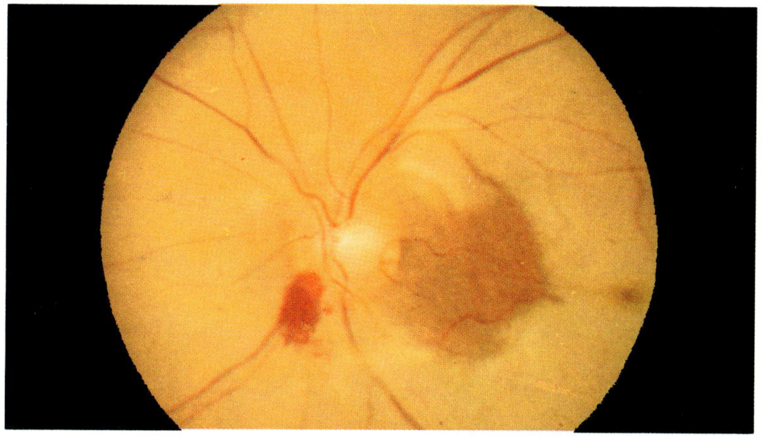

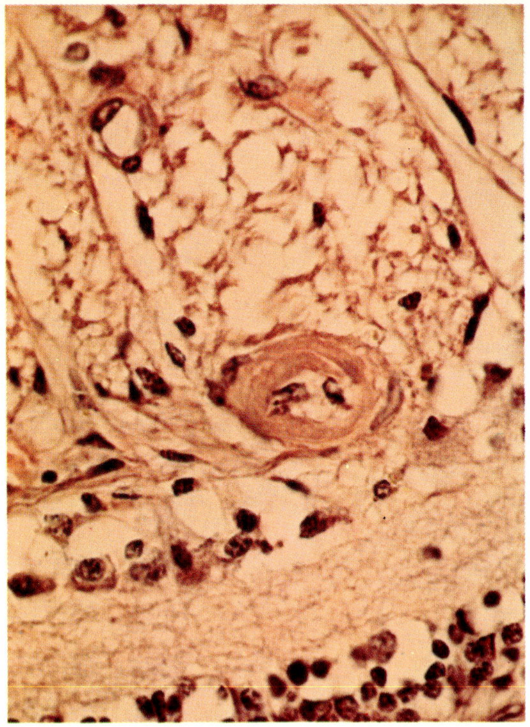

Plate 40. Arteriole of retina. Narrowing of lumen. Intimal and medial thickening and hyalinization (PTAH, × 400).

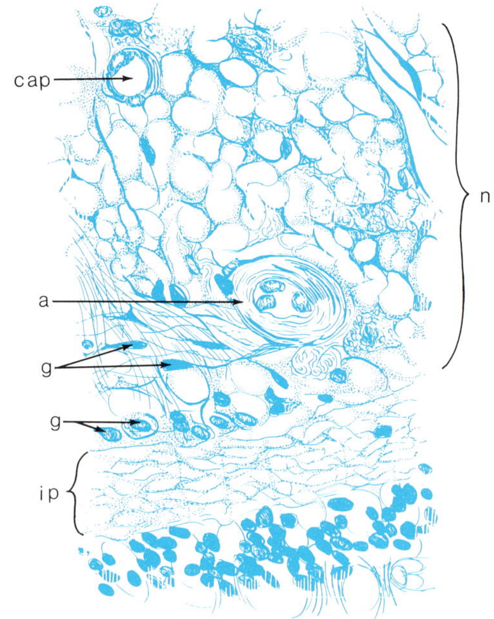

Drawing 40. Plate 40 (cap, capillary; a thick–walled arteriole; nf, nerve fiber layer; g, ganglion cells; ip, inner plexiform layer).

Alteration of the A–V ratio from the normal 2:3 relationship to 1:2 or 1:3 is an expected result of retinal arteriolar narrowing. Since engorgement of venules can produce the same ratio change, the clinical use of this ratio is not meaningful unless the caliber of the arteriole or venule is individually described. Furthermore, the A–V ratio may be misleading unless two vessels of comparable order of division are selected for comparison.[90]

Straightening of arterioles, according to Leishman,[81] is found in children or young adults with hypertension (Plate 38 and Drawing 38).

PATHOLOGY OF ARTERIOLAR NARROWING

The irreversibility of retinal arteriolar narrowing in long standing hypertension is understandable in view of the vascular pathology commonly found in that disease. The arteriolar changes are characterized by endothelial hyperplasia, intimal and medial hyalinization, medial hypertrophy, and luminal narrowing (Plate 40 and Drawing 40). The concept that

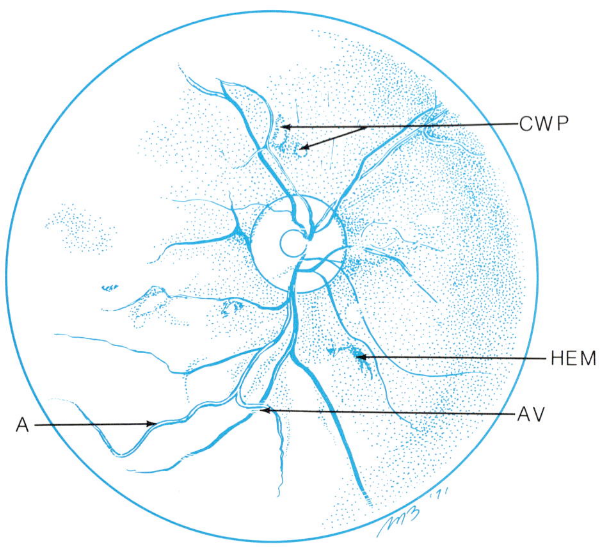

Drawing 41. Plate 41 (A, "copper and silver wire" change; AV, arteriovenous compression; CWP, cotton wool patch; HEM, hemorrhage).

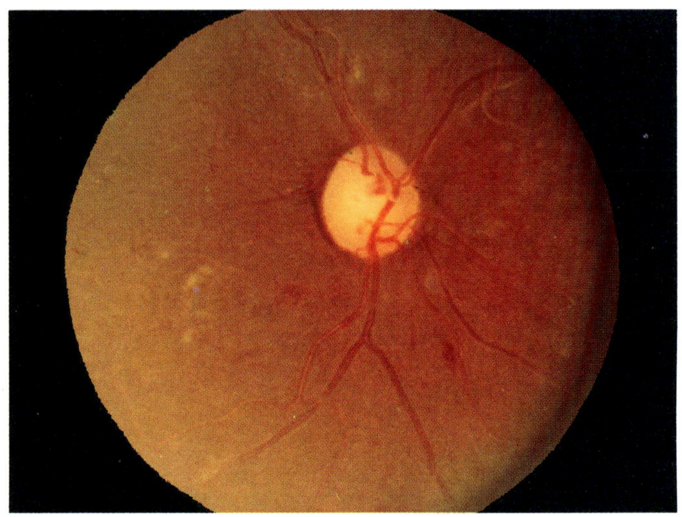

Plate 41. O.D. (1) Tortuous inferior temporal arteriole. (2) Widened central light streak of inferior and superior temporal arterioles. (3) "Copper wire" merging into "silver wire" change of inferior temporal arteriole. (4) Arteriovenous compression of inferior temporal vessels. (5) Hemorrhages at 5 and 7 o'clock one disc diameter from disc (see Chapter III). (6) Cotton wool patches at 12, 3, and 9 o'clock (see Chapter III). (7) Hard exudates at 7 o'clock, below the macula (see Chapter III). (8) Dark pigmented background color in a black patient.

correlates these pathological vascular alterations with retinal arteriolar narrowing, either diffuse or segmental, was proposed originally by H. Friedenwald[91] and J. S. Friedenwald[92] and is currently accepted by most authorities in ophthalmology.

WIDENING AND TORTUOSITY OF RETINAL ARTERIOLES

According to Seitz[93] and Leishman[81] increased width of arterioles is a manifestation of arteriolar disease and occurs in benign hypertension. Seitz[93] attempts to correlate such changes with histologic evidence of a thickened sclerotic arteriolar media with hyperplasia of elastic tissue surrounding it. The adventitia and the wall–to–lumen ratio remain normal. Leishman[81] describes a form of patchy fibrosis of arterial and arteriolar walls which he believes is an aging process. He refers to this change as involutionary sclerosis and considers this lesion different from other forms of arteriosclerosis.[81] Although involutionary sclerosis may be present in patients with hypertension, Leishman does not believe that they are causally related. According to this concept, arterioles with this histologic abnormality have lost their elasticity in the segments involved. Hence, if hypertension develops, these abnormal segments dilate passively, in contrast to the normal segments which constrict, and the blood column appears wider in the involved areas. Eventually, the normal vascular segments will develop replacement fibrosis and the entire vessel will appear to be diffusely widened and tortuous (Plate 41 and Drawing 41). Leishman[81] describes a normal wall–to–lumen ratio in the involved vessels. He, however, in contrast to Seitz,[93] describes the histology of the wall as thin and fibrotic.

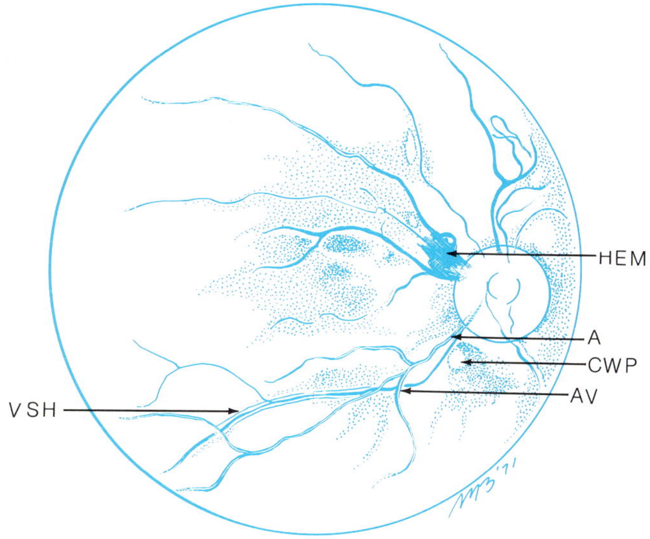

Drawing 42. Plate 42 (A, "silver wire" change; AV, arteriovenous compression; VSH, venous sheathing; HEM, hemorrhage; CWP, cotton wool patch).

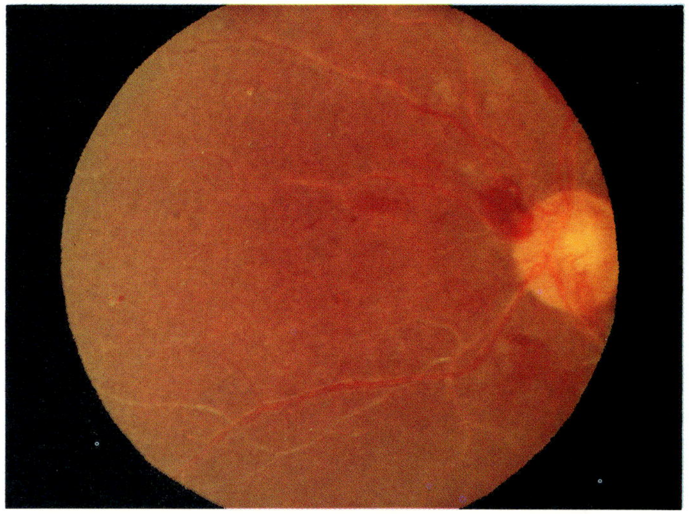

Plate 42. O.S. (1) Numerous small blood vessels on the optic disc (neovascularization) (see Chapter VI). (2) "Copper wire" arteriole, superior nasal. (3) "Silver wire" inferior nasal arteriole. (4) Sheathing of inferior and superior nasal venule (see Chapter IV). (5) A–V compression, inferior temporal vessels. (6) Flame-shaped hemorrhage overlying the disc at 11 o'clock, other hemorrhages at 6 and 9 o'clock. (7) Microaneurysm (small, round, red dot) at 9 o'clock, 1½ disc diameters from disc (see Chapter V). (8) Dark pigmented background of a black patient.

Alterations of Central Light Streak

As previously mentioned, the central light streak is believed to result from the reflection of the light of the opthalmoscope as it strikes the interface of the column of blood and the vessel wall. It appears as a narrow, bright, white streak in the center of the vessel along its long axis. With hyalinization of the arteriolar wall, the reflection of light increases and the light streak is broadened (Plates 41 and 42 and Drawings 41 and 42). The progression of the arteriolar disease with hypertension is associated with further widening of the light reflex, and the entire vessel assumes a red–brown color, the "copper wire" change[83, 92] (Plates 41 and 42 and Drawings 41 and 42). The same correlation was observed in experimental hypertension in the monkey.[94] Further progression of the vascular disease leads to the development

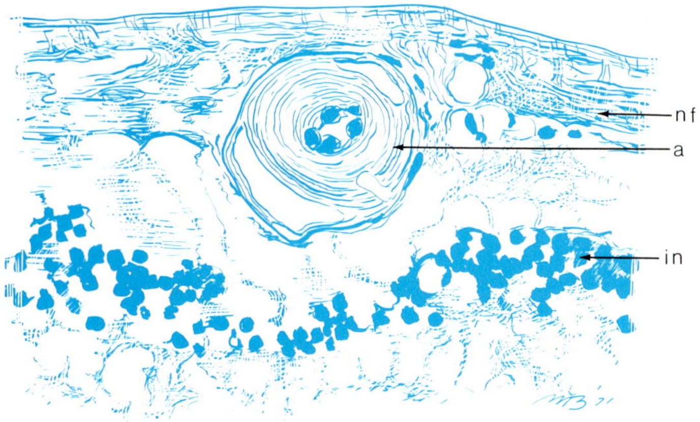

Drawing 44. Plate 44 (a, thick–walled arteriole; in, inner nuclear layer; nf, nerve fiber layer).

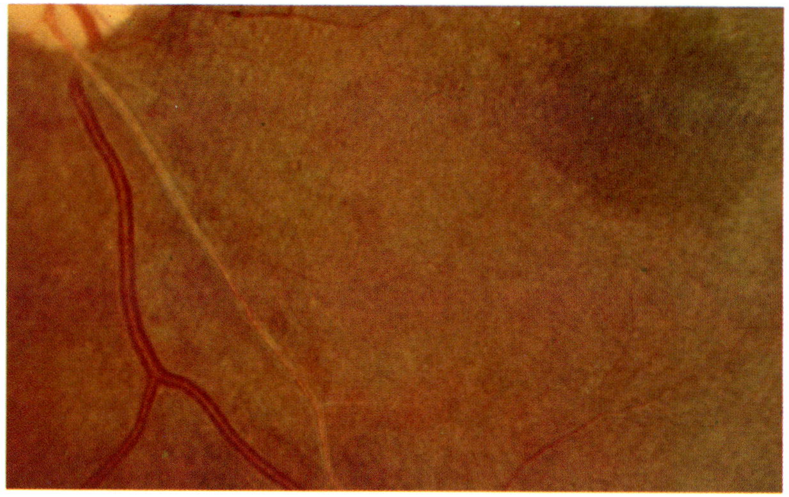

Plate 43. O.S. Magnified view. (1) Dark, oval area is the macula. (2) "Silver wire" inferior temporal arteriole. Blood column is visible in part of that arteriole. (3) A small arteriole at 7 o'clock also shows "silver wire" change.

Plate 44. Note small lumen, hyalinization of entire vessel wall, and increased thickness (PTAH, × 300).

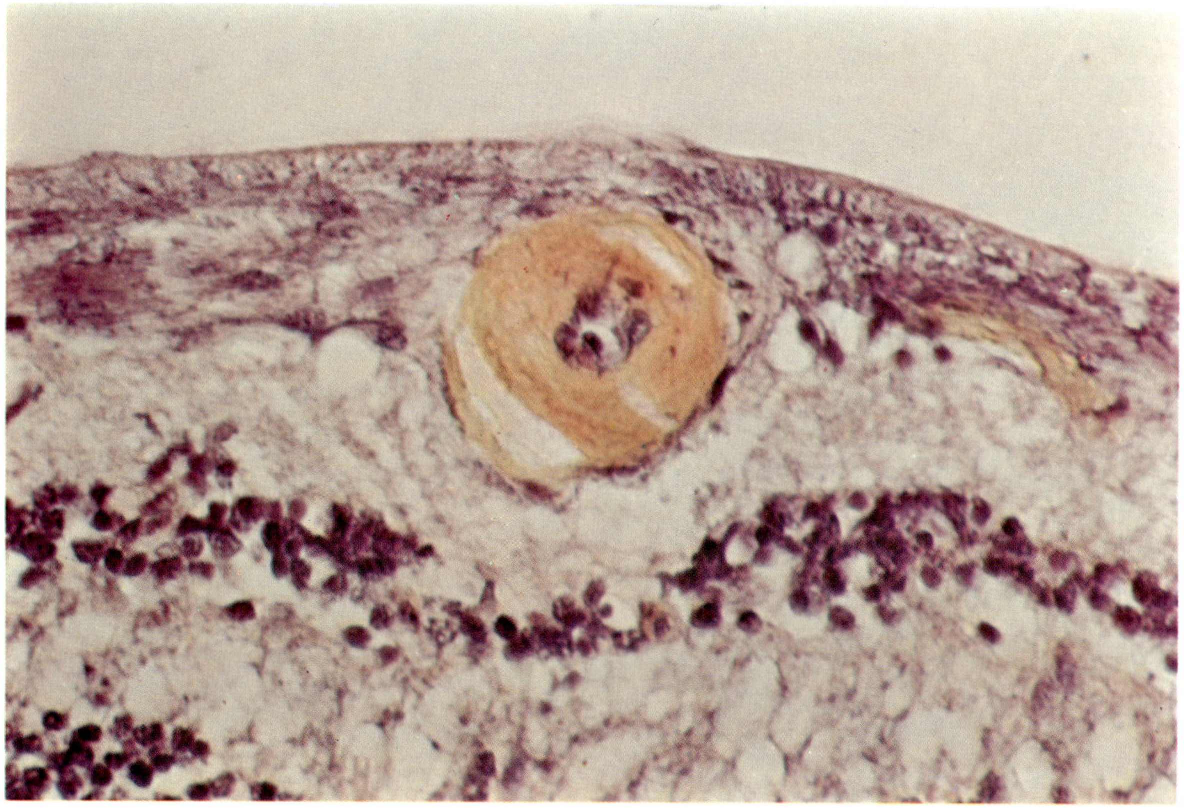

of a narrow white vessel which contains no visible blood column, the "silver wire" change (Plates 42 and 43).

All three of the above clinical manifestations of arteriolar disease may be observed in one or more vessels in varying combinations. Of the three, the "silver wire" change is the most reliable and is most frequently associated with severe diastolic hypertension. It may, however, be observed in all four arteriolar branches following occlusion of the central retinal artery or singly with arteriolar branch occlusion.

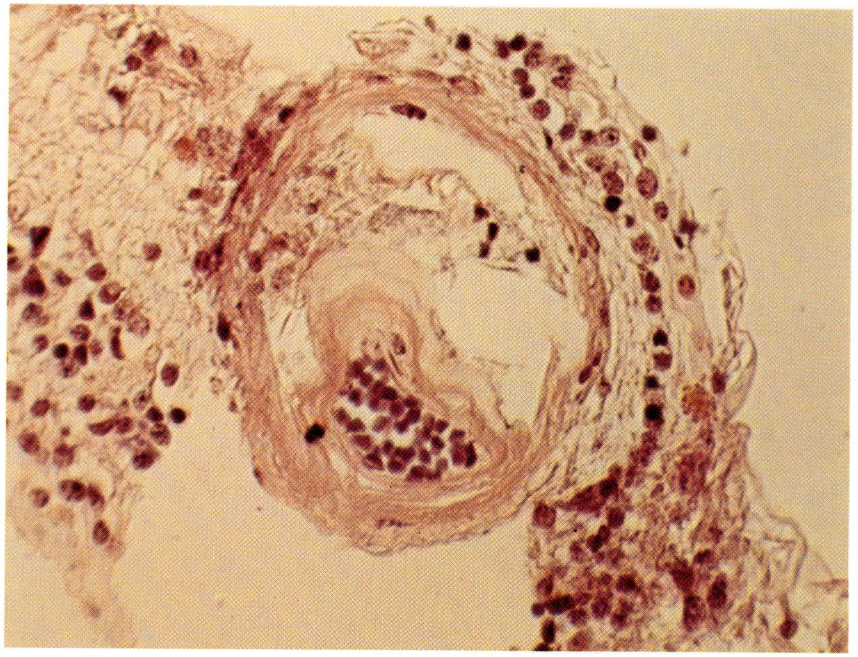

Plate 45. Note recanalized arteriole. This section was made through a "silver wire" arteriole (PTAH, × 400).

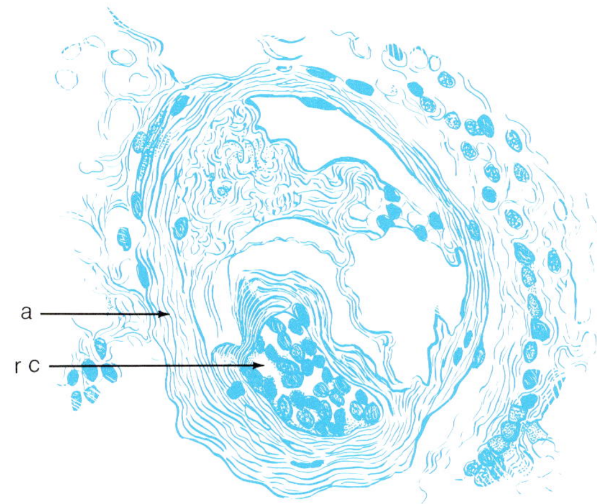

Drawing 45. Plate 45 (a, thick–walled arteriole; rc, recanalized arteriole).

PATHOLOGY

The basic arteriolar histologic changes common to all of the above clinical findings consist of endothelial hyperplasia, intimal hyalinization, medial hypertrophy, and hyalinization (Plate 44 and Drawing 44). Adventitial thickening may also be present. However, the quantitative differences which account for the change from increased central light streak to the "copper wire" appearance are not apparent. On the other hand, the "silver wire" change correlates well with progressive vascular disease which includes an extremely small or occluded lumen[92] (Plates 44 and 45 and Drawings 44 and 45) and/or fibrinoid necrosis of the vessel wall, chiefly in the media (necrotizing arteriolitis, Plate 46 and Drawing 46).

Drawing 46. Plate 46 (a, fibrinoid necrosis of arteriole; nf, nerve fiber layer).

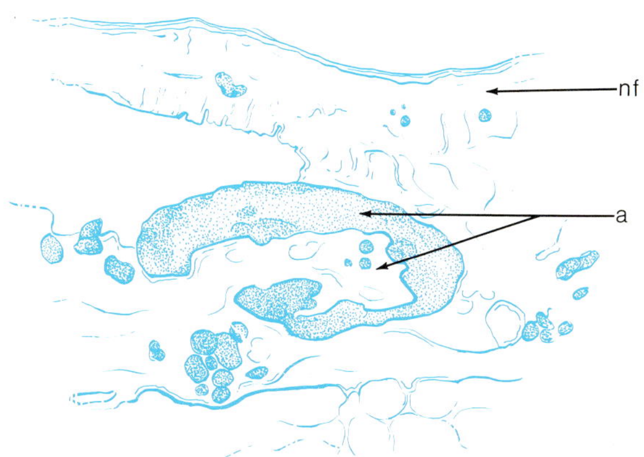

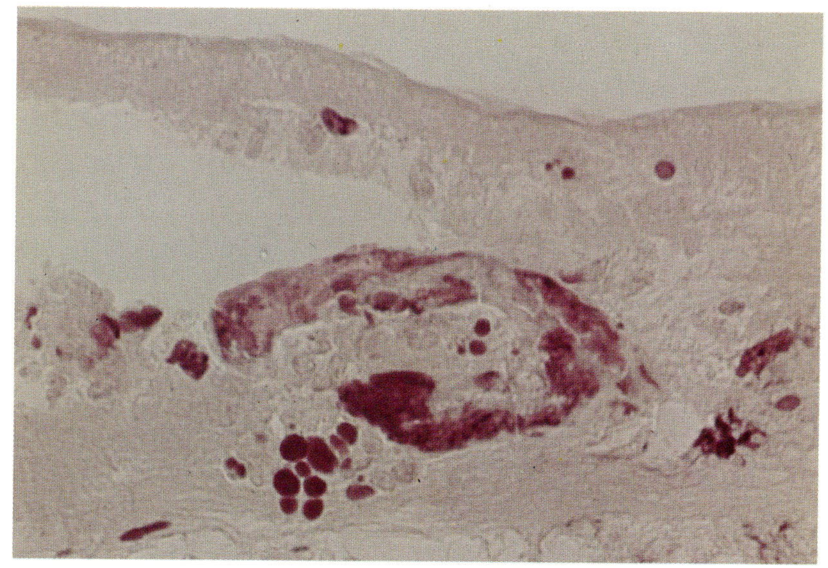

Plate 46. Fibrinoid change in arteriolar wall. The tear in the vessel wall may be an artefact (PTAH, × 400).

Plate 47. Magnified view. Parallel sheathing. Note bilateral white streak parallel with "copper wire" arteriole. In addition, note: (1) Circular white area behind an arteriole. It is an obvious defect in the retina, and choroid. Its cause is not obvious. (2) Pipe–stem sheathing of two venular branches.

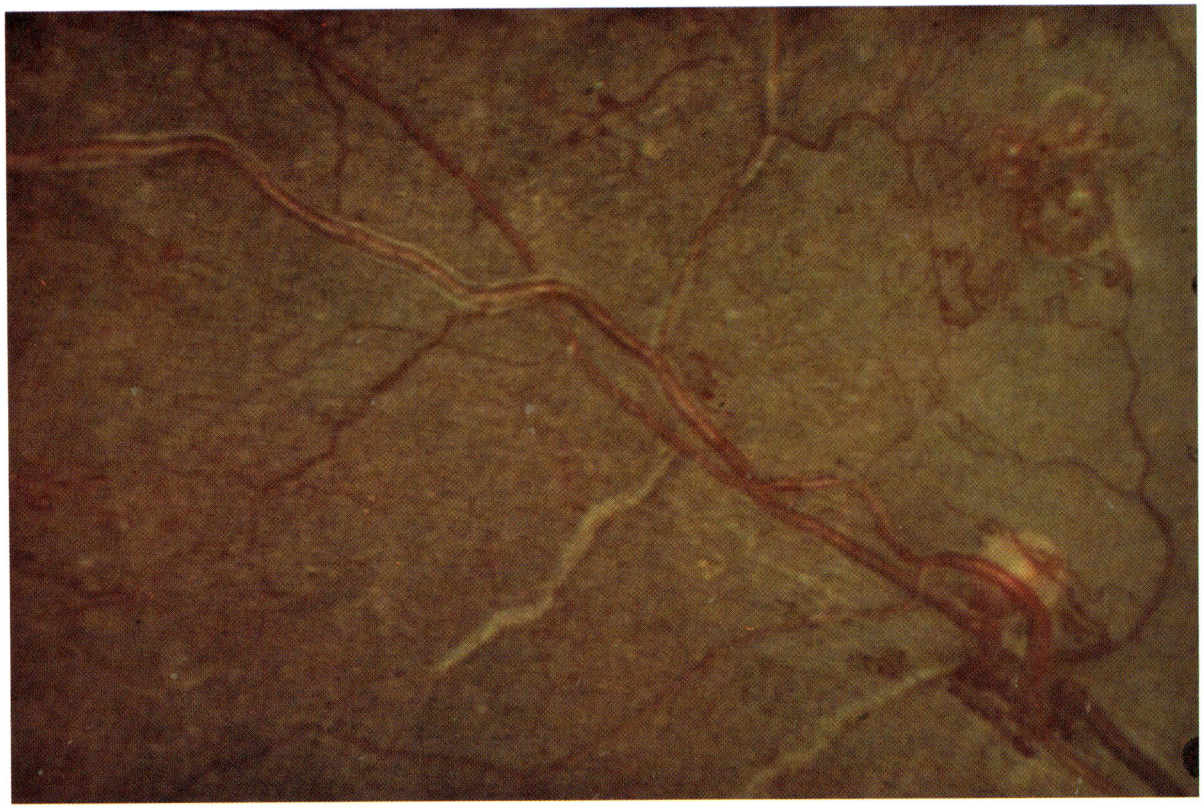

Drawing 47. Plate 47 (SH, sheathing; A, arteriole; V, vein; OV, occluded vein).

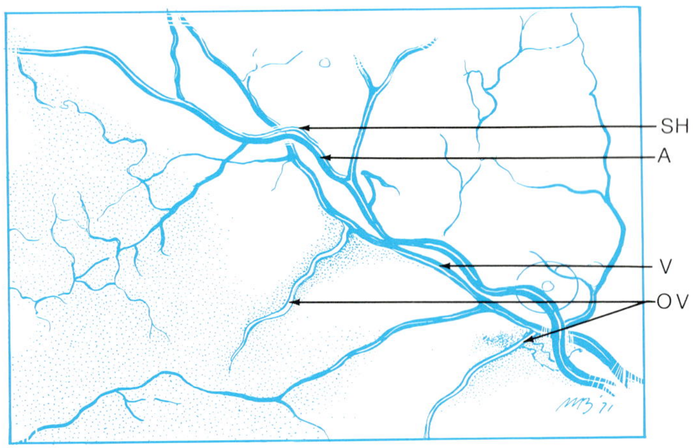

Sheathing

Arteriolar sheathing is characterized by the appearance of a white line immediately adjacent to the vessel. In so–called parallel sheathing, the axial reflex and column of blood are visible and the white stripe is found along one or both sides of the arteriole (Plate 47 and Drawing 47). If the column of blood is not visible and the entire vessel becomes a broad white strand, it is designated as pipe–stem sheathing (Plate 48 and Drawing 48). Parallel sheathing occurs in leukemia,[95] polyarteritis nodosa,[4 (p. 94)] and other forms of vasculitis.[96] In hypertension both parallel and pipe–stem sheathing may be present.

PATHOLOGY

Histologic findings are characterized by the presence of adventitial disease resulting from leukemic infiltration, and inflammatory or sclerotic changes. The latter are found in malignant hypertension and are frequently associated with marked medial sclerosis (Plate 49 and Drawing 49).

Cellular infiltrates are found in polyarteritis nodosa[97] and other forms of vasculitis.[96] Infiltration of the blood vessel wall and the perivascular tissue with abnormal white blood cells occurs in leukemia.[95] Congenital sheathing has been described along the large vessels of the optic disc.[4 (p. 93)]

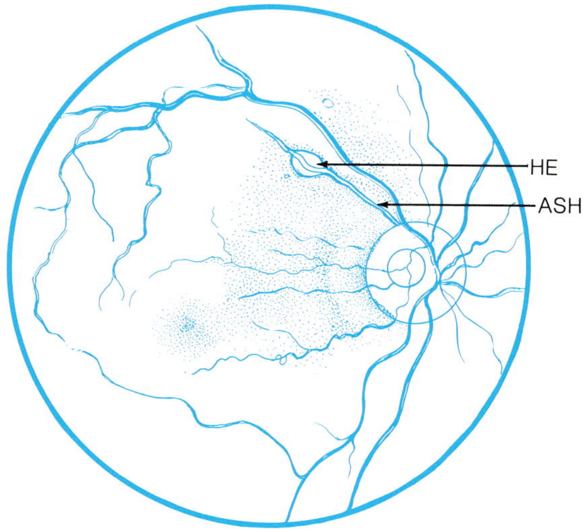

Drawing 48. Plate 48 (ASH, arteriolar sheathing; HE, hard exudate).

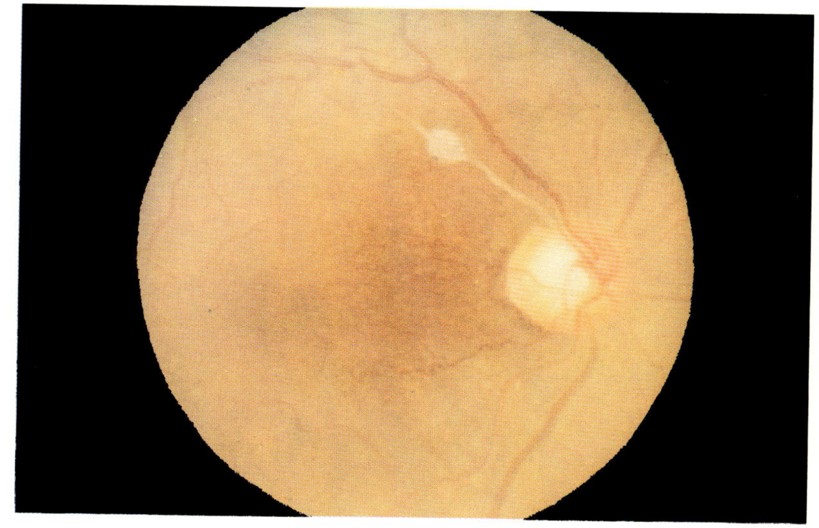

Plate 48. O.D. Pipe–stem sheathing. Note that entire vessel is white and broad. The oval white lesion at 11 o'clock is behind the pipe–stem vessel. It is probably a hard exudate (see Chapter III).

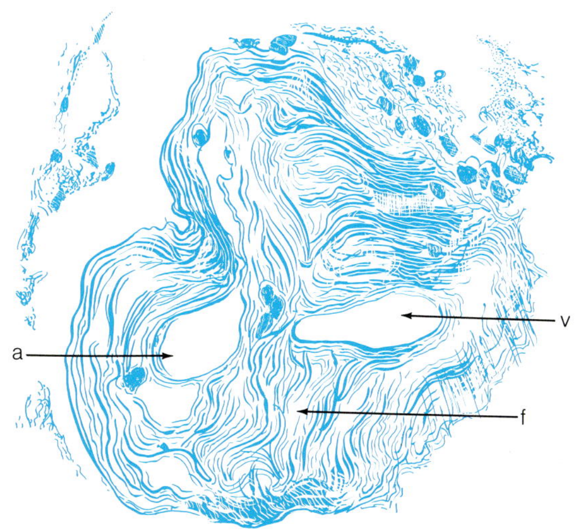

Drawing 49. Plate 49 (a. arteriole; v, vein; f, perivascular fibrosis and adventitial thickening).

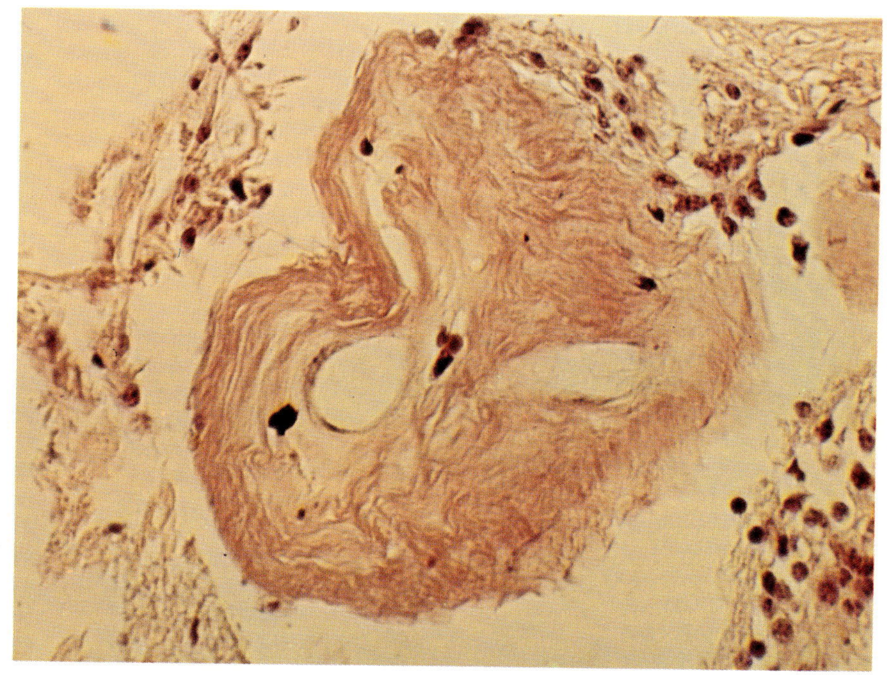

Plate 49. Marked thickening of adventitia of arteriole and venule. Perivascular fibrosis is also present (H&E, approx. × 400).

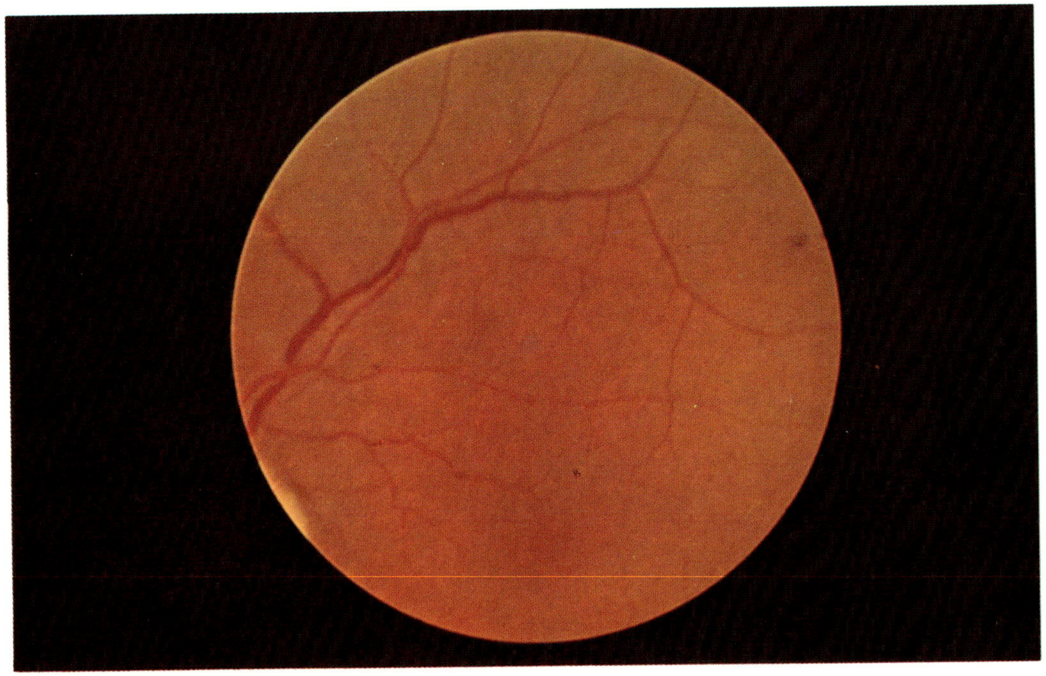

Plate 50. O.S. Note deflection of venule at second crossing of superior temporal arteriole and venule.

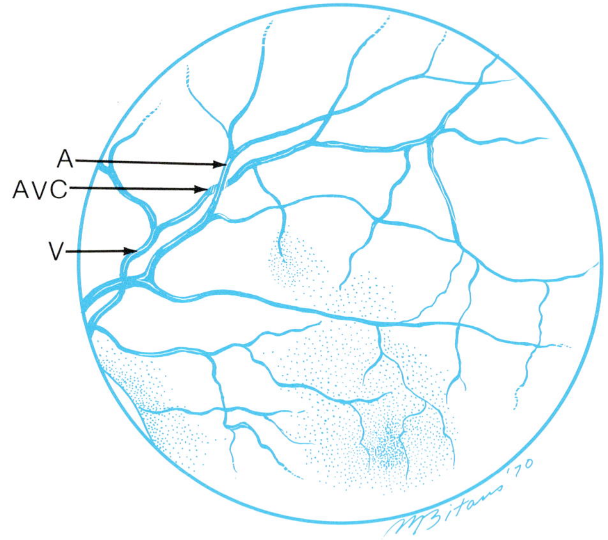

Drawing 50. Plate 50 (A, arteriole; V, venule; AV, arteriovenous displacement).

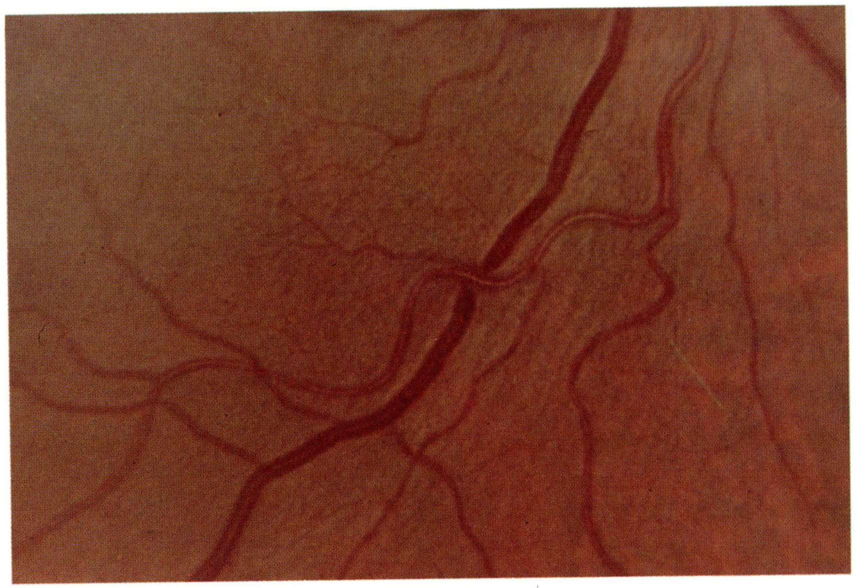

Plate 51. Magnified view. Note tapering of venule at either side of the crossing.

Drawing 51. Plate 51 (A, arteriole; V, venule; AV, arteriovenous compression).

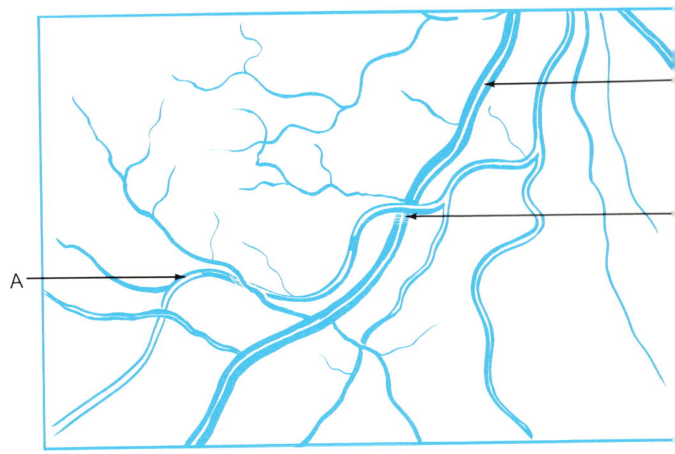

Arteriolar–Venular Compression (Arteriovenous Compression) (A–V nicking)

As previously stated, arteriolar–venular crossing occurs frequently in the retina. Generally the arteriole crosses the venule; less frequently the reverse occurs. In the normal fundus, the blood column of the underlying venule, which retains its normal caliber and position at the site of the crossing, is visible through the arteriole. Arteriovenous compression may appear as venular displacement (Plate 50 and Drawing 50), kinking, or interruption. The last is frequently characterized by tapering of the venule at the site of the crossing (Plate 51 and Drawing 51). When the segment of the venule distal to the A–V compression becomes engorged and tortuous the change is designated as "banking" (Plate 52 and Drawing 52).

Drawing 52. Plate 52 (A, arteriole; V, venule; AV, arteriovenous compression).

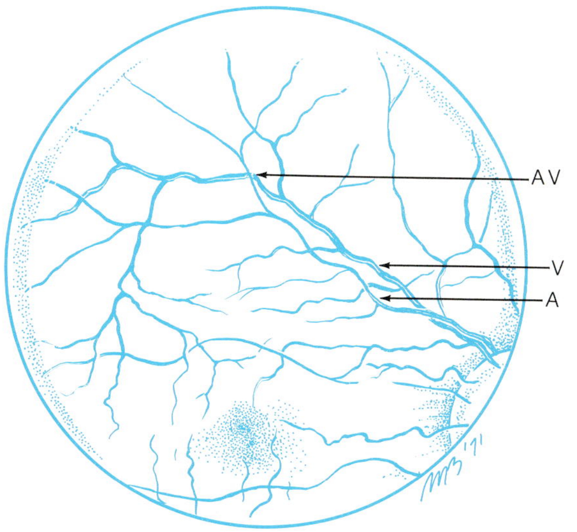

Plate 52. O.D. The macula can be identified as a dark oval area slightly inferior and temporal to edge of the disc. A–V compression is produced by the superior temporal arteriole at the first and second crossing. Note the venous engorgement and tortuosity distal to both sites of compression ("banking").

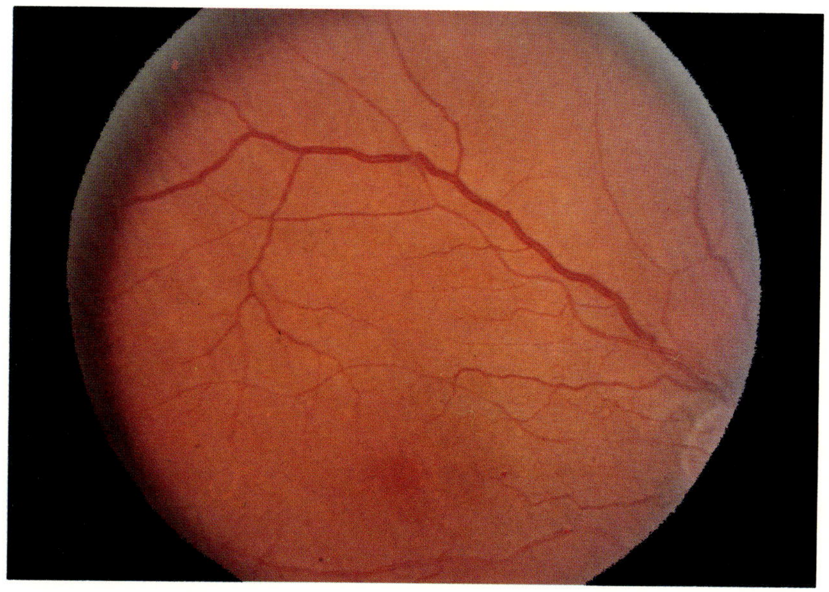

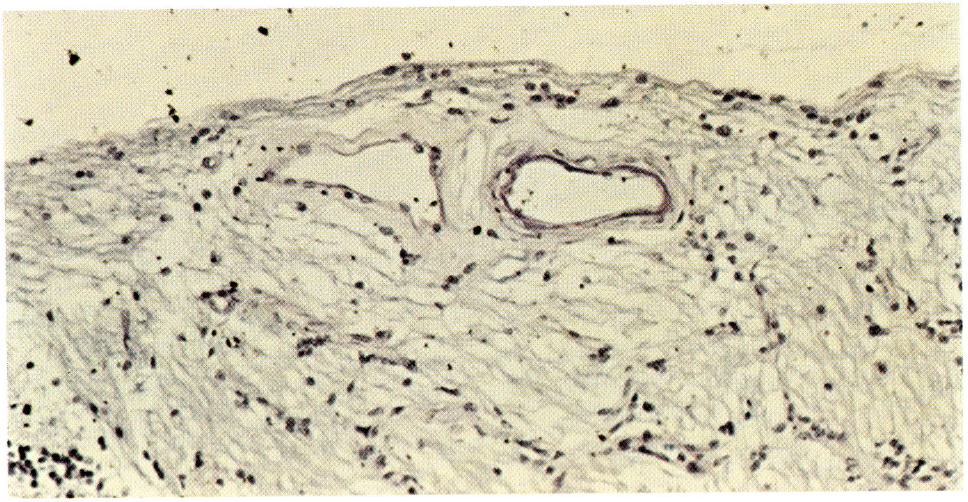

Plate 53. Histology of normal A–V crossing. Note common adventitial sheath shared by the arteriole and venule (LFB. × 120).

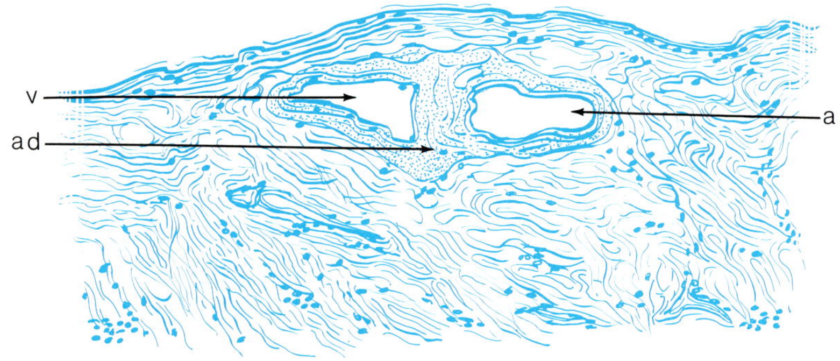

Drawing 53. Plate 53 (a, arteriole; v, venule; ad, common adventitia).

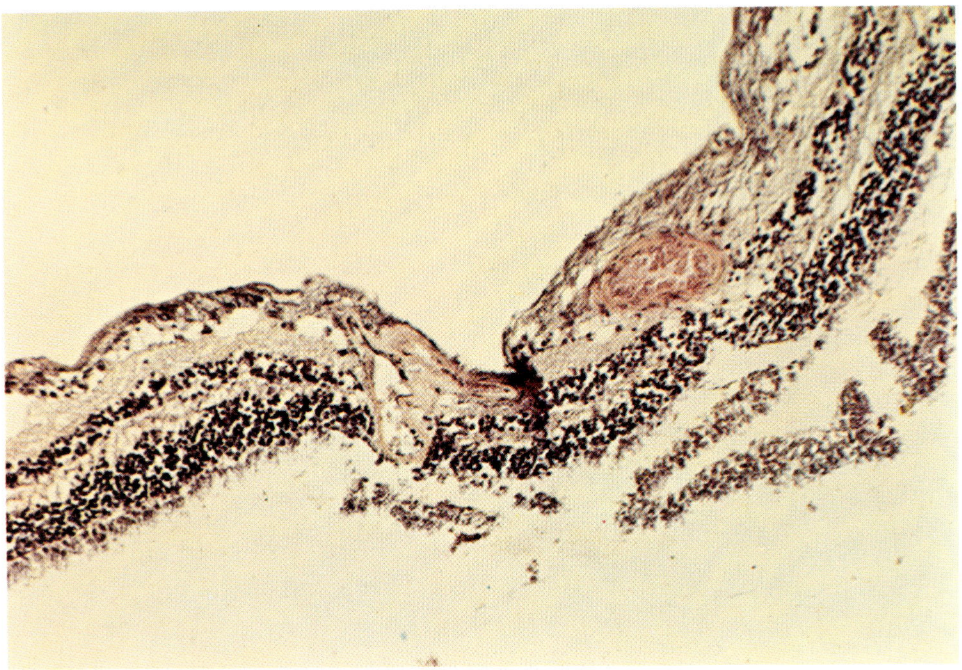

Plate 54. Arteriovenous compression and displacement. A thick-walled arteriole shares a common adventitia with the underlying venule. The latter is compressed and displaced into the outer nuclear layer (PTAH, × 80).

Drawing 54. Plate 54 (im, internal limiting membrane; a, thick-walled arteriole; v, compressed and displaced venule; on, outer nuclear layer).

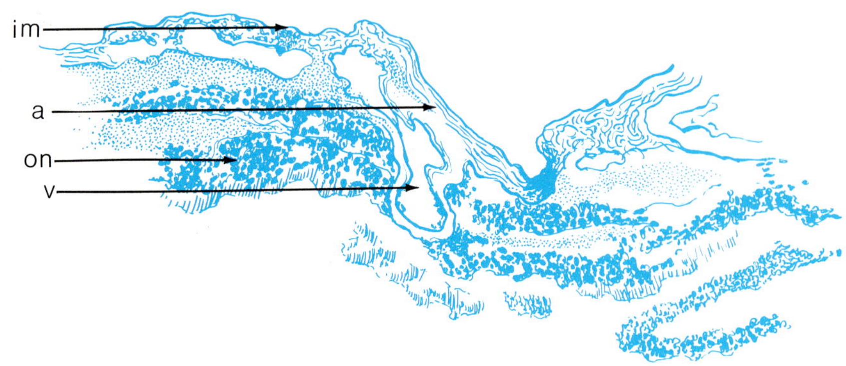

PATHOLOGY AND PATHOGENESIS

Histologic studies of the normal retina demonstrate the presence of a common adventitial sheath for both of the vessels at the site of crossing (Plate 53 and Drawing 53). This anatomical relationship has served as the basis for one or more of the explanations offered for arteriovenous compression in the presence of arteriolar disease. There is considerable evidence to support the concept that the venous compression is produced by the thick–walled arteriole within the adventitial envelope shared by both vessels at the crossing site[2 (p. 501), 83] (Plates 54 and 55 and Drawings 54 and 55). It also seems likely that the sclerotic change of the arteriolar wall may obstruct the view of the underlying venule. Invasion of the venous wall by the sclerotic process may provide another mechanism for the loss of the venular blood column at the site of the crossing.[2 (p. 501)] The dilatation and tortuosity of the venule distal to the crossing suggests impairment of venous return consistent with the concept of venous compression. In accord with that idea is the observation that venous branch occlusions commonly occur distal to an arteriovenous crossing.[2 (p. 503)]

After careful histologic study of numerous serial sections of the retina, Seitz[93 (pp. 61-64)] denies that evidence for venous compression exists. He describes histologic alterations such as hypertrophy and thickening of the adventitia and perivascular glia at the crossing site. According to his concept, such tissue is opaque and will obscure the underlying vessel. He admits that arteriolar medial hyalinization could also participate in the loss of the underlying venular blood column.

It has also been suggested that the disappearance of the venule at the site of the crossing is the result of dipping of the latter (Plate 56 and Drawing 56) and loss of transparency of the retina resulting from edema.[4 (pp. 95-96)] According to that concept, the above mechanism can be invoked in hypertensive retinopathy before severe arteriolar changes develop. More significance is placed on the retinal edema than on the posterior venous displacement.

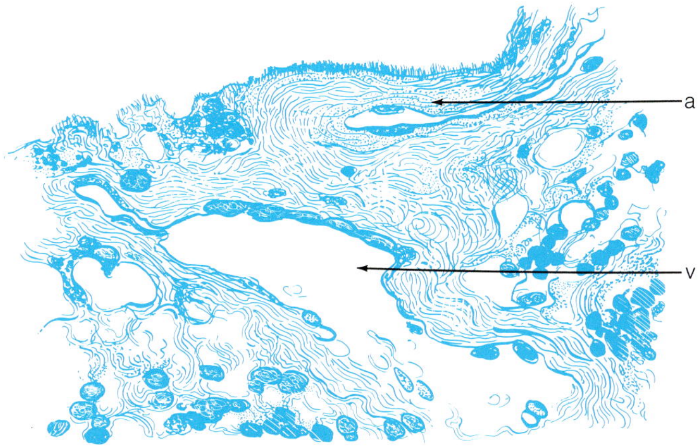

Drawing 55. Plate 55 (a, thick–walled arteriole; v, compressed and displaced venule).

Drawing 56. Plate 56 (a, thick–walled arteriole; v, displaced venule).

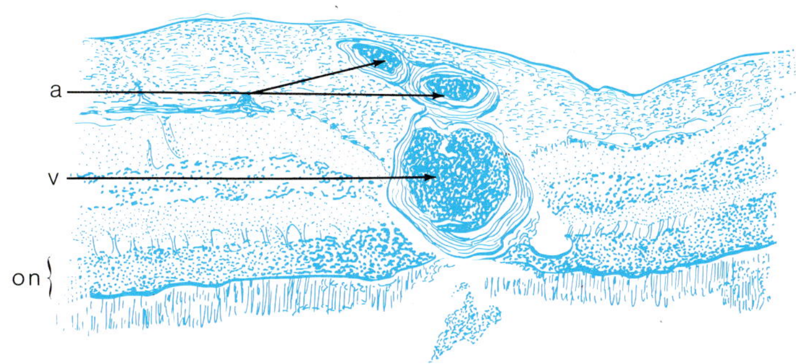

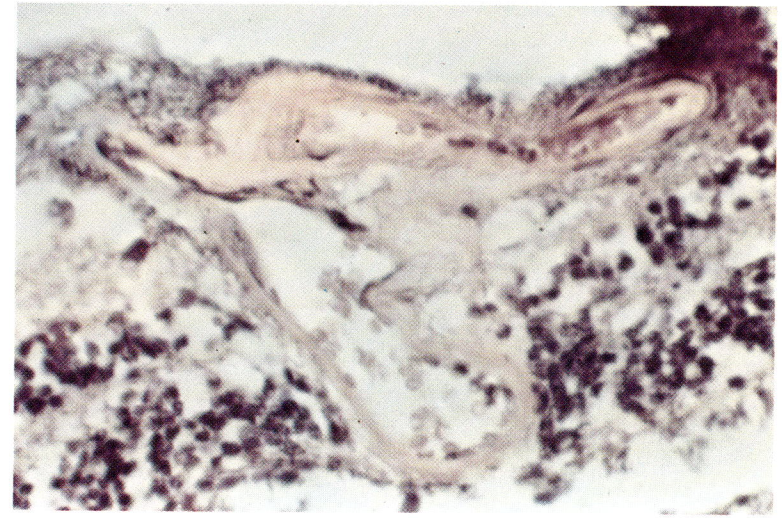

Plate 55. Magnification of arteriole and venule described in Plate 54. Note the thick–walled arteriole and its narrow lumen. The arteriole overlies the venule, shares its adventitia with the venule, and compresses it (PTAH, × 320).

Plate 56. Note displacement of the venule by a thick–walled arteriole into the outer plexiform layer (PTAH, × 80).

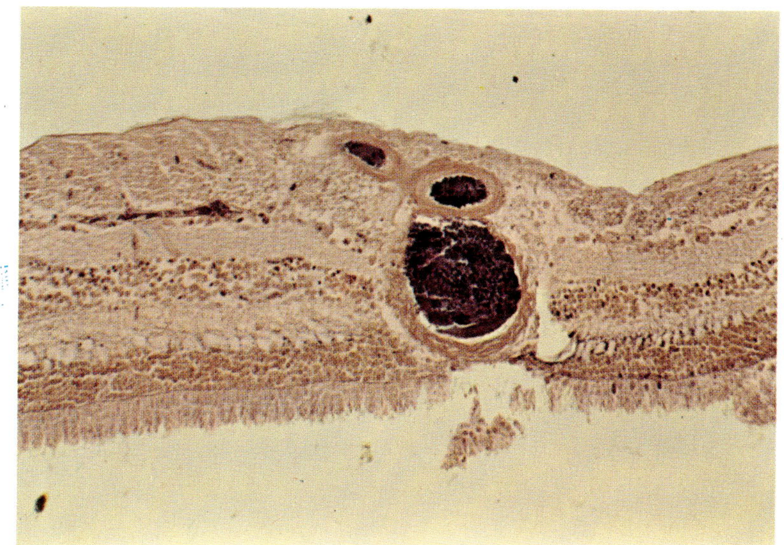

SIGNIFICANCE OF ARTERIOVENOUS COMPRESSION (A–V NICKING)

A–V nicking is believed to be significant if it occurs either more than one disc diameter from the disc or at the second vascular crossing. That clinical maxim is based on the knowledge that the branches of the central retinal artery develop the structure of arterioles at those sites. Since the proximal portions of those vessels may retain their thick and continuous media until they reach the above landmarks, a normal artery could conceivably obscure the underlying vein at either the first crossing or close to the disc.

A–V nicking, like other forms of arteriolar disease, is generally associated with hypertension and is considered to be evidence of long standing disease. When A–V nicking is present in diabetes mellitus, hypertension is generally present as well. A–V nicking is usually associated with one or more of the previously described signs of arteriolar disease such as narrowing and "copper" and "silver wire" change.

According to Seitz[93 (p. 73)] A–V compression may occur with so-called senile sclerosis in the absence of hypertension.

SUMMARY AND SIGNIFICANCE OF CLINICAL MANIFESTATIONS OF RETINAL ARTERIOLAR DISEASE

The funduscopic changes of arteriolar narrowing, "silver wire" change, sheathing, and arteriovenous compression are readily recognized. These clinical findings are supported by correlative pathological changes and can be accepted as reliable signs of arteriolar disease. As previously indicated, it may be misleading to express arteriovenous ratio without signifying whether the arterioles are narrowed or the venules are dilated. Since, as pointed out by Friedenwald,[91] the width and brightness of the vascular light reflex are significantly influenced by the size of the pupil and illuminating system of the ophthalmoscope, such signs as a broadened central light streak and "copper wire" change are difficult to evaluate.

The prime example of arteriolar disease is the hypertensive state. In fact, the degree of retinal arteriolar change and the presence or absence of extravascular lesions such as hemorrhage, cotton wool patches, hard exudates, and neuroretinal edema help separate benign from malignant hypertension. In the former, retinal arteriolar narrowing and arteriovenous compression are rarely associated with extravascular lesions. In the malignant or accelerated form of the disease, sheathing and "silver wire" change are frequently superimposed upon the previously described arteriolar changes and extravascular lesions are invariably present.

ANNOTATED BIBLIOGRAPHY

Central Retinal Artery Occlusion

Ballantyne, A. J. and Michaelson, I. C.: *Textbook of the Fundus of the Eye,* 2nd ed., pp. 191–202, Williams & Wilkins, Baltimore, 1970. A good brief presentation of diseases of the central retinal artery.

Duke–Elder, W. S. and Dobree, J. H.: *Diseases of the Retina,* in: Duke–Elder, W. S. (ed.): *System of Ophthalmology,* Vol. X.: pp. 66–97, Mosby, St. Louis, 1967. An excellent review of retinal arterial disease.

Gunning, A. J., Pickering, G. W., Robb–Smith, A. H. T., and Russell, R. R.: *Mural Thrombosis of the Internal Carotid Artery and Subsequent Embolism,* Q. J. Med., **33:** 155, 1964. A good presentation of carotid artery disease and its role in embolism of cerebral and retinal arteries.

Hollenhorst, R. W.: *Significance of Bright Plaques in the Retinal Arterioles,* JAMA, **178:** 23, 1961. A very good discussion of the relationship of occlusive disease of the carotid arteries and embolic occlusion of the central retinal artery and its branches.

Arteriolar Disease

Friedenwald, J. S.: *Disease Processes Versus Disease Pictures in Interpretation of Retinal Vascular Lesions,* Arch. Ophthalmol., **37:** 403, 1947. A good clinical pathological correlation of anteriolar disease.

Hogan, M. J. and Zimmerman, L. E. (eds.): *Ophthalmic Pathology. An Atlas and Textbook,* 2nd ed., pp. 495–506, Saunders, Philadelphia, 1962. A clear and concise presentation of the pathology of retinal arterioles.

Marr, W. G.: *Ophthalmoscopic Signs of Cardiovascular Disease,* Modern Concepts of Cardiovascular Disease, **31:** 763, 1962. A clear and concise presentation of the interpretation of retinal arteriolar disease.

Scheie, H. G.: *Evaluation of Ophthalmoscopic Changes of Hypertension and Arteriolar Sclerosis,* Arch. Ophthalmol., **49:** 117, 1953. A good clinical pathological correlation of arteriolar disease.

Seitz, R.: *The Retinal Vessels; Comparative Ophthalmoscopic and Histologic Studies on Healthy and Diseased Eyes,* translated by F. C. Blodi, Mosby, St. Louis, 1964. A detailed, carefully developed study of the pathology of the retinal vasculature.

Test Plates (unlabeled retinal photographs and unlabeled retinal photomicrographs)

Questions and Answers A1–A6

Plate A1

Clinical findings: A 33–year–old male who has had hypertension for four years. Bl. P. range 190/152 — 170/130 mm Hg. BUN — 21mg/100 ml creatinine — 1.2 mg/100 ml. A1 — Plate — O.D. — nasal .

QUESTIONS — A1

Question 1. List variations from normal (see answer, p. 51).

Question 2. What is the mechanism for the production of the pigmented crescent?

Question 3. What is its significance?

Question 4. What is the tigroid or tessellated fundus?

Question 5. Is arteriolar narrowing always a permanent change?

PLATE A1

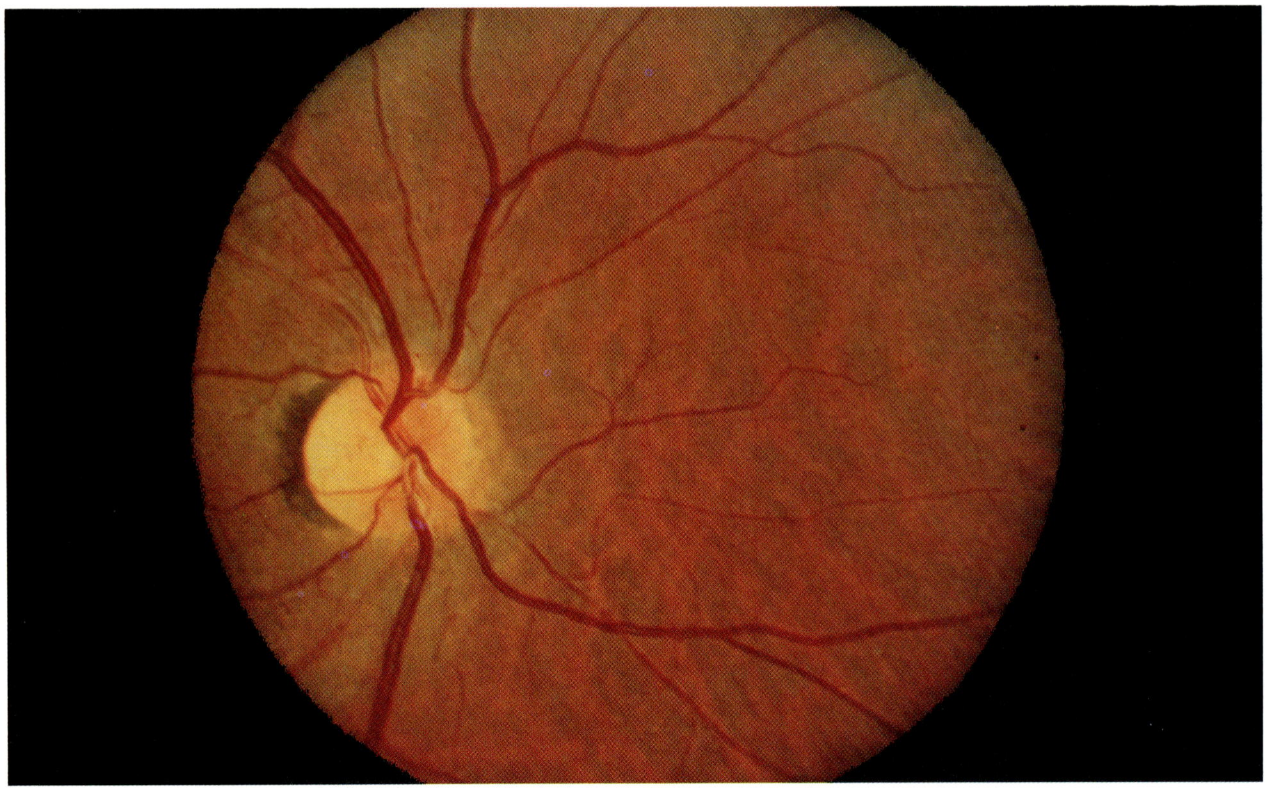

ANSWERS — A1

Answer 1. Normal disc with temporal pigment ring. Tigroid (tessellated) fundus. Arterioles are narrow. The venules are normal. There are no extravascular lesions.

Answer 2. See p. 20.

Answer 3. It is generally a normal variant. However, it may accompany the scleral ring of myopia (see p. 20).

Answer 4. See p. 22.

Reference

Hogan, M. J. and Zimmerman, L. E. (eds.): *Ophthalmic Pathology. An Atlas and Textbook,* 2nd ed., pp. 114–117, Saunders, Philadelphia, 1962.

Answer 5. No (see p. 37).

References

Duke–Elder, W. S. and Dobree, J. H.: *Diseases of the Retina,* in: Duke–Elder, W. S. (ed.): *System of Ophthalmology,* Vol. X: pp. 350–356, Mosby, St. Louis, 1967.

Wagener, H. P. and Keith, N. M.: *Diffuse Arteriolar Disease with Hypertension and the Associated Retinal Lesions,* Medicine, **18:** 317, 1939.

Plate A2

Clinical findings: A 40–year–old man who suddenly developed blindness of his left eye two years ago. There was neither associated headache nor pain in the eye. Bl. P. — 220/140 mmHg. Visual acuity: O.D. — 20/30; O.S. — total blindness. Pupil O.S. was dilated and larger than pupil O.D. There was no pupillary response to light — O.S. Funduscopic examination. — Plate A2 — O.S. — inferior nasal.

QUESTIONS — A2

Question 1. List abnormalities in Plate A2 (see answer, p. 53).

Question 2. Is the optic nerve normal?

The patient's chart which contains the record of his illness of two years ago becomes available to you. Examination at that time disclosed: Bl. P. — 230/150 mmHg; the left pupil was dilated and did not constrict with direct stimulation of light; funduscopy — O.S. — normal disc. Arterioles were very narrow and the retina was pale. In the temporal portion of the retina, 1½ disc diameters from the disc, a round, red area is visible. O.D. — normal disc. "Silver wire" arterioles and arteriovenous compression at several second crossings were observed. There were several discrete white patches between the macula and the disc. Blood vessels crossed over those lesions.

Question 3. What happened to the left eye two years ago?

Question 4. What are the histo–pathologic changes in this entity?

Question 5. How can you relate the optic atrophy to the central retinal artery occlusion?

Question 6. What vascular anomaly may allow the patient to retain some of his vision after occlusion of the central retinal artery?

Question 7. Review funduscopic changes recorded two years ago when the patient developed blindness in his left eye. What does the red spot represent and why does it have that characteristic appearance?

Question 8. What are the pathological changes which correspond with:

a. the narrowed arterioles;
b. the "copper wire" change;
c. the "silver wire" change as noted in Plate A2.

PLATE A2

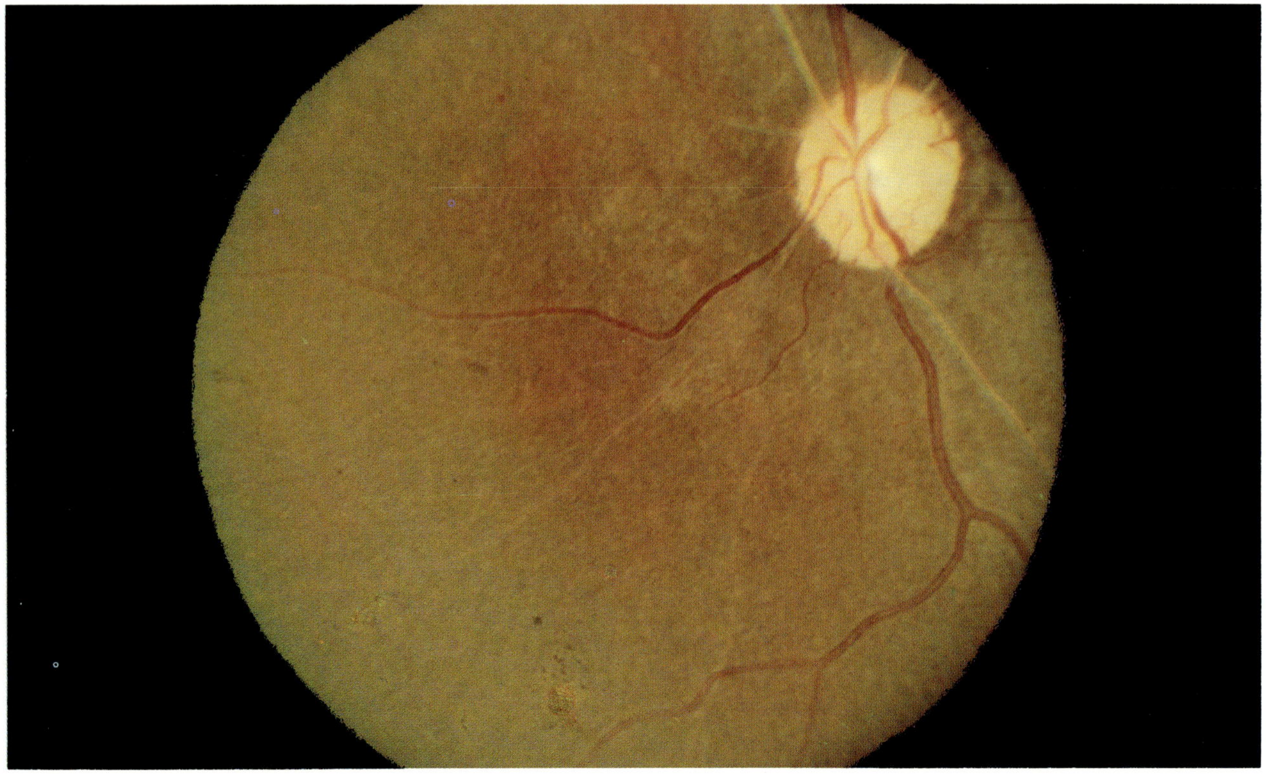

ANSWERS — A2

Answer 1. The disc is pale and its margins are sharp and slightly irregular. A small number of small tortuous vessels overlap the margins of the disc. Arterioles are narrow and show "copper" and "silver wire" change. There is slight venular tortuosity.

Answer 2. This is an abnormal optic disc. It is white, pale, and its margins are very sharp. Few small vessels cross its margins. Those abnormalities, the loss of vision of that eye, and the pupillary changes are the classic findings of optic atrophy (see pp. 184–186).

Answer 3. Occlusion of central retinal artery (see pp. 30–36).

Answer 4. See pp. 33–34.

Answer 5. See pp. 33, 193.

Answer 6. A cilioretinal artery which supplies the macular area (see p. 30).

Answer 7. Cherry–red spot of the fovea (see macula, p. 8).

Reference — central retinal artery occlusion

Ballantyne, A. J. and Michaelson, I. C.: *Textbook of the Fundus of the Eye,* 2nd ed., pp. 191–201, Williams & Wilkins, Baltimore, 1970.

Answer 8. See pp. 38, 41.

Reference

Scheie, H. G.: *Evaluation of Ophthalmoscopic Changes of Hypertension and Arteriolar Sclerosis.* Arch. Ophthalmol., **49:** 117, 1958.

PLATE A3

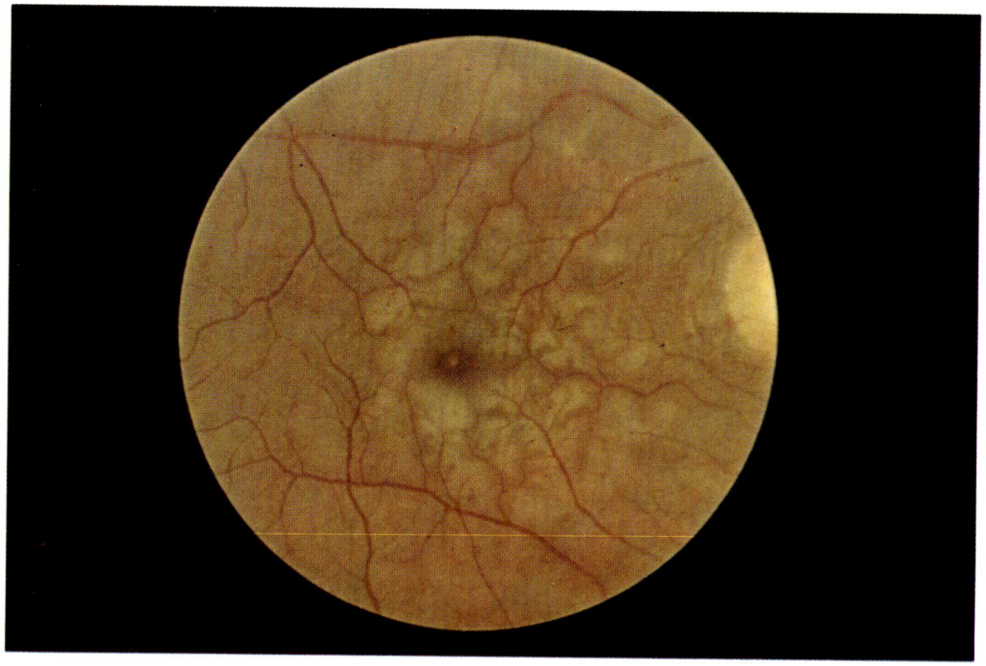

Plate A3

Clinical findings: A 50–year–old male with chronic obstructive disease of the lungs. Bl. P. 180/80 mmHg. Sudden loss of vision of the right eye developed fifteen days prior to time retinal photograph A3 was taken. Plate A3 — O.D. — temporal.

QUESTIONS — A3

Question 1. List abnormalities (see answer p. 55).

Question 2. In view of the clinical history and the funduscopic changes, what is your diagnosis?

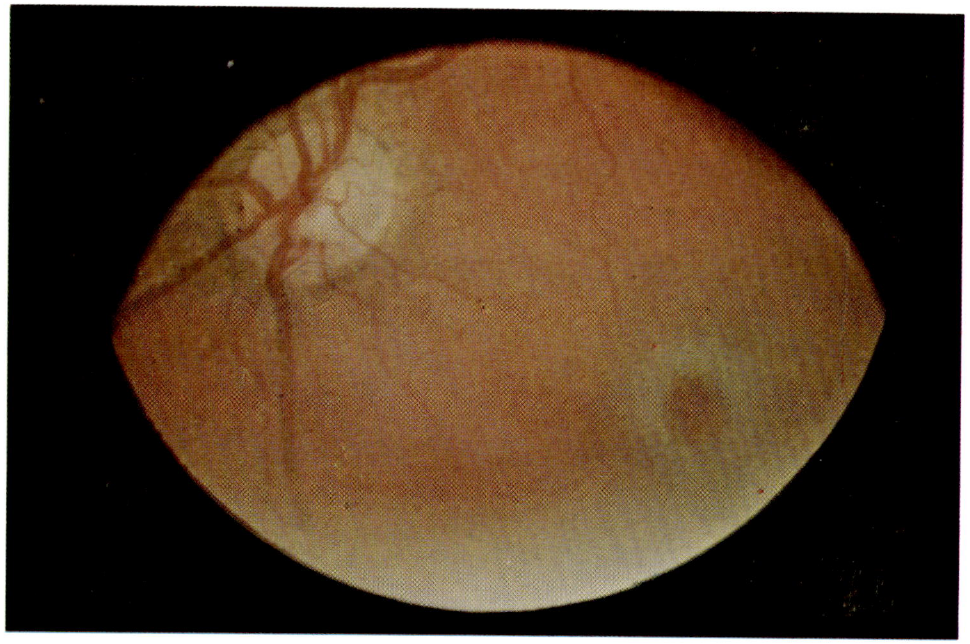

PLATE A4

Plate A4

Clinical findings: A two–year–old female. Product of full term uncomplicated pregnancy. Visual impairment was noted at 3 months. She needed assistance to sit up at 12 months. Neurological examination confirmed the poor vision and the patient's extreme difficulty lifting her head and shoulders off the bed. Plate A4 — O.S. — central and temporal.

QUESTIONS — A4

Question 1. State abnormality (see answer, p. 55).

Question 2. What diagnostic procedure would be helpful?

Question 3. Diagnosis?

ANSWERS — A3

Answer 1. The temporal portion of the disc is normal. The arterioles are narrow. The venules are normal. There are numerous pale areas surrounding the macula. The fovea and macula stand out as a brown area.

Answer 2. Occlusion of the central retinal artery.

ANSWERS — A4

PLATE A4

Answer 1. Normal disc, arterioles, and venules; red circular area surrounded by a white halo temporal and inferior to the disc.

Answer 2. Rectal biopsy. Ganglion cells of Meissner's and Auerbach's plexus are laden and distended with glycolipid material.

Answer 3. Amaurotic familial idiocy (Tay–Sachs disease). The retinal lesion is the cherry–red spot. Compare with Plate A3.

References

Ballantyne, A. J. and Michaelson, I. C.: *Textbook of the Fundus of the Eye,* 2nd ed., pp. 357–362, Williams & Wilkins, Baltimore, 1970. The lipidoses.

Frederickson, D. S. and Tram, E. G.: *Ganglioside Lipidosis: Tay–Sachs Disease,* in: Stanbury, J. B., Wyngaarden, J. B., and Fredrickson, D. S. (ed): *The Metabolic Basis of Inherited Disease,* 2nd ed., pp. 523–538, McGraw–Hill, New York, 1966.

Plate A5

Microscopic section stained with PTAH × 100. Note — thick walled fragmented arteriole in nerve fiber layer (see Drawing A5).

QUESTION — A5

Question. What clinical arteriolar change would be expected in this patient? (See answer, this page.)

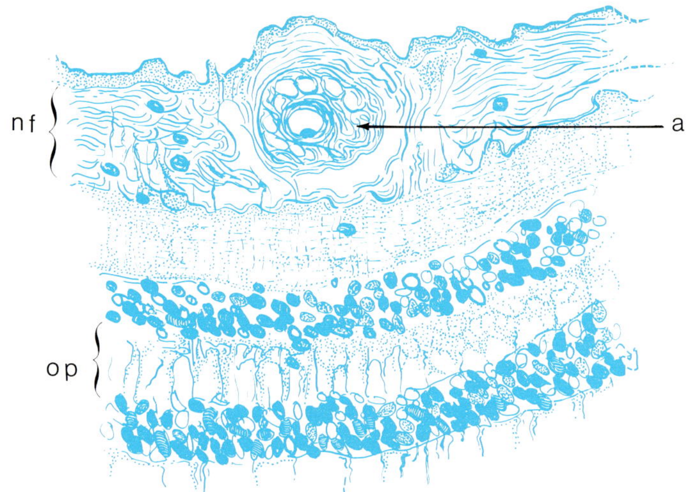

Drawing A5. Plate A5 (nf, nerve fiber layer; a, arteriole (thickened and fragmented wall); op, outer plexiform layer).

ANSWER — A5

Answer. Arteriolar medial thickening and fragmentation would be associated clinically with arteriolar narrowing, increased central light streak, and probably "copper wire" change (see pp. 36–40).

PLATE A5

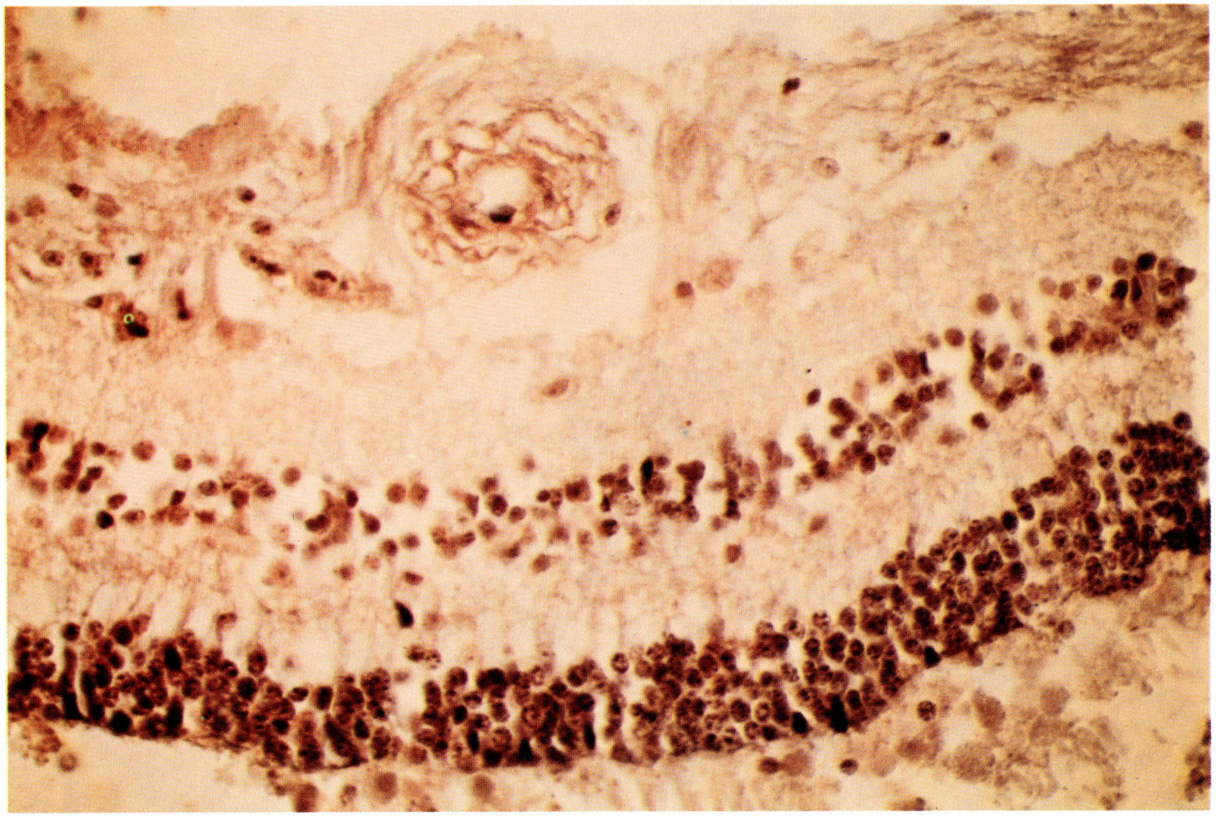

Plate A6

Microscopic section—Luxol fast blue stain × 100 (approx.) Note that arteriole in nerve fiber layer shares a common adventitia with the underlying venule. The latter has a thick and fragmented wall and is displaced into the outer nuclear layer (see Drawing A6).

QUESTION — A6

Question. What sign of arteriolar disease would be expected? (See answer, this page.)

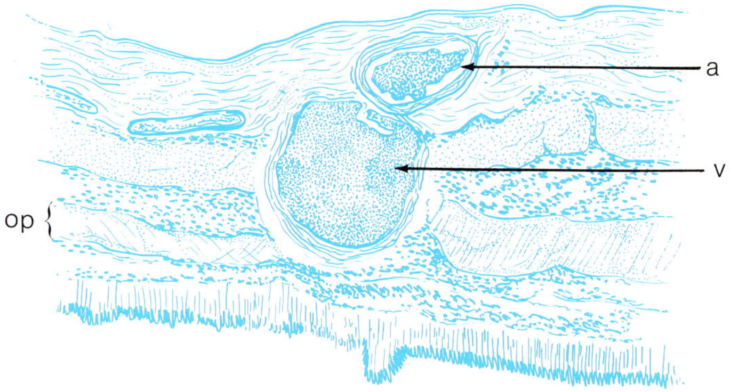

Drawing A6. Plate A6 (a, thick–walled arteriole; v, displaced venule; op, outer plexiform layer).

ANSWER — A6

Answer. Arteriovenous displacement — a form of A–V compression (see pp. 45–48).

Reference

Seitz, R.: *The Retinal Vessels; Comparative Ophthalmoscopic and Histologic Studies on Healthy and Diseased Eyes,* translated by F. C. Blodi, pp. 20–74, Mosby, St. Louis, 1964.

PLATE A6

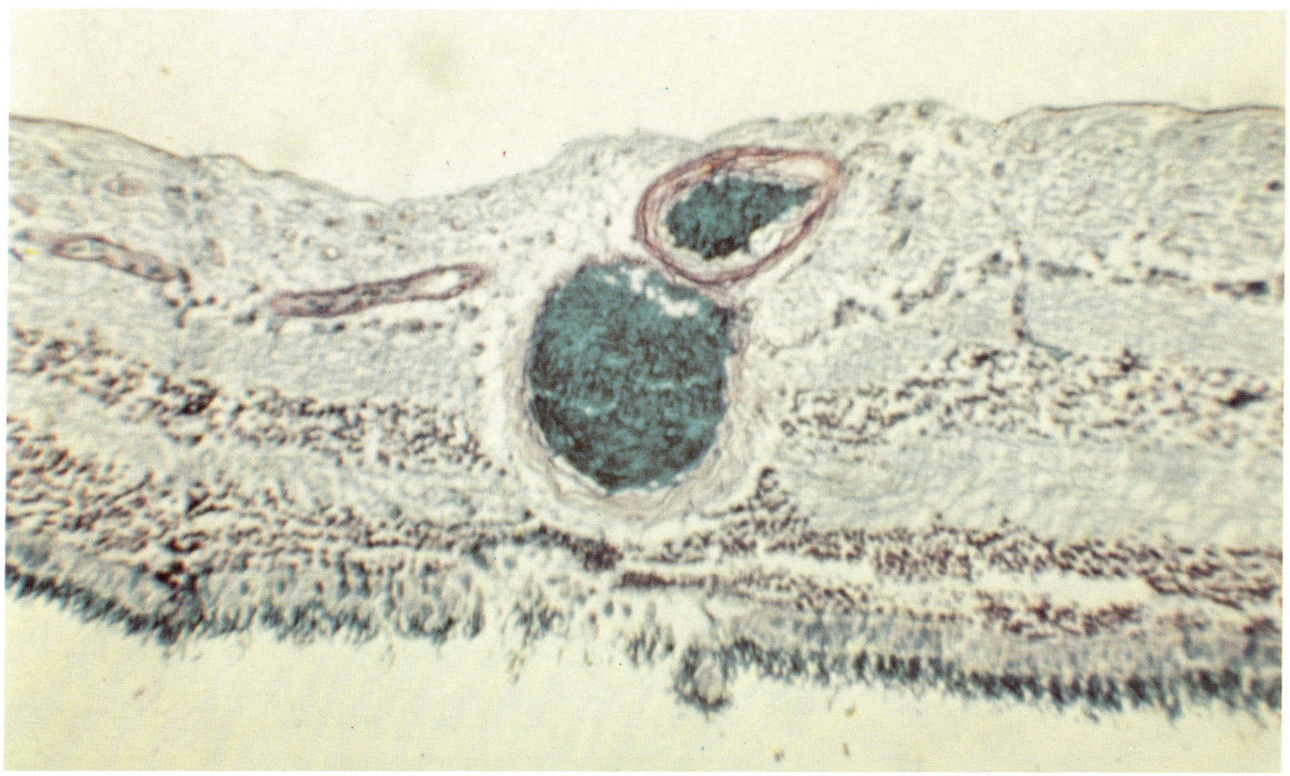

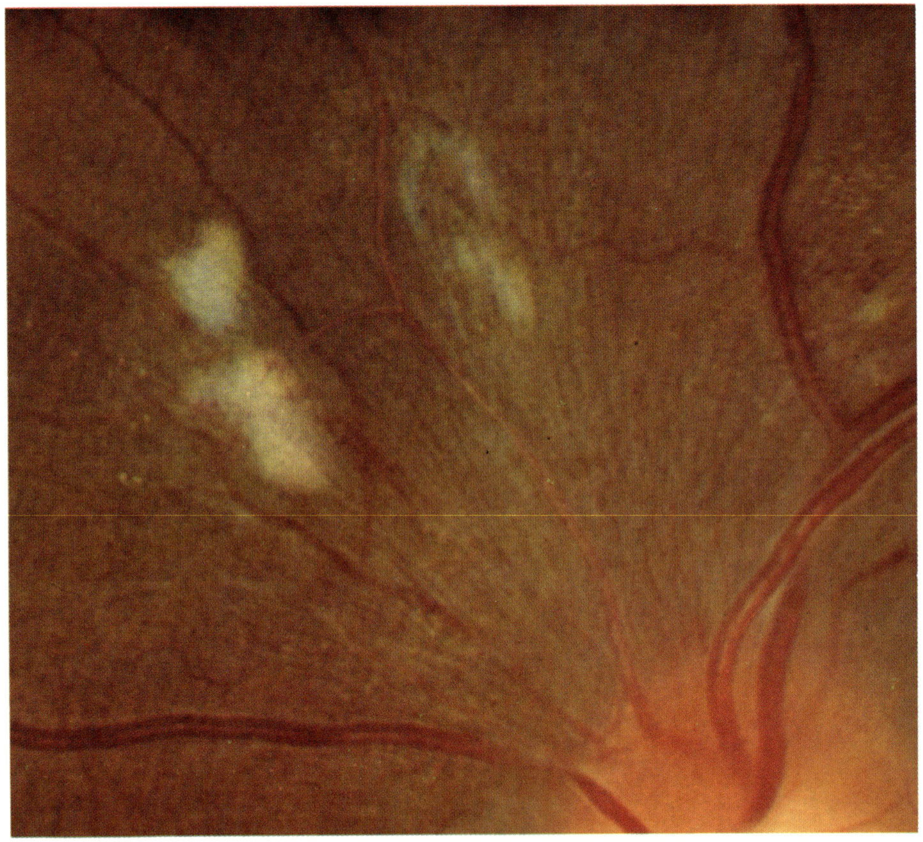

Plate 57. Magnified view. Note three white feathery lesions.

Drawing 57. Plate 57 (O, optic nerve; CWP, cotton wool patch).

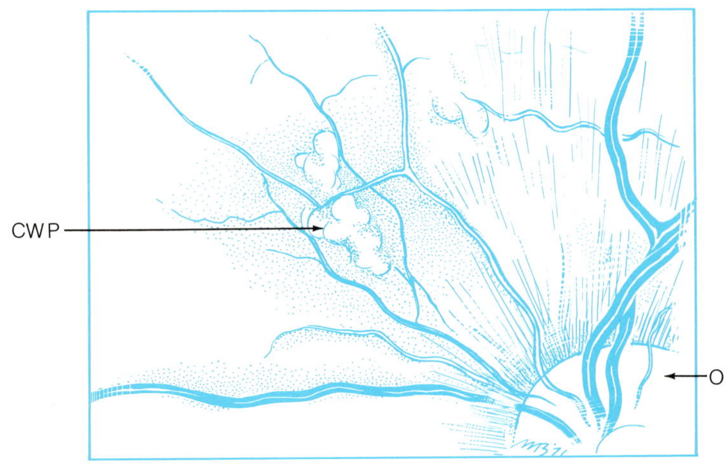

Chapter III

EXTRAVASCULAR LESIONS OF THE RETINA

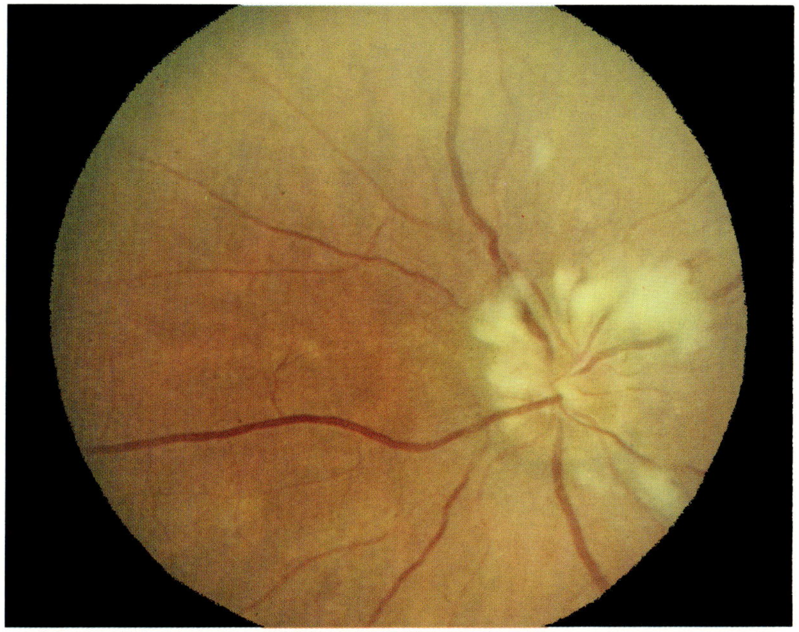

Plate 58. O.S. Central and nasal. Note multiple cotton wool lesions close to the disc. Observe that they overlie blood vessels.

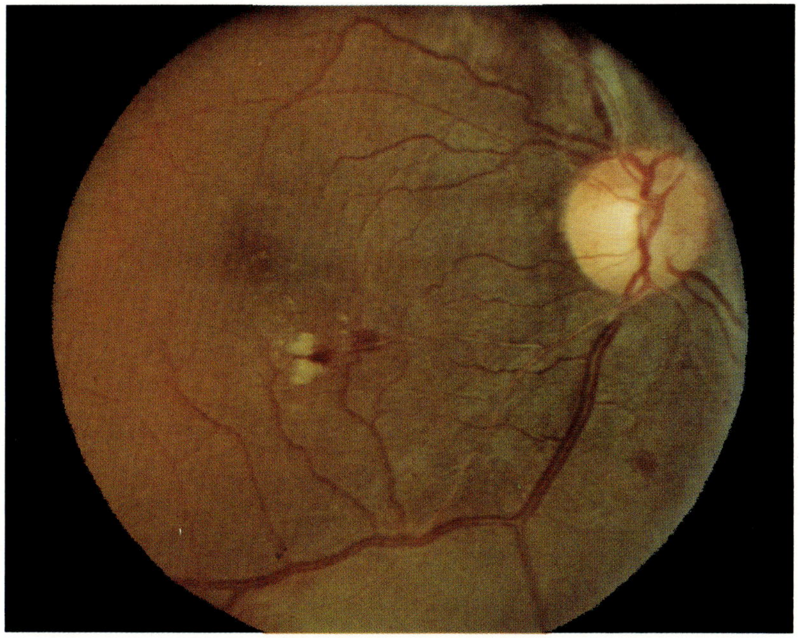

Plate 59. O.D. Inferior and temporal. Note hemorrhage and cotton wool patch below the macula. Did you notice the "silver wire" arteriole?

The retinal lesions associated with arteriolar disease are the cotton wool patch (soft exudate), the hard exudate, and hemorrhage.

THE COTTON WOOL PATCH

Clinical Appearance

The cotton wool patch, often referred to as the soft exudate, appears as a white, gray, or yellow area of degeneration in the retina (Plate 57 and Drawing 57). Although it may occur singly, there are generally multiple lesions situated close to the optic disc varying in size from 1/10 to 1/3 of that structure (Plate 58). Characteristically these lesions have a feathery appearance and resemble a patch of absorbent cotton. Since they form in the nerve fiber layer they often have striate borders radiating in the direction of the affected fibers and they overlie or deflect the retinal vessels which traverse that layer of the retina. Linear or flame–shaped hemorrhages may occur within or around any part of such a lesion (Plate 59). Cotton wool patches often produce irregular sector visual defects. However, when the macular area is involved central vision may be lost.

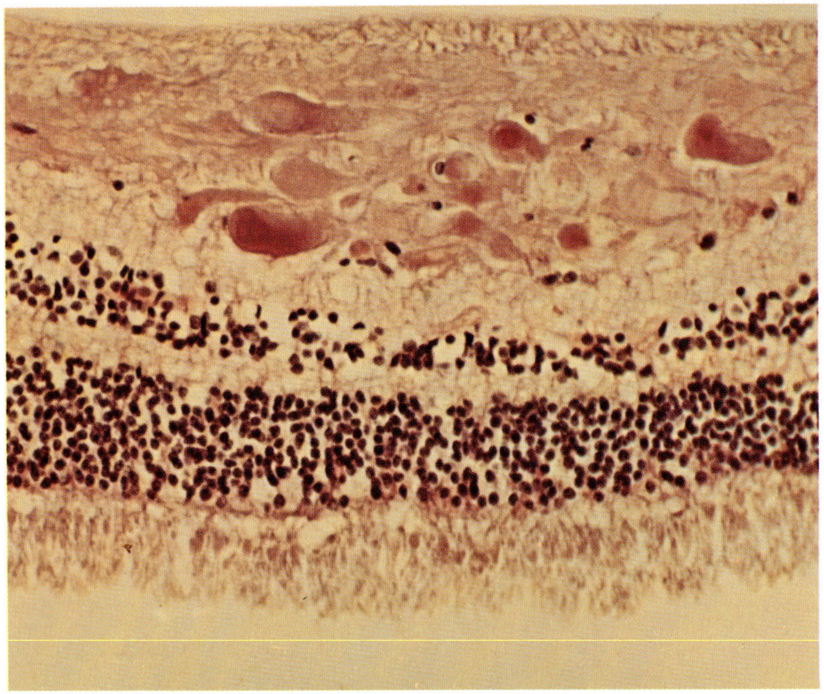

Plate 60. Cluster of eosinophilic, elliptical, swollen axis cylinders in nerve fiber layer of retina. Note that the cluster forms a nodule which dips into the inner plexiform layer (H&E, × 80).

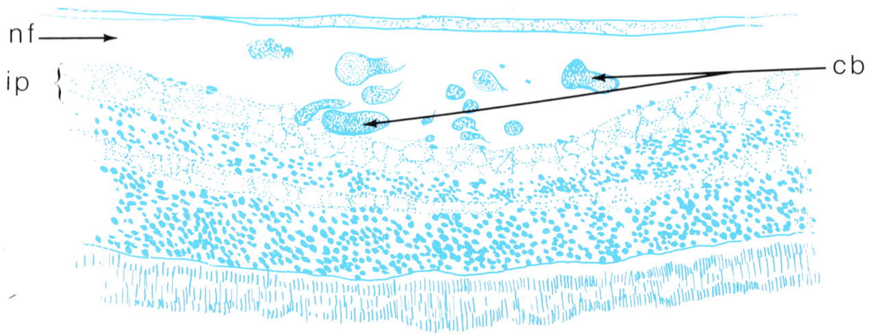

Drawing 60. Plate 60 (cb, cytoid bodies; nf, nerve fiber layer; ip, inner plexiform layer).

Plate 61. Cluster of ovoid, eosinophilic bodies in nerve fiber and ganglion cell layers of retina (H&E, × 100).

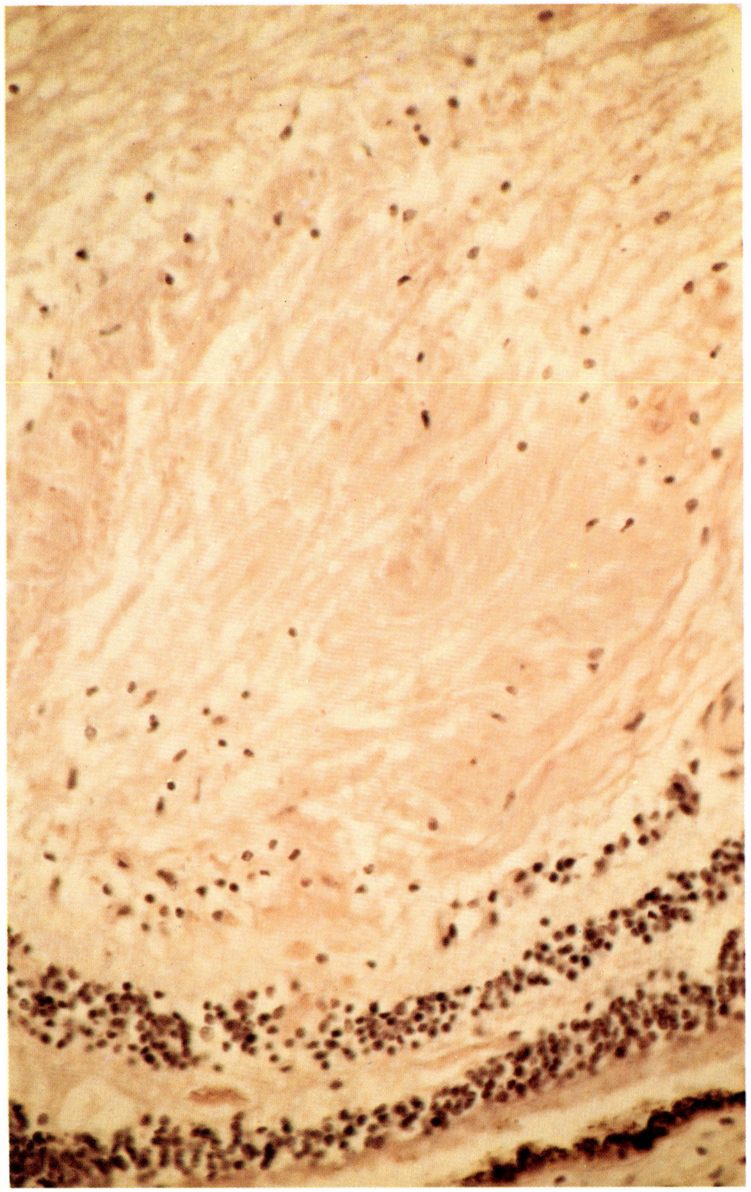

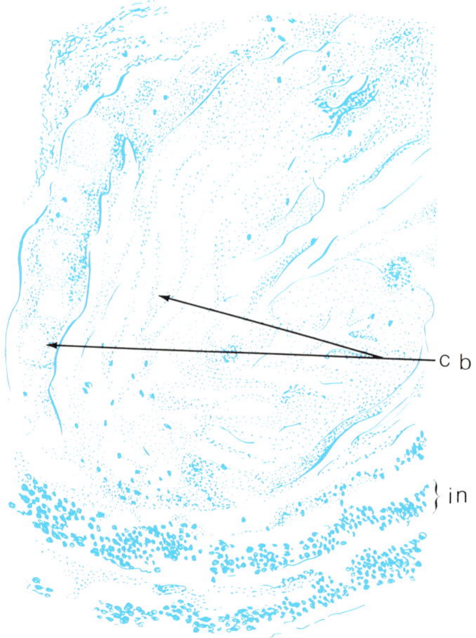

Drawing 61. Plate 61 (cb, cytoid bodies; in, inner nuclear layer).

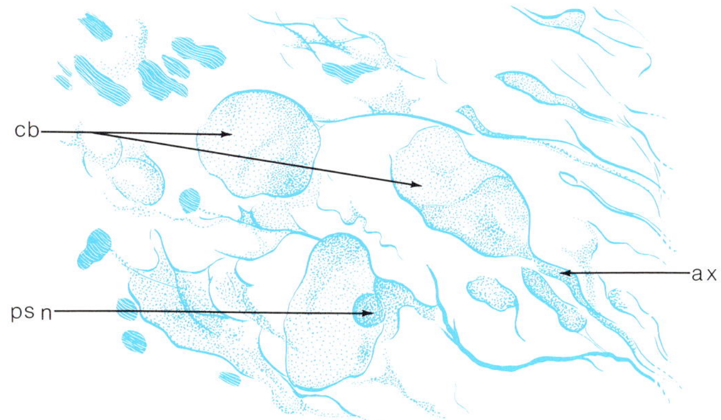

Drawing 62. Plate 62 (ax, axon; cb, cytoid bodies; psn, pseudonucleus).

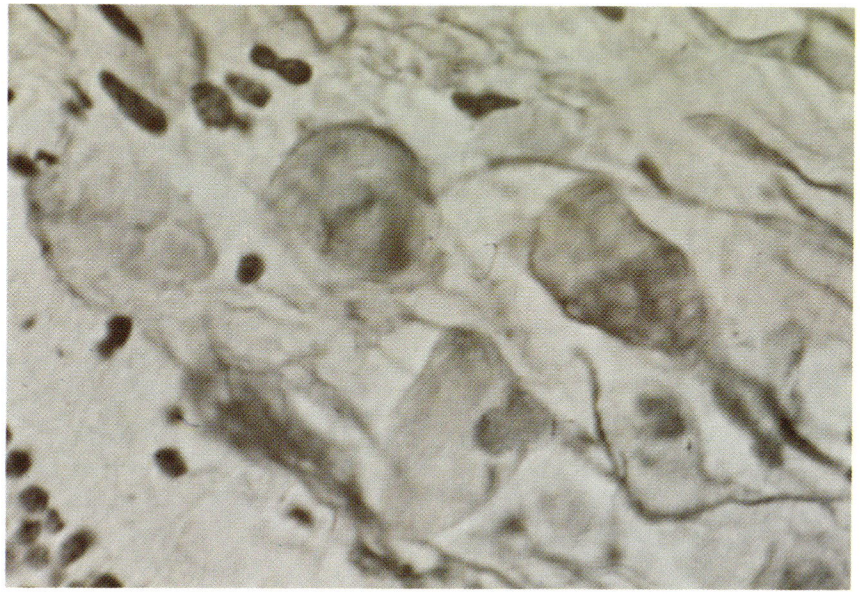

Plate 62. Cytoid bodies, swollen axis cylinders (Bodian silver stain, approx. × 450).

Pathology

The histologic equivalent of the cotton wool patch consists of microinfarcts in the nerve fiber layer of the retina. The areas of infarction are composed of clusters of ovoid, cell-like structures called cytoid bodies (Plates 60 and 61 and Drawings 60 and 61). The latter measure 10 to 20 micra and may contain an eccentric or central darker area called the pseudonucleus. When stained with hematoxylin and eosin the cytoid bodies are eosinophilic. If silver stains are used, these abnormal structures are identified as the terminal swellings of Cajal at the site of axonal interruption[98, 99] (Plate 62 and Drawing 62). Hemorrhage may partially surround or intermingle with such lesions (Plate 63 and Drawing 63).

Drawing 63. Plate 63 (cb, cluster of cytoid bodies; hem, hemorrhage; im, internal limiting membrane; in, inner nuclear layer).

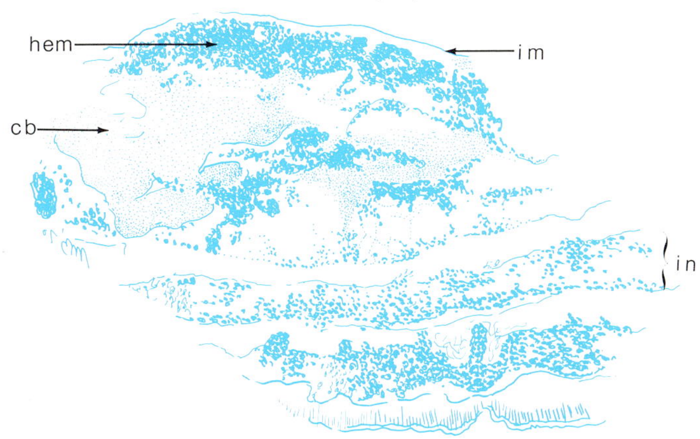

Plate 63. Hemorrhage and cytoid bodies (PTAH, approx. × 80).

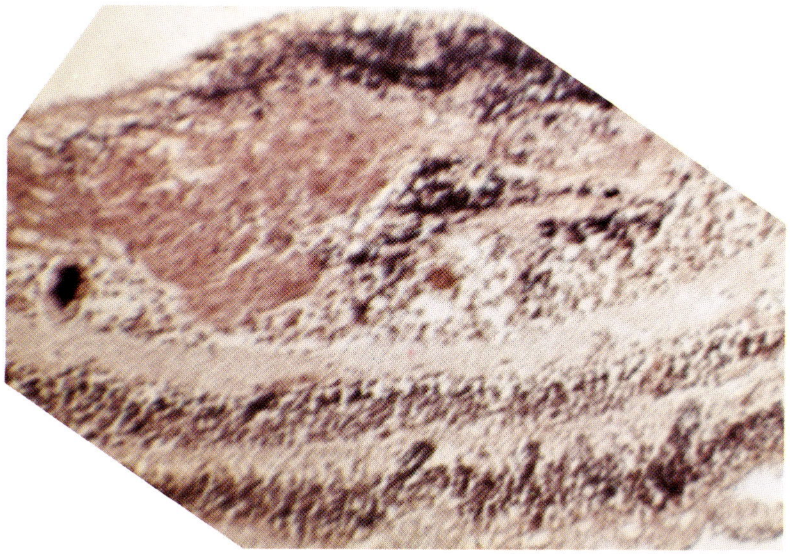

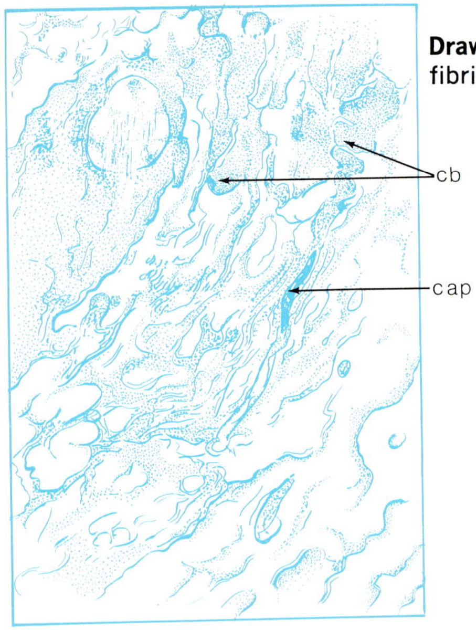

Drawing 65. Plate 65 (cb, cytoid bodies; cap, fibrin–occluded capillary).

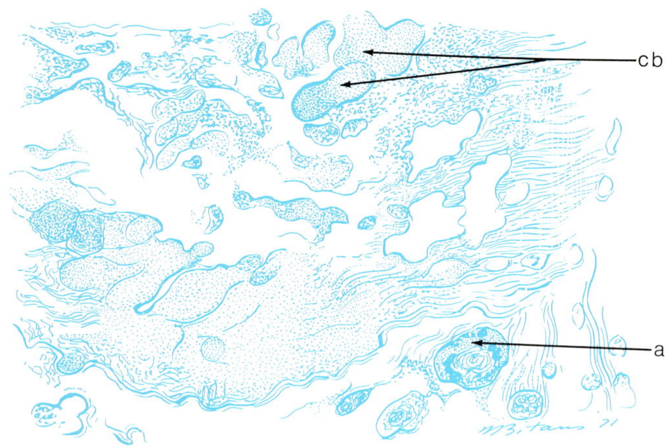

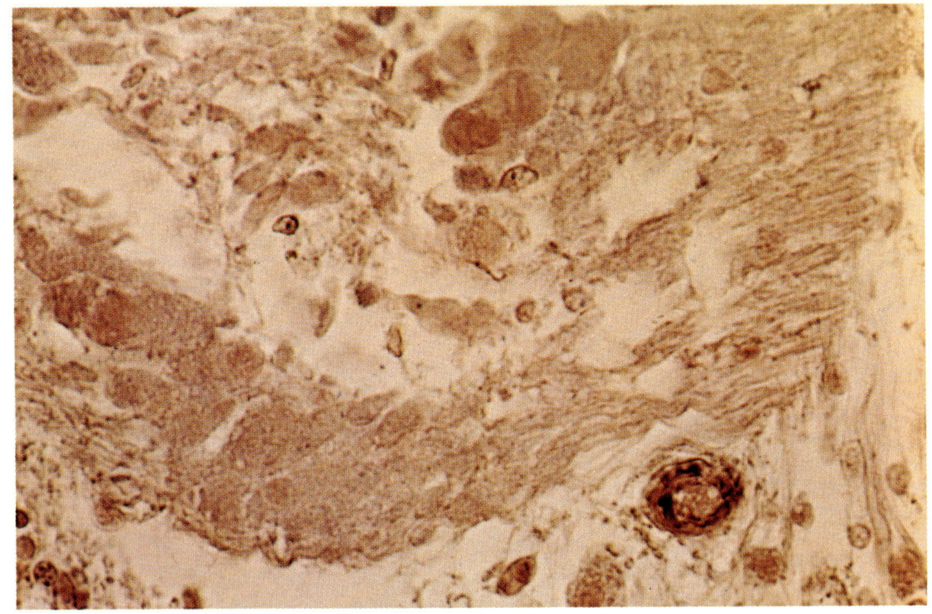

Drawing 64. Plate 64 (cb, cytoid bodies; a, occluded arteriole).

Plate 64. Arteriolar occlusion and cytoid bodies (PTAH, × 400).

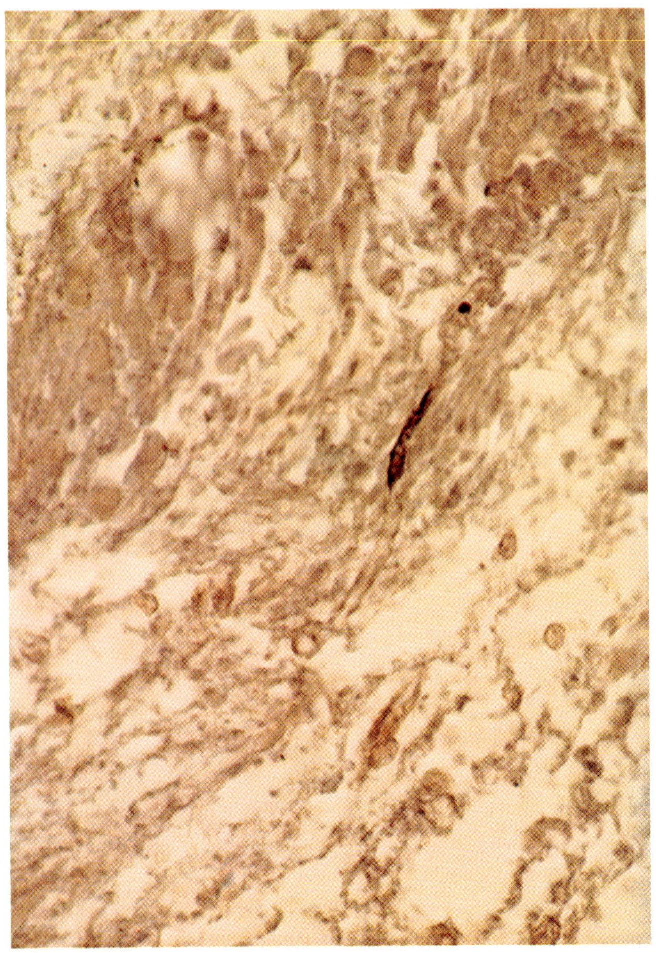

Plate 65. Fibrinoid occlusion of capillary within a cluster of cytoid bodies (PTAH, × 400).

Plate 66. Retinal digest. Fibrin occlusion of capillaries (PTAH, approx. × 80).

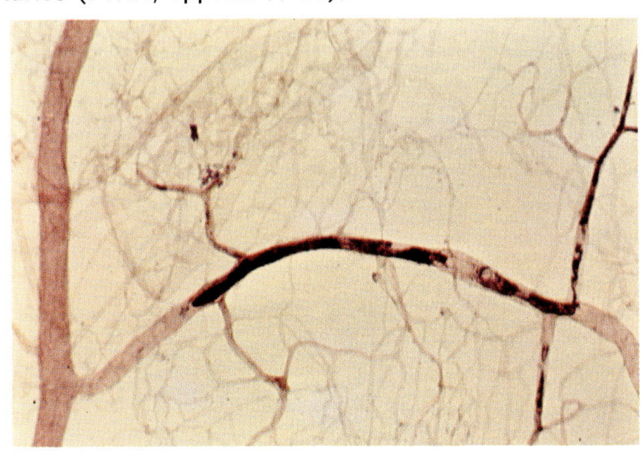

Pathogenesis of Cotton Wool Patch and Cytoid Body Formation

Friedenwald[100] considered these lesions to be microinfarcts but was unable to demonstrate the presence of vascular occlusion. Subsequently Ashton,[101] Klien,[102] and others were able to demonstrate the presence of occluded arterioles and/or capillaries within or close to the zones of infarction in accelerated hypertension and scleroderma (Plates 64 and 65 and Drawings 64 and 65). In malignant hypertension, fibrinoid necrosis of arteriolar walls and fibrin thrombi are present in diseased areas (Plate 65 and Drawing 65). Adding further support to the concept of infarction secondary to vascular occlusion[103] (Plate

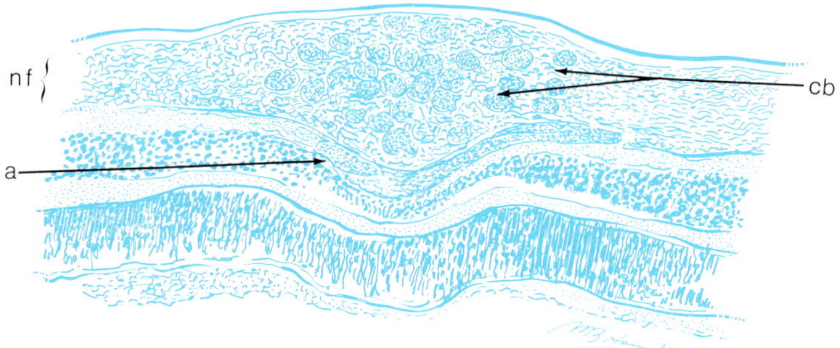

Drawing 67. Plate 67 (nf, nerve fiber layer; cb, cytoid bodies; a, lipid–occluded arteriole).

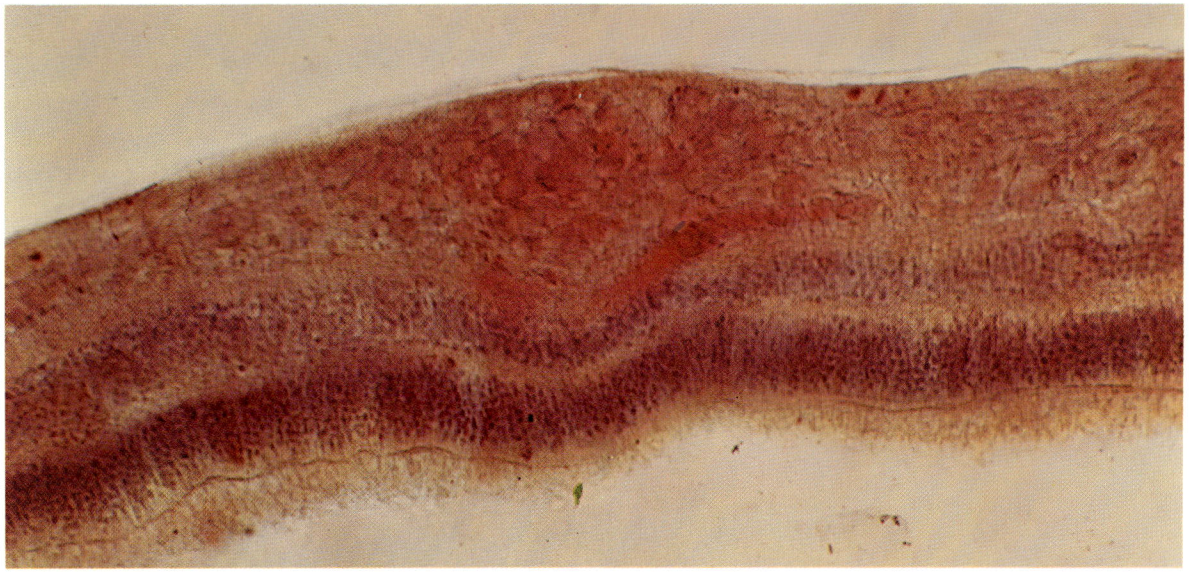

Plate 67. Section of retina embedded in gelatin. Note arteriolar occlusion with lipid within cluster of cytoid bodies (Scharlach R, × 80).

Plate 68. Retinal digest. Lipid occlusion of precapillary arteriole and capillaries (Scharlach R, × 80).

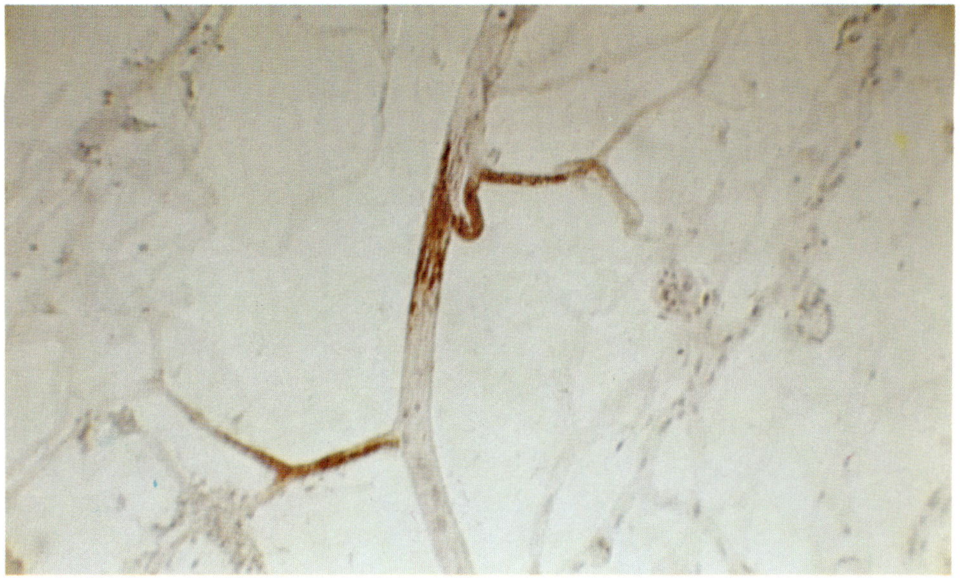

66) is the presence of focal areas of fibrin–occluded capillaries, often associated with microaneurysms, in flat mounts of trypsin–digested retinas from patients with malignant hypertension. In addition, Chester and Banker[104] have presented evidence which relates the formation of cytoid bodies and microaneurysms in diabetes mellitus to lipid occlusion of arterioles and capillaries (Plates 67 and 68 and Drawing 67).

Experimentally cotton wool patches and cytoid bodies have been reproduced in the cat by occlusion of retinal arterioles with glass beads by Ashton and Henkind[105] and in the pig by Dollery *et al.*, [106] and Shakib and Ashton.[107]

At the site of experimentally occluded retinal arterioles in the pig, Shakib and Ashton[107] observed swelling of axons in the nerve fiber and inner plexiform layers of the retina in 1 hour. Within 24 hours the axonal swelling became marked and degeneration of ganglion cells was noted. By the third day the expanded axons of the nerve fiber layer became round or oval structures. The latter became more numerous and were accompanied by macrophages on the seventh day. By the fourteenth day, few oval bodies were present and many of the damaged ganglion cells had disappeared. Macrophages, in such areas, contained basophilic granules in their cytoplasm. Although some normal nerve fibers were observed after 25 days, the majority had been replaced by glial cells and macrophages; ganglion cells were absent. Thus the healing process resulted in loss of the normal architecture in the affected area. In the same study, the authors observed that the cytoid bodies may be well advanced in intact axons and are not dependent upon axonal interruption as proposed by Wolter.[99] However, they do not deny that ultimately a break occurs in the nerve fibers and that the distal stump attached to the ganglion cell develops a bulblike swelling which may be the cytoid body, while the proximal fiber atrophies.

The experimental studies of Margolis and Brown[108] and the clinical observations of Ashton *et al.*[109] suggest that ischemia, even in the absence of vascular occlusion, may be responsible for the development of cytoid bodies of the retina. Margolis and Brown[108] found cytoid bodies in the retinas of 12 dogs that had breathed 100% oxygen at 3 atmospheres for 4 hours or longer. They suggested that the hyperoxia inhibited the enzyme reactions of visual cells and that death of retinal tissue resulted. It is equally possible that the hyperoxia produced vasoconstriction. In that event, the resulting anoxia could account for the injury to the retina. In man, although exposure to hyperbaric oxygen produced marked retinal venular and arteriolar constriction, no extravascular lesions were observed, Saltzman *et al.*[110] Ashton *et al.*[109] observed the development of cotton wool patches in a patient following massive gastrointestinal bleeding and hypotension. Histologic studies of the retina disclosed cytoid bodies in the absence of vascular occlusion.

In summary, there appears to be substantial evidence, both in the study of disease in man and in the experimental animal, to support the concept that the microinfarcts in the nerve fiber layer of the retina, represented by the clusters of cytoid bodies, are the result of retinal ischemia, most often associated with vascular occlusion.

The Cotton Wool Patch and Disease States

Although the cotton wool lesion is found most commonly in hypertension[82, 91] and diabetes mellitus,[15, 111, 112] it may be associated with a variety of other diseases. These include the various connective tissue diseases such as lupus erythematosus,[113, 114] polyarteritis nodosa,[115] dermatomyositis,[116, 117] and scleroderma.[102, 118] It can occur as well in multiple myeloma,[119] macroglobulinemia of Waldenström,[120, 121] and sickle cell disease.[122] Vascular occlusive phenomena may occur in all the above diseases, thus lending further support to that concept of the genesis of the lesion under discussion. No adequate explanation is available for the development of the cotton wool patch in various anemias. The cotton wool patch is described in leukemia.

[119, 123] Both cytoid body formation and leukemic infiltration of the retina may be the pathologic counterpart of that lesion.[119] Hollenhorst[124, 125] has pointed out the frequency of the cotton wool lesion in association with thrombosis of the internal carotid artery.

Clinical Course of the Cotton Wool Patch

In a clinical study of the cotton wool patch in patients with accelerated hypertension, Hodge and Dollery[126] observed that such lesions may appear in 1–2 days in an apparently normal area. However, with careful observation, a faint gray–white pallor of the involved area could be recognized before the characteristic lesion appeared. At this stage, fluorescein angiograms disclosed fluorescence of the involved area, presumably the result of increased vascular permeability. The fluorescence often persisted after the funduscopically visible lesion disappeared. In some patients the fluorescence was lost before the lesion disappeared clinically; in others the absence of fluorescence coincided with the disappearance of the lesion by direct funduscopy.

(continued on p. 66)

At times, this technique also demonstrated defects in capillary filling and microaneurysms before the cotton wool patch developed. The latter lesion then evolved rapidly, reaching its maximum size in a few days to two weeks. Complete ophthalmoscopic disappearance of the cotton wool lesion is frequently observed within several weeks after successful treatment of accelerated hypertension[82, 88] (Plates 69–73). In anemia such lesions may disappear even in the absence of improvement of the hematologic changes. As the lesion regresses it decreases in size, assumes a granular appearance, and blood vessels can be observed growing into it. Within several months the involved area of the retina appears to be normal ophthalmoscopically.

The changes described in the retina following experimental occlusion of retinal arterioles of the pig with glass microspheres corroborated, with few exceptions, the findings in human disease.[106] In the pig within 3 to 45 minutes after induced embolization, a grayish–white discoloration appeared distal to the obstructed retinal arteriole. During the next 24 hours to 4 days, the typical cotton wool patch developed at that site. In 7 days, the lesion had almost completely faded; and in 4 to 6 weeks that area appeared to be normal. Hemorrhage was less frequently associated with the cotton wool patch than it was in human disease. In the pig, fluorescein angiograms demonstrated initial absence of dye in capillaries distal to the occluded vessel. Such capillaries filled with dye later than the rest of the retina via retrograde flow. Microaneurysms were not observed.

Serial retinal photographs in patient with accelerated hypertension.

Plate 69. Note cotton wool patches surrounding optic disc.

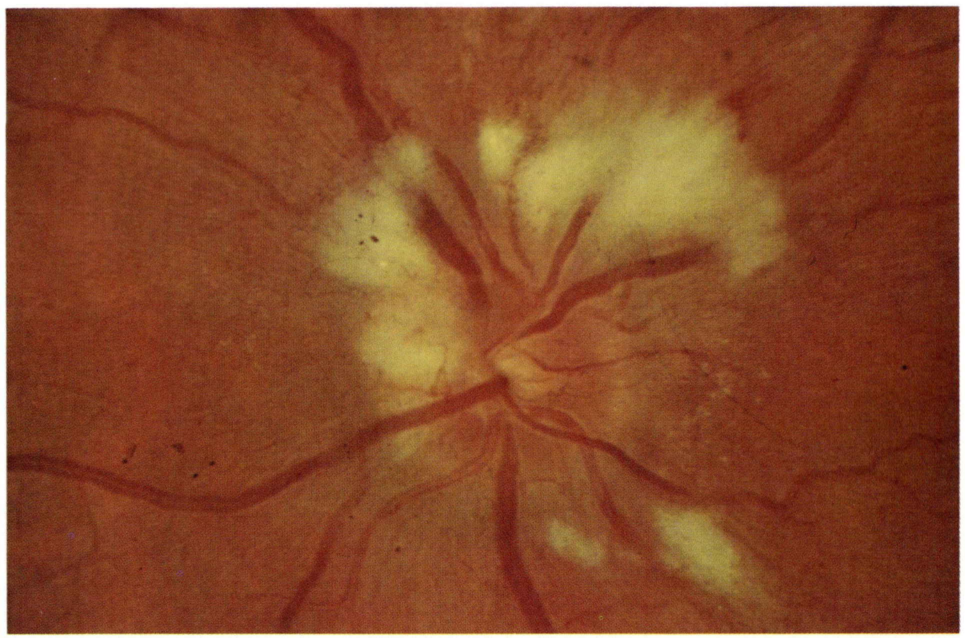

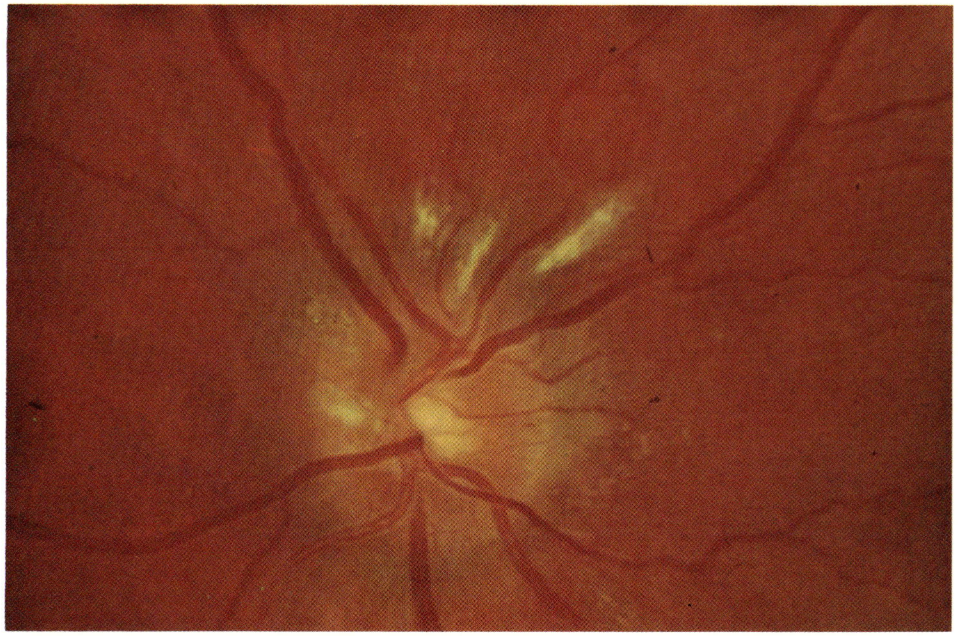

Plate 70. Note almost complete resolution of the cotton wool lesions (1 month later) after successful treatment of hypertension.

Plate 71. Note complete resolution of the cotton wool lesions (8 months later). Treatment of hypertension continued.

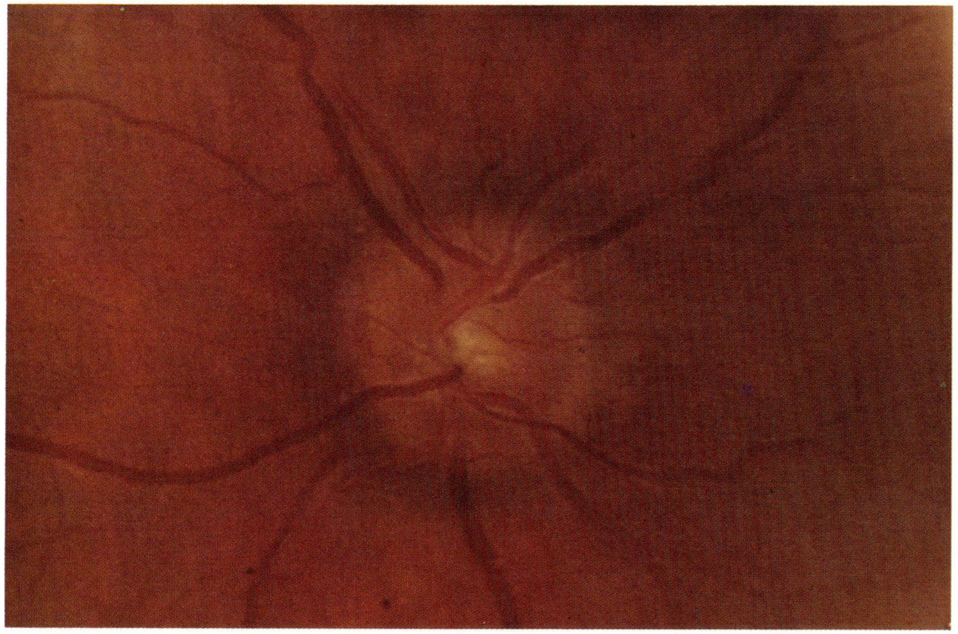

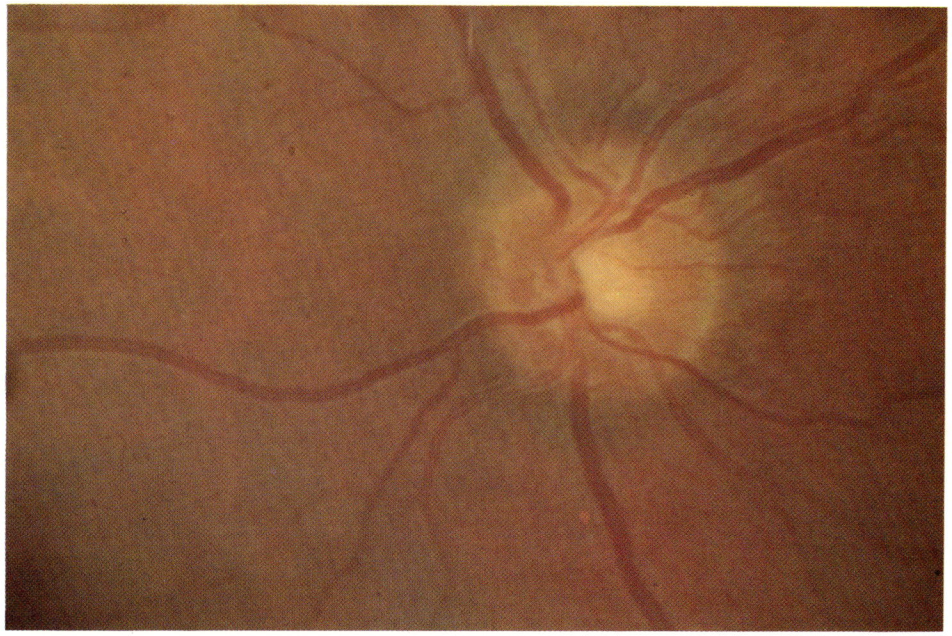

Plate 72. Sixteen months later.

Plate 73. Four years later.

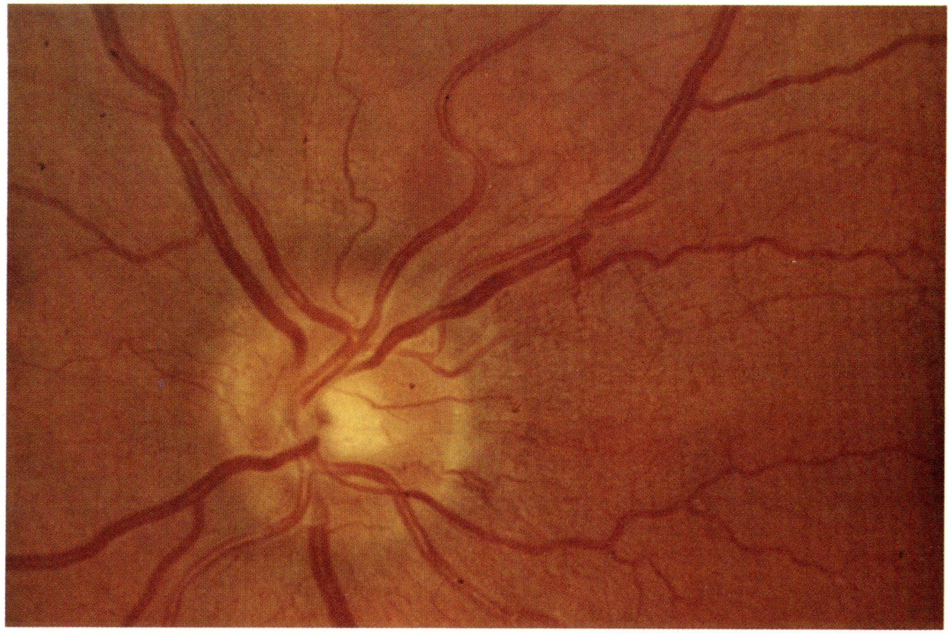

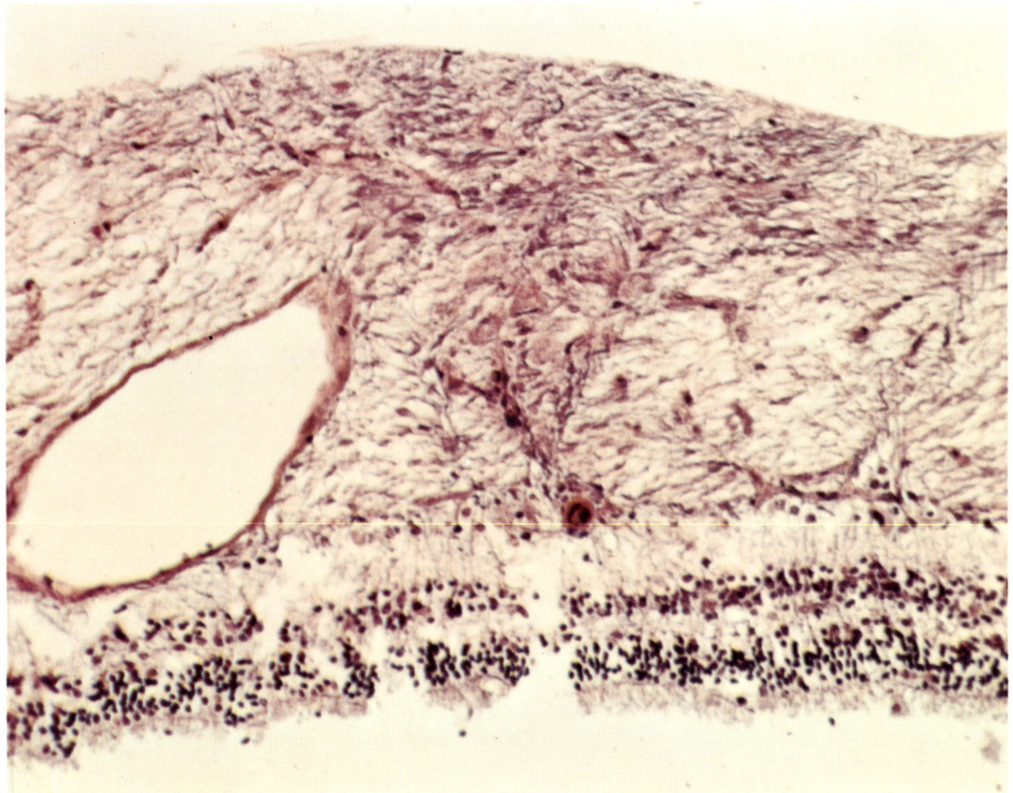

Sections of Retina—Photomicrographs.

Plate 74. Microinfarct in the nerve fiber layer of the retina demonstrating a fibrin–occluded arteriole, cytoid bodies, glial response, and distortion of the normal architecture. Breaks in the nuclear and plexiform layers are artefacts (PTAH, × 100).

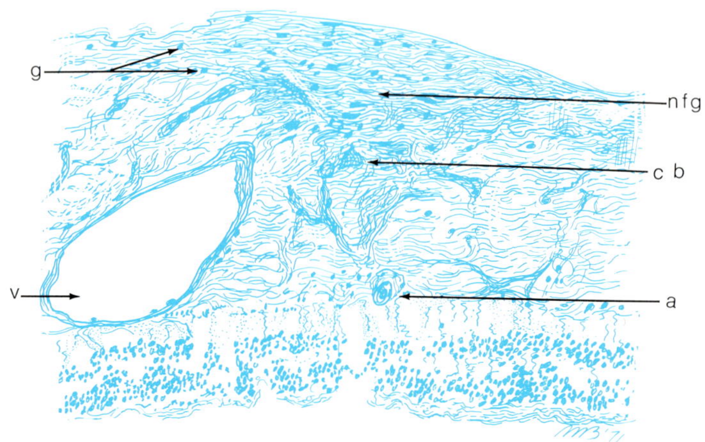

Drawing 74, Plate 74 (nfgl, nerve fiber layer gliosis; g, ganglion cells; a, occluded arteriole; cb, cytoid bodies; v, vein).

The Histologic Residua of the Cotton Wool Patch

After embolization of retinal arterioles of the pig with glass microspheres Shakib and Ashton[107] were able to identify histological residua of the healed cotton wool patches. As previously described, the microscopic changes consisted of gliosis in the nerve fiber layer with loss of its normal architecture, the presence of macrophages, and the absence of ganglion cells. Comparable changes have been found in human retinas after documentation of healed cotton wool patches (Plates 74–76 and Drawings 74–76).

Significance of the Cotton Wool Patch

The cotton wool patch is an indication of progression of the underlying disease. In connective tissue disorders, diabetes mellitus, and hypertension it is the result of retinal arteriolar or capillary occlusion. Acceleration of hypertension and the onset of the malignant form of that disease may be heralded by the development of the cotton wool patch. In anemia it is a reflection of increased severity and/or the presence of a serious underlying hematologic disorder.

The potential reversibility with adequate treatment of the cotton wool patch in anemia and other hematologic disorders, the connective tissue diseases such as polyarteritis and lupus erythematosus, eclampsia, accelerated hypertension, and carotid artery insufficiency serves as an excellent reminder of the need to recognize the retinal abnormality, to relate it to the basic underlying disease, and to offer adequate treatment as rapidly as possible.

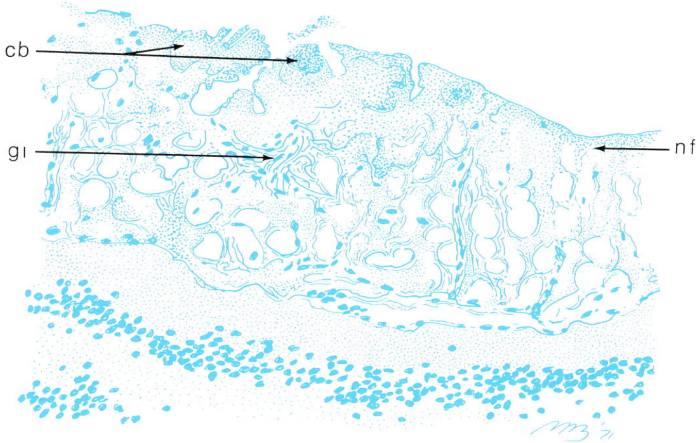

Drawing 75. Plate 75 (nf, nerve fiber layer; cb, cytoid bodies; gl, gliosis).

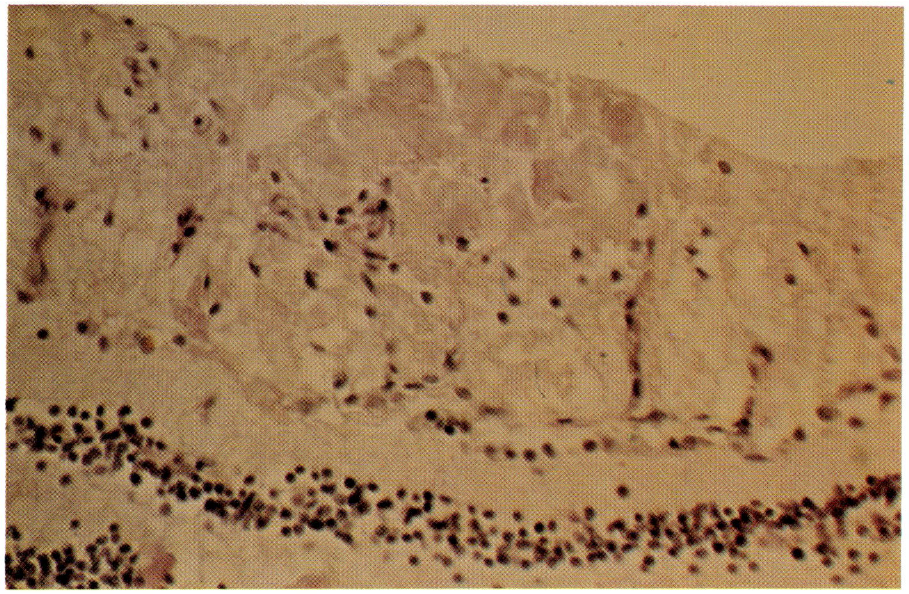

Plate 75. Cytoid bodies in the nerve fiber layer of the retina have evoked a glial response. Two deposits of PAS positive amorphous material are present in the outer plexiform layer. The break in the continuity of the nerve fiber layer is an artefact (periodic acid—Schiff stain, PAS, × 200).

Plate 76. Residual gliosis and distortion of architecture of the nerve fiber layer of the retina. Few cytoid bodies and ganglion cells can be identified (H&E, × 200).

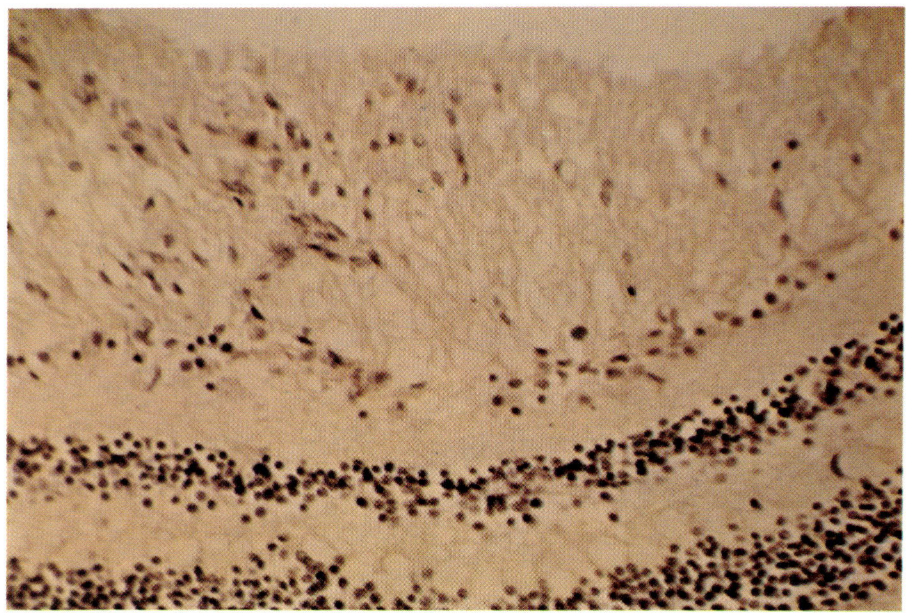

Drawing 76. Plate 76 (nf, nerve fiber layer; gl, gliosis).

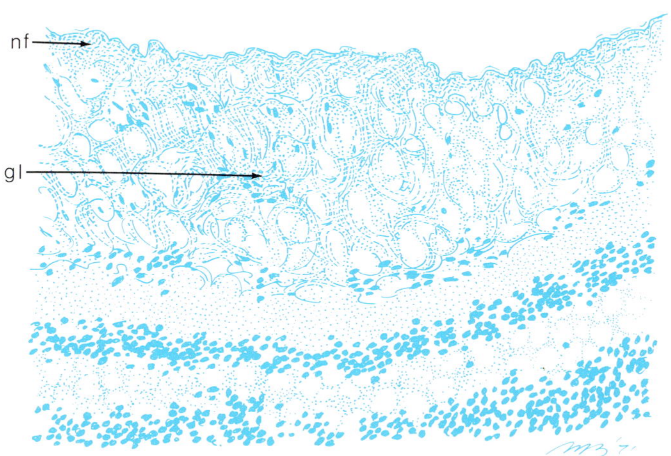

Plate 77. Magnified view. There are two discrete lesions. Tortuous venules cross over them.

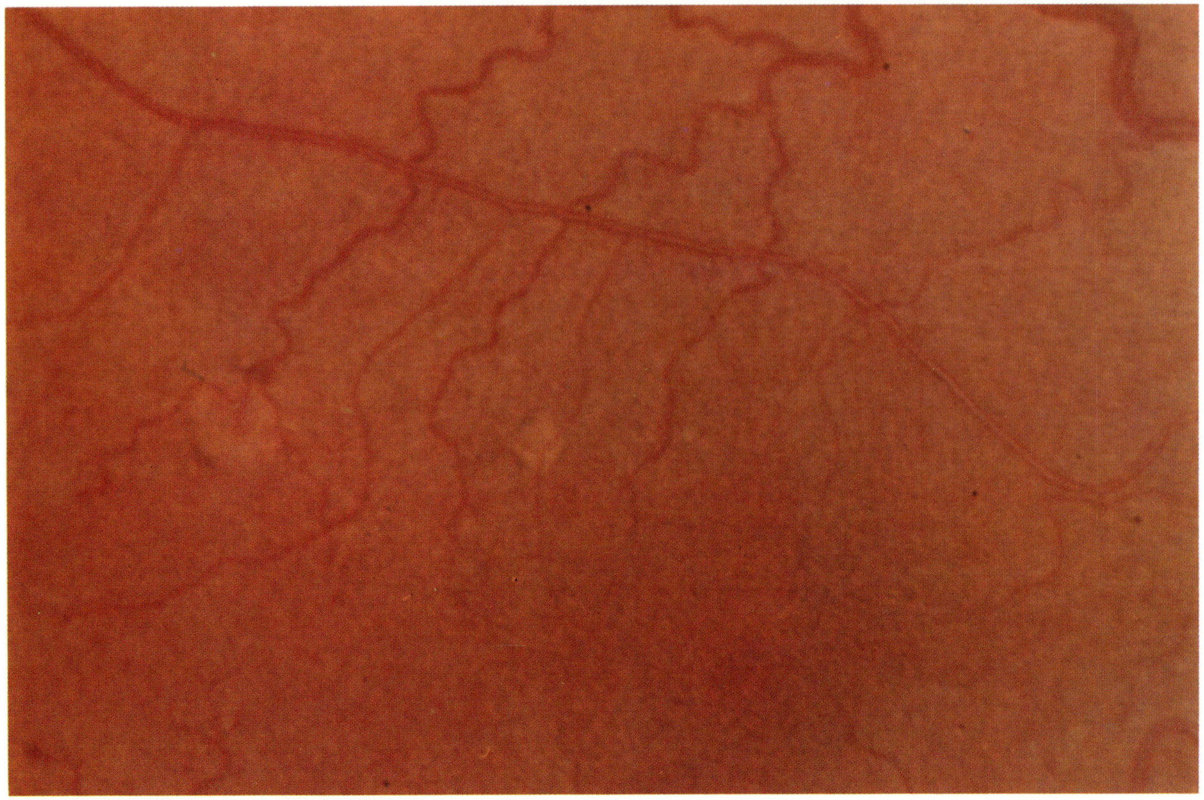

THE HARD EXUDATE

Clinical Appearance

The hard exudate is yellow or white in color and may appear as either discrete punctate lesions (Plate 77) or conglomerate masses (Plate 78). Characteristically the lesions are posterior to the retinal vessels. If present in the macular region they form a cluster of linear lesions radiating toward the central fovea like the spokes of a wheel (Plate 79). Such a lesion is called a macular star.

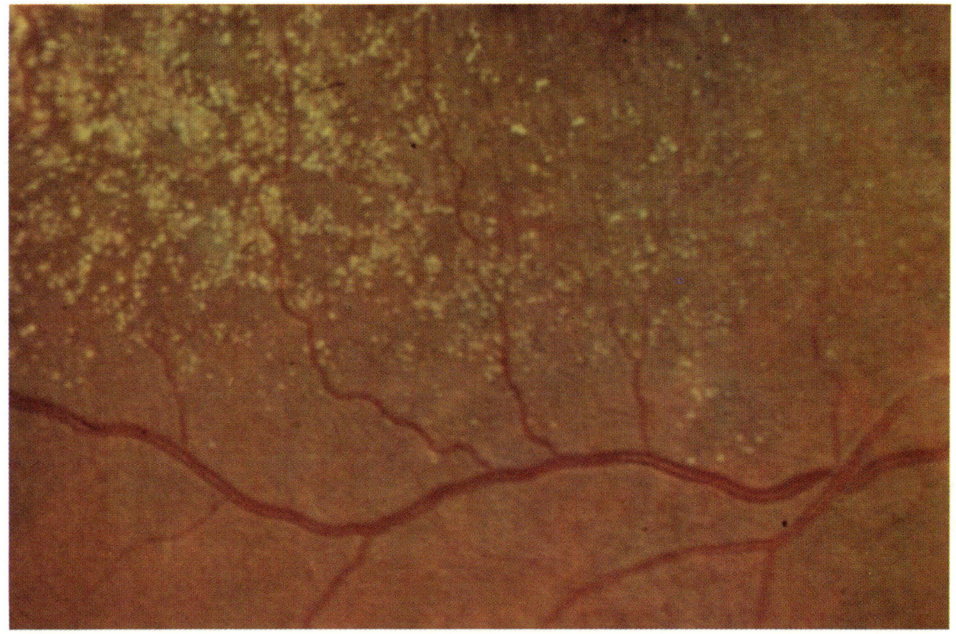

Plate 78. Conglomerate hard exudates are situated behind the retinal blood vessels. Magnified view. Did you notice the A–V compression?

Plate 79. O.S. Temporal. Macular star. Note star-like pattern of linear lesions radiating toward the fovea. In contrast, several cotton wool patches overlie blood vessels. Did you notice the retinal hemorrhages near the macula?

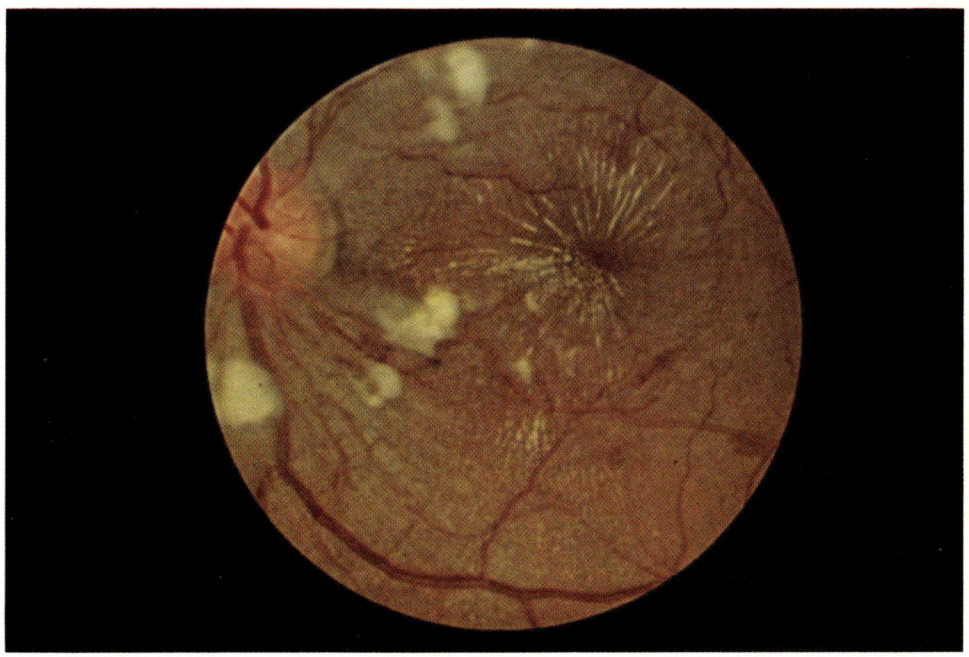

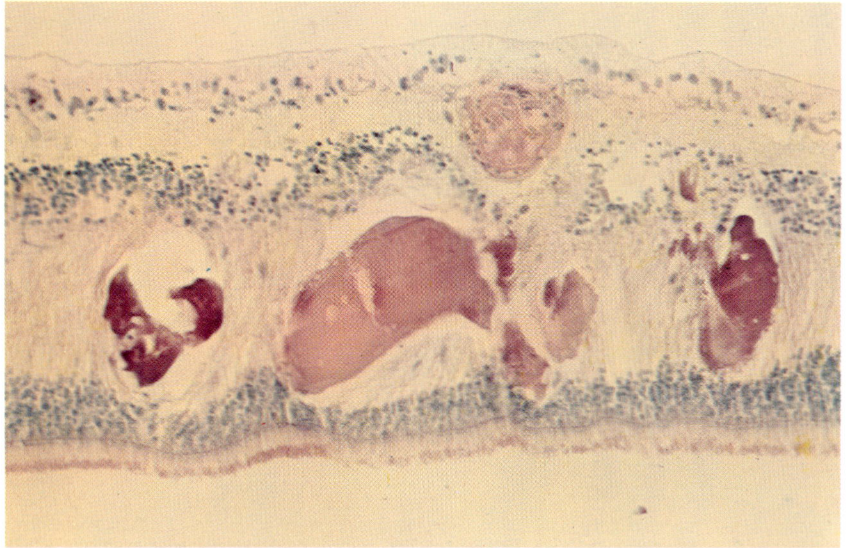

Outer plexiform lesions.

Plate 80. PAS positive deposits in the outer plexiform layer. Note the macrophages within the lesions (PAS, × 250).

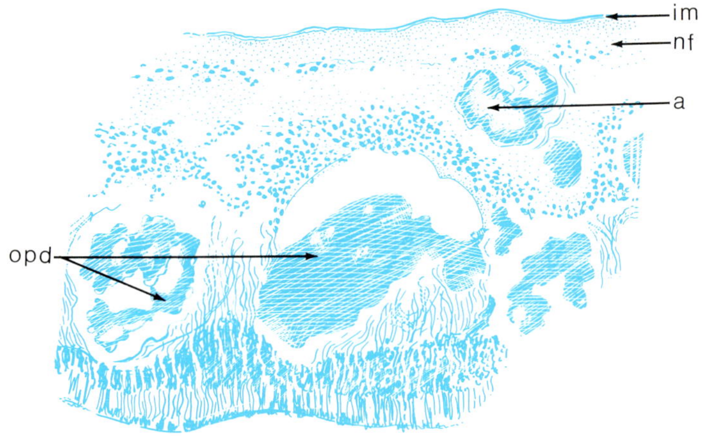

Drawing 80. Plate 80 (nf, nerve fiber layer; a, arteriole; opd, outer plexiform layer deposit; im, internal limiting membrane).

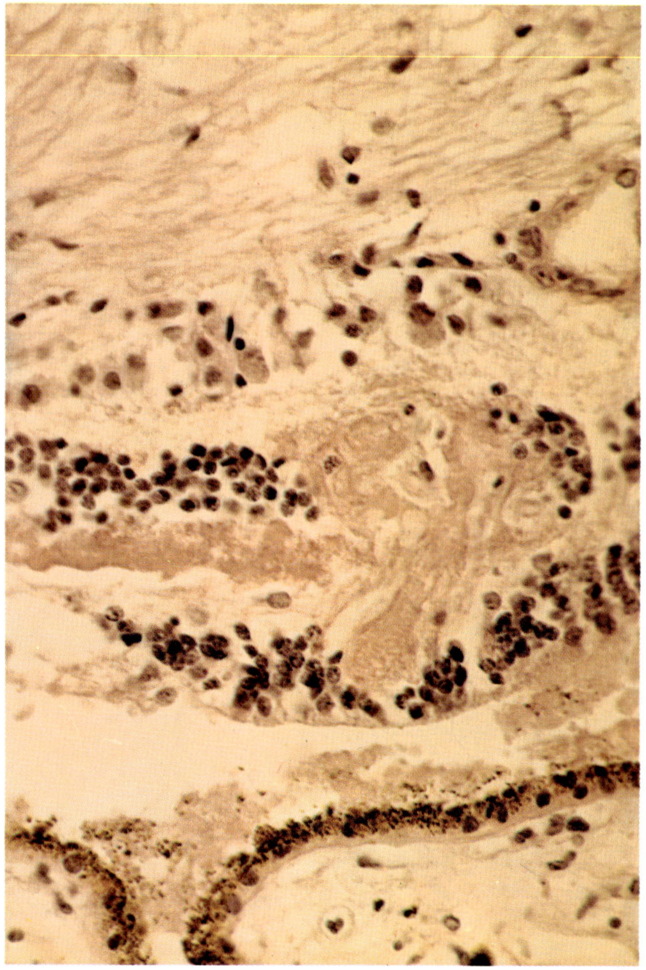

Plate 81. Eosinophilic deposits (H&E, × 400).

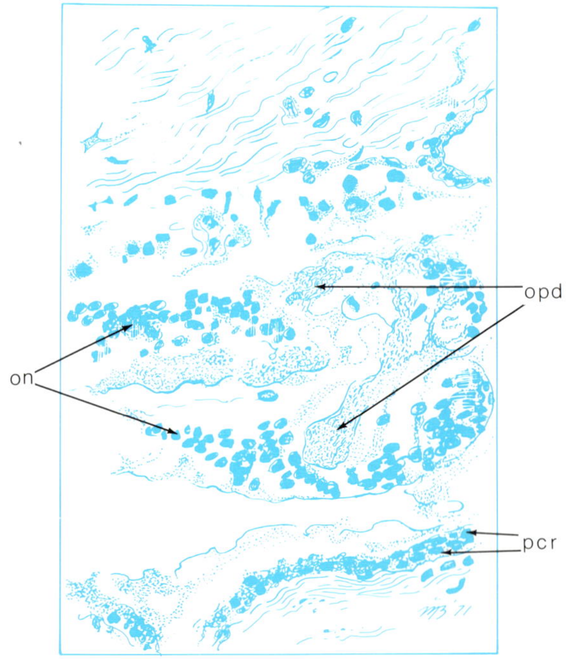

Drawing 81. Plate 81 (opd, outer plexiform layer deposit; pcr, pigment cell layer of retina; on, outer nuclear layer).

Pathology

The histologic equivalent of the hard exudate consists of discrete deposits or conglomerate masses, generally in the outer plexiform layer and often extending into one or more of the nuclear layers (Plates 80–83 and Drawings 80–83). The lesions often displace or destroy the nerve fibers of the outer plexiform layer. These lesions may be eosinophilic (Plate 81), and they may contain pools or strands of fibrin (Plate 82), neutral fat, and fatty acids (Plate 83). Macrophages may be found within the lesions (Plate 80). Hemorrhage in one or more retinal layers and cytoid bodies may accompany these changes.

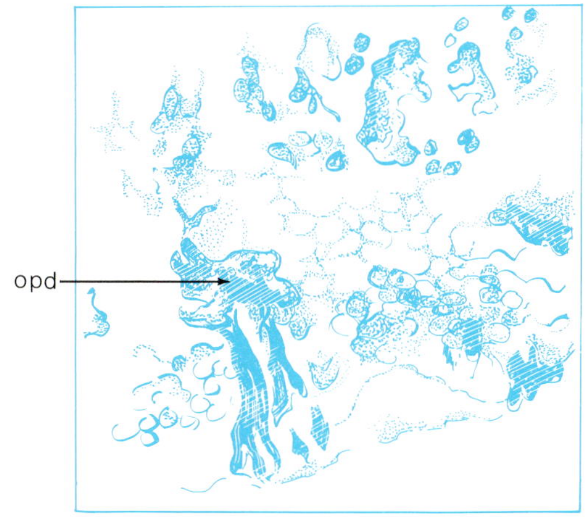

Drawing 82. Plate 82 (opd, outer plexiform deposit of strands of fibrin).

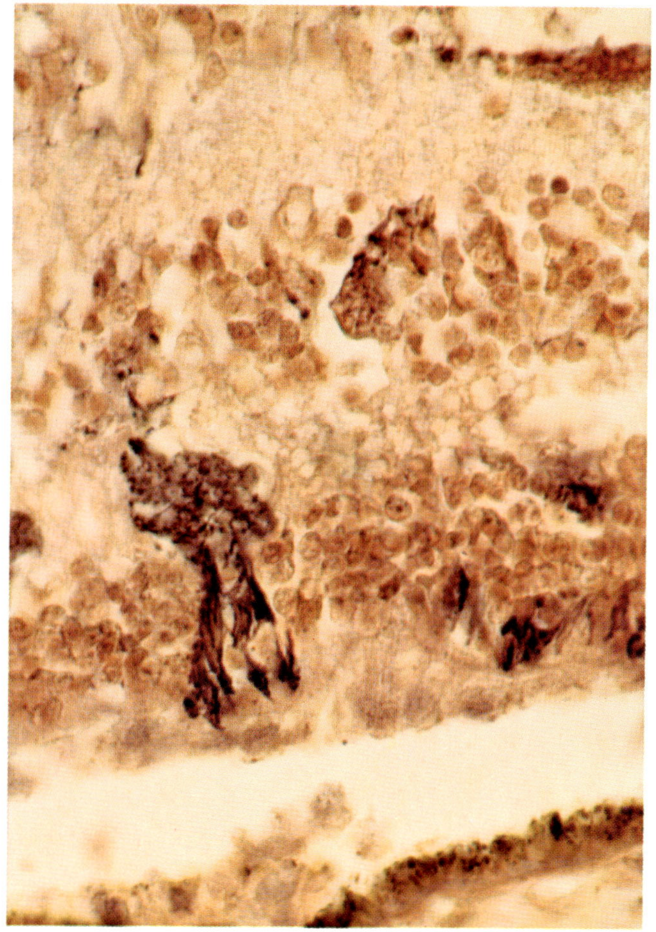

Plate 82. Fibrin deposits (PTAH, × 400).

Drawing 83. Plate 83 (opd, outer plexiform lipid deposits).

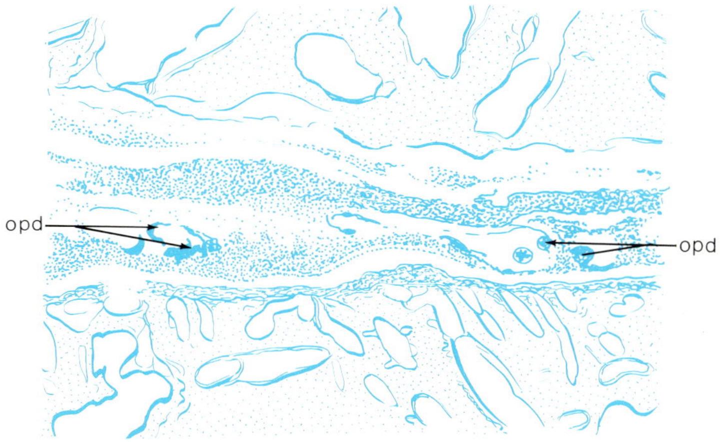

Plate 83. Deposits of sudanophilic material (lipid, Scharlach R, × 120).

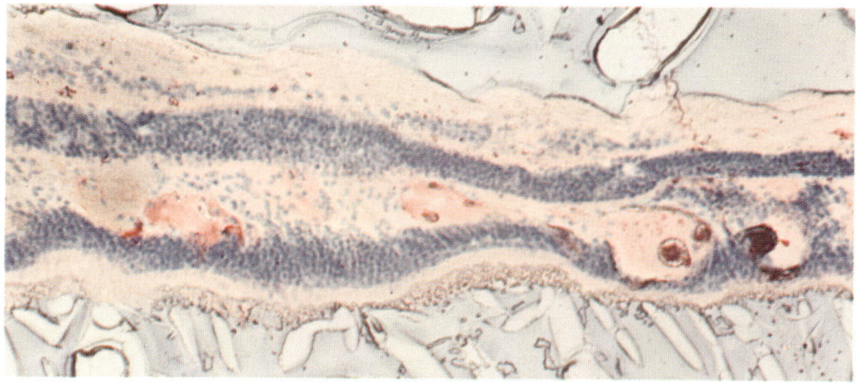

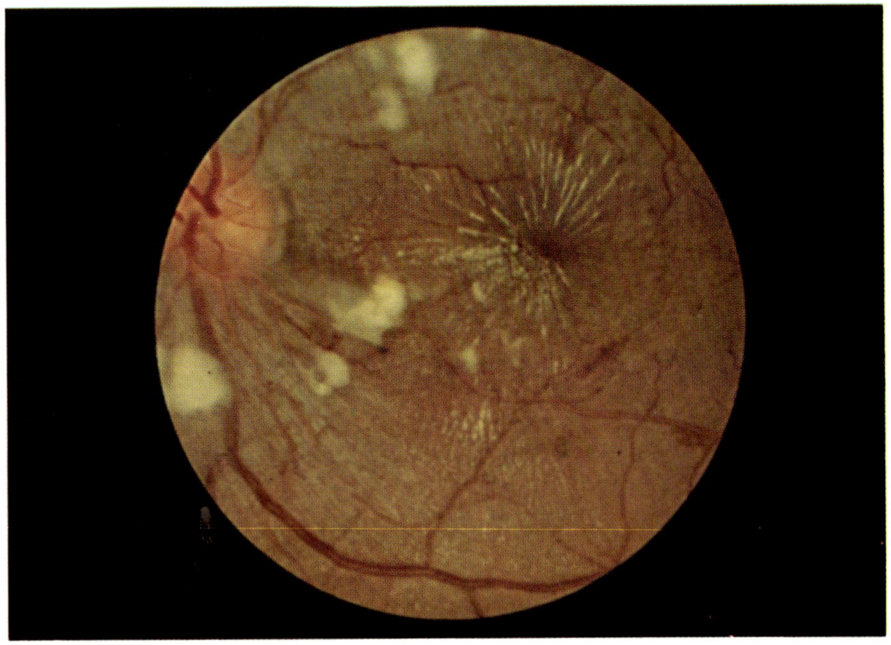

Plate 79. O.S. Temporal — Macular Star. Note star–like pattern of linear lesions radiating toward the fovea.

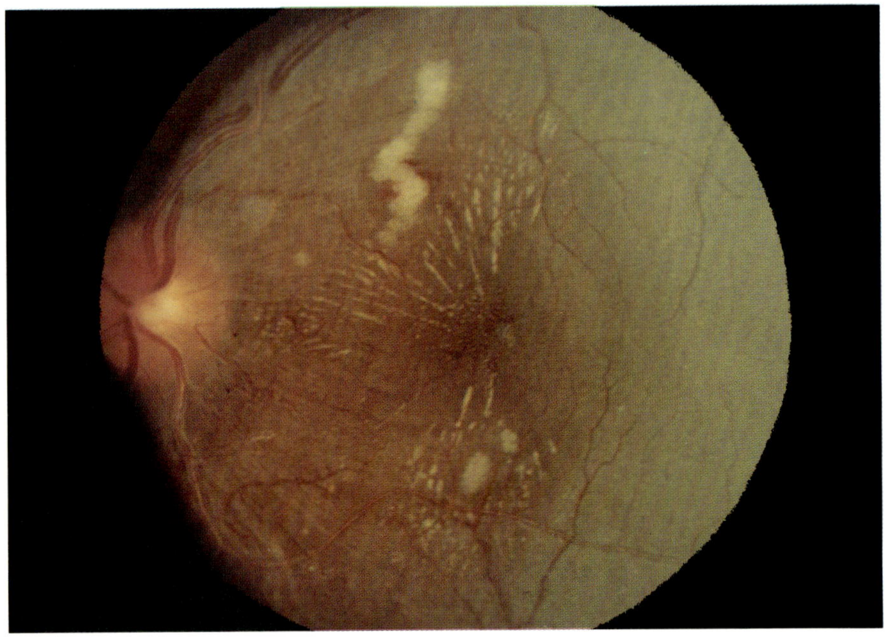

Plate 84. O.S. Macular star. Note linear hard exudates which radiate from a central area of the macula to produce a star-like figure. The lesions are sharply defined and are posterior to the retinal vessels. Note cotton wool patches above and below the macula. Did you notice the small hemorrhage within the large cotton wool patch?

Drawing 84. Plate 84 (O, optic nerve; CWP, cotton wool patches; MS, macular star).

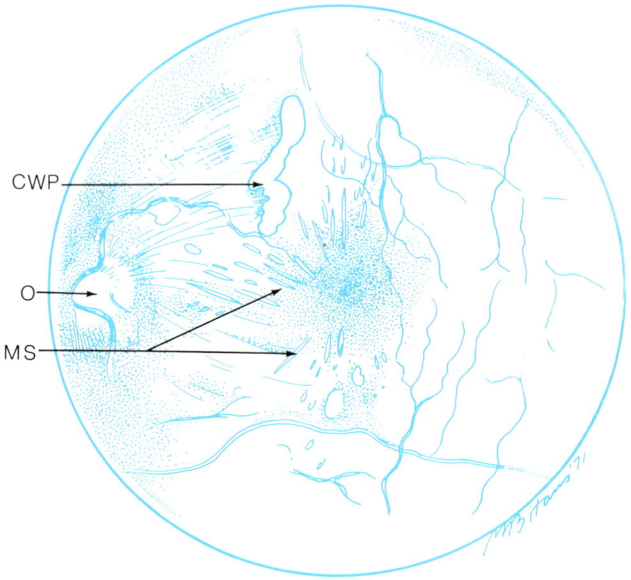

Macular Star

When outer plexiform lesions develop in the macular region, a starlike lesion results (Plates 79, 84, and 85, and Drawing 84). Its clinical appearance is determined by the anatomic arrangement of the macula (see p. 8). Because the outer plexiform layer (called Henle's layer in the macula) radiates toward the central fovea, hard exudates that develop in that area conform with the anatomic pattern and the lesion appears as noted in Plates 79, 84, and 85.

The hard exudate exemplifies the effect of location of a lesion upon its clinical appearance. The pressure applied by the vertically arranged fibers of the outer plexiform layer determine the form of such lesions and account for their sharply defined borders. Since the lesions are found in layers posterior to the branches of the central retinal artery, the hard exudates are seen behind the retinal vessels when the fundus is examined.

Pathogenesis of the Hard Exudate

The pathogenesis of the outer plexiform lesion is unknown. According to Hogan and Zimmerman,[2 (p. 504)] the lesion originates as edema which collects in pools in the various layers of the retina and produces degeneration of nervous tissue. Ultimately, according to that concept, the fluid undergoes change and accumulates as lipid, fibrin, and cellular debris. Ballantyne and Michaelson[4 (p. 49)] state that the capillary plexus at the junction of inner nuclear and outer plexiform layers serves as the source of the original transudate deposited in that area. Gass,[127] utilizing fluorescein angiograms in patients with hypertensive retinopathy, failed to demonstrate either leakage of the dye from macular

Plate 85. An enlarged view of the macular star demonstrated in Plate 84.

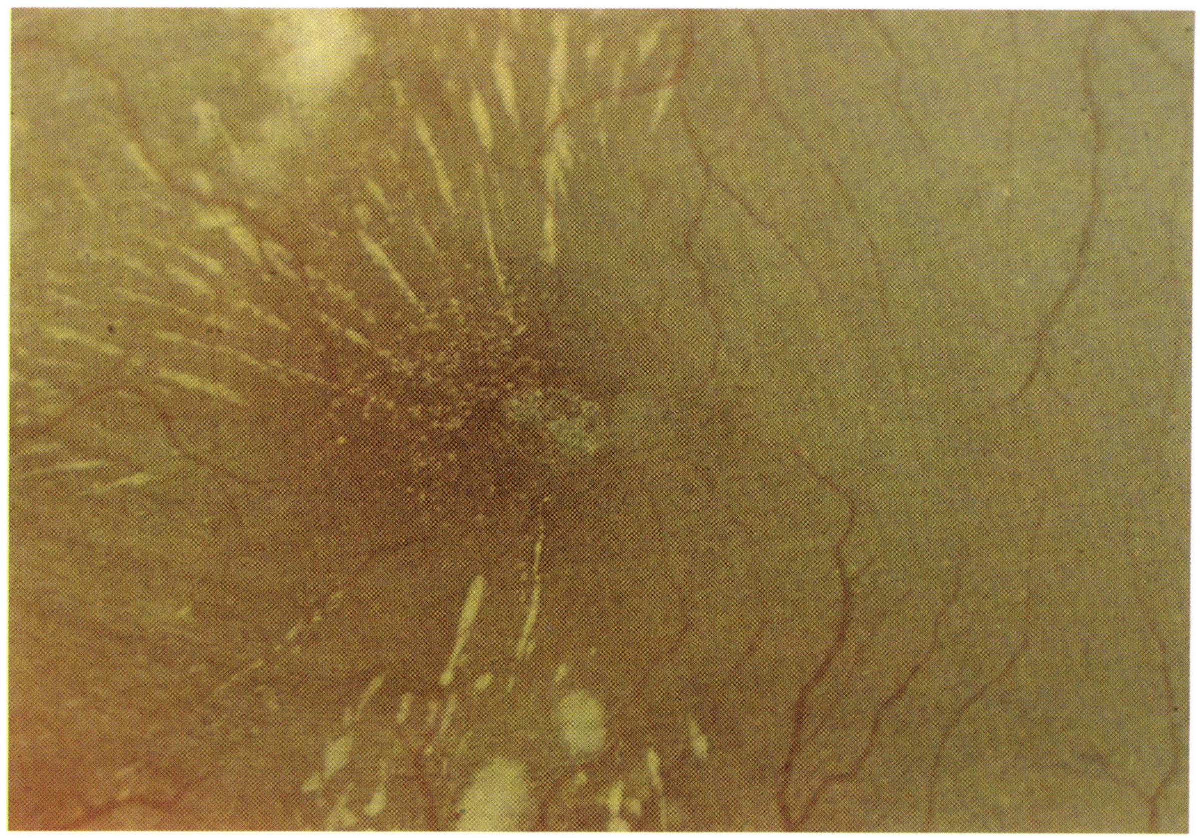

capillaries or fluorescence of the outer plexiform macular lesions. Based upon these observations, he suggested that the macular lesions were products of retinal tissue breakdown rather than serous exudate derived from retinal vessels. The observations of Shakib and Ashton[107] appear to support the concept of primary nervous tissue damage as a cause of the outer plexiform lesion. In the study of the effects of experimental retinal arteriolar embolization, they observed outer plexiform changes in addition to the cytoid bodies in the nerve fiber layer. The alterations of dendrites and axons in the outer plexiform layer ultimately led to a complete loss of architecture of that portion of the retina. These findings suggest that retinal arteriolar occlusion may be the common denominator for the production of outer plexiform lesions as well as those in the nerve fiber layer. The frequent association of cotton wool patches and hard exudates and their respective pathological equivalents, namely, cytoid bodies and outer plexiform deposits in malignant hypertension[2 (pp. 503-505)] and diabetes mellitus,[110] is well documented. In both of those diseases occlusion of retinal arterioles and/or capillaries has been demonstrated and is considered to be the mechanism for the production of the microinfarcts of the nerve fiber layer resulting in the formation of cytoid bodies and the clinical equivalent, the cotton wool patch. Although one is tempted to relate occlusive retinal arteriolar and capillary disease to the production of the outer plexiform lesion, current concepts indicate that the outer layers of the retina receive their nourishment from the choriocapillaries by diffusion through Bruch's membrane rather than via the central retinal artery and its branches. However, it is conceivable that retinal capillaries which extend to the junction of the inner nuclear and outer plexiform layers play a role in the nourishment of the latter area. In any event, choriodal vascular disease may be an important additional causal factor in the formation of the outer plexiform lesions. In support of this concept, fibrinoid necrosis of choroidal arteries has been observed in association with outer plexiform lesions and cytoid bodies in malignant hypertension.[103, 128, 129]

Countering that evidence are the results of Gass,[127] who failed to find either ophthalmoscopic or angiographic change in the macular pigment epithelium in most hypertensives. According to Gass, this lack of change denies the importance of choroidal vascular insufficiency in macular dysfunction. Despite his observations, there appears to be sufficient evidence to postulate that obstructive disease of retinal arterioles and capillaries when combined with severe choroidal vascular disease, at least in malignant hypertension, may be causally related to the formation of outer plexiform lesions. There is an obvious need for careful study of the choroidal vascular system in other diseases in which hard exudates are found.

The Hard Exudate and Clinical Disease States

Like the cotton wool patch, the hard exudates are most commonly found in accelerated hypertension[2 (pp. 503-505), 4 (pp. 139-144)] and diabetes mellitus.[110] Hard exudates are also described in polyarteritis nodosa,[130] scleroderma,[131] and anemia.[132]

Clinical Course

Unlike the cotton wool patch, the hard exudate resolves slowly, if at all. In successfully treated accelerated hypertension, the lesions generally last months, disappearing much later than hemorrhage and cotton wool patches. Recent reports indicate that the hard exudate of diabetic retinopathy may regress with rigid dietary restriction[133-135] and with the administration of hypolipidemic agents.[136]

Clinically two lesions resemble the hard exudate. They are drusen (colloid) bodies and chorioretinitis.

DRUSEN (COLLOID) BODIES

Clinical Findings

The drusen bodies appear as small, round, yellow lesions posterior to the retinal vessels (Plate 86). Although usually discrete, they may coalesce and appear as a confluent mass larger than the optic disc. As a rule the lesions are observed in older individuals who have no other significant funduscopic changes. In the absence of other retinal changes, drusen bodies are readily distinguished from the hard exudate; on the other hand, when associated with other retinopathies it is virtually impossible to make that distinction clinically. Vision may be seriously affected when drusen bodies invade the macula.

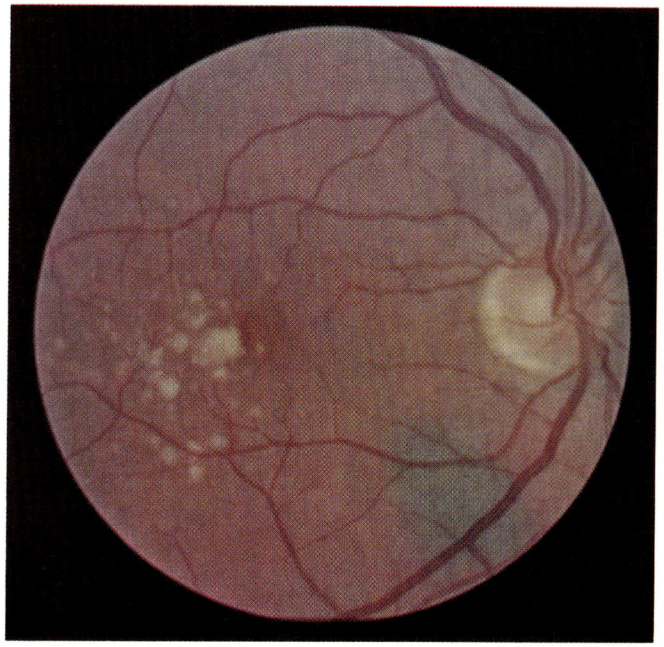

Plate 86. Temporal. Drusen bodies. Observe the well–defined lesions behind retinal vessels in the macular area. Note the absence of arteriolar, venous disease, and extravascular lesions other than the drusen bodies. The dark, pigmented area temporal and inferior to the disc is a choroidal nevus.

Drawing 87. Plate 87 (db, drusen bodies; bm, Bruch's membrane; ch, choroid; on, outer nuclear layer of retina).

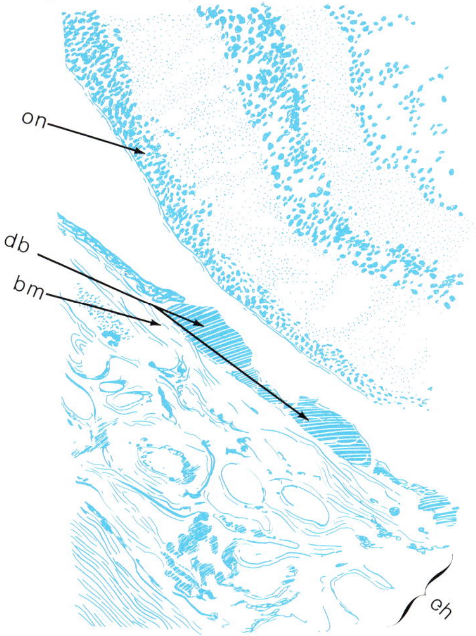

Plate 87. Note dome–shaped excrescences extending anteriorly from Bruch's membrane. The lesions are purple–red. They disrupt the pigment cell layer of the retina (PAS, × 80).

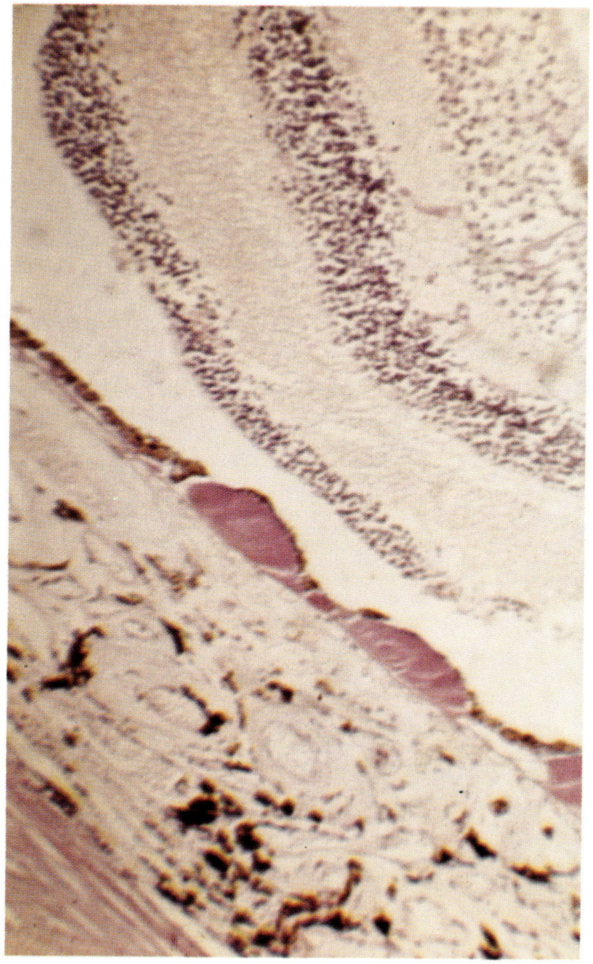

Pathology

Microscopically, the drusen bodies are dome–shaped excrescences which project anteriorly from Bruch's membrane and displace or elevate the pigment cells of the retina (Plate 87 and Drawing 87). Histochemically, they are eosinophilic with hemotoxylin and eosin. They are purple–red with the periodic acid–Schiff stain; they are often sudanophilic, and may become calcified. In a recent study, Farkas *et al.*[137] have identified two substances in the drusen bodies. The first of these, a PAS positive substance, was determined to be sialomucin, a mucopolysaccharide. The other component was identified as cerebroside, a lipid.

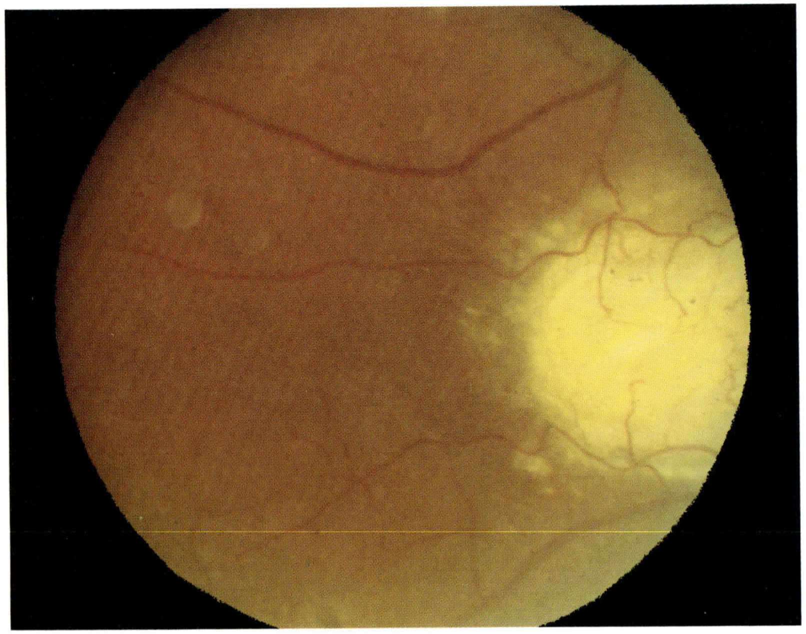

Plates 88 and 89. Note white oval lesions behind retinal vessels. Some either contain or are surrounded by clumps of brown–black pigment. In Plate 89, the striate lesions resemble part of a macular star. It is difficult to be certain that they are not hard exudates.

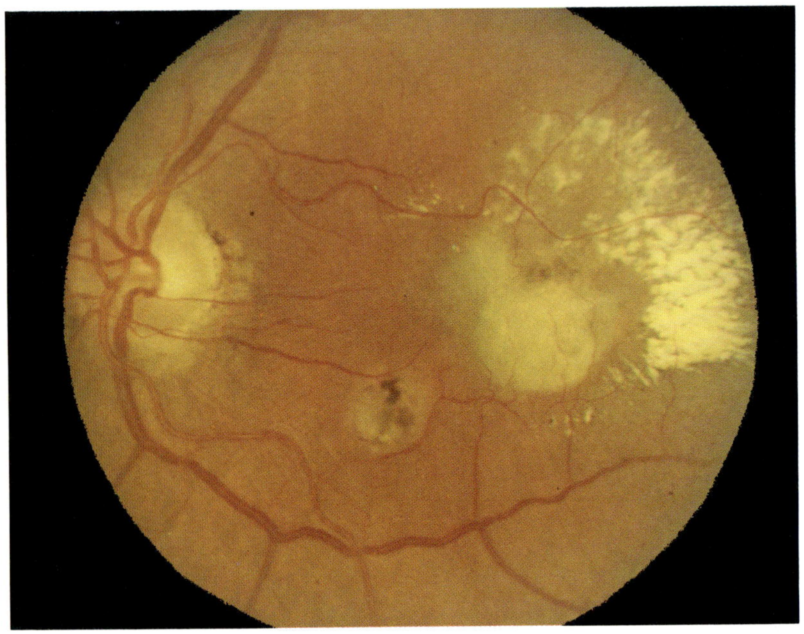

Drawing 89. Plate 89 (CHR, chorioretinitis; PD, pigment deposit).

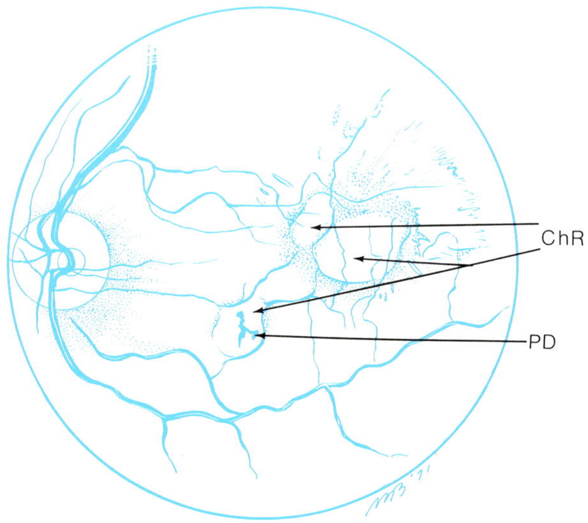

Pathogenesis

Although the pathogenesis of drusen bodies is not clear, there is evidence which suggests that they are the by–products of degeneration of the pigment cells of the retina.[138]

Clinical States and Drusen Bodies of Bruch's Membrane

Although drusen bodies are generally observed in elderly patients, a less common, dominantly inherited form which begins in childhood is also described.[139] Colloid bodies are observed in pseudoxanthoma elasticum.[140]

CHORIORETINITIS

Clinical Findings

Early in the course of chorioretinitis the funduscopic examination discloses one or more yellow or white oval lesions, at times with frayed borders, situated posterior to the retinal vessels (Plate 88). Over a period of several months the lesions become more sharply outlined and are accompanied by pigmentary changes. Generally, the end result is a sharply circumscribed oval, white lesion surrounded by or invaded with brown–black pigment and situated behind the retinal blood vessels (Plate 89 and Drawing 89). Occasionally choroidal vessels are visible within the lesion.

In contrast to the hard exudate, the lesion of chorioretinitis is not primarily associated with arteriolar disease, cotton wool patches, hemorrhage, or microaneurysms. In addition, the pigmentary changes which are characteristic of chorioretinitis do not occur with the hard exudate (Plate 90).

Visual disturbances occur when the disease is extensive, particularly when the macula is involved.

Plate 90. O.S. Central and inferior. There is a large, irregular, and deeply pigmented lesion at 6 o'clock. The upper portion is surrounded by pigment. A branch of the inferior temporal arteriole crosses over the lesion. The arterioles and venules are normal. There are no other retinal abnormalities.

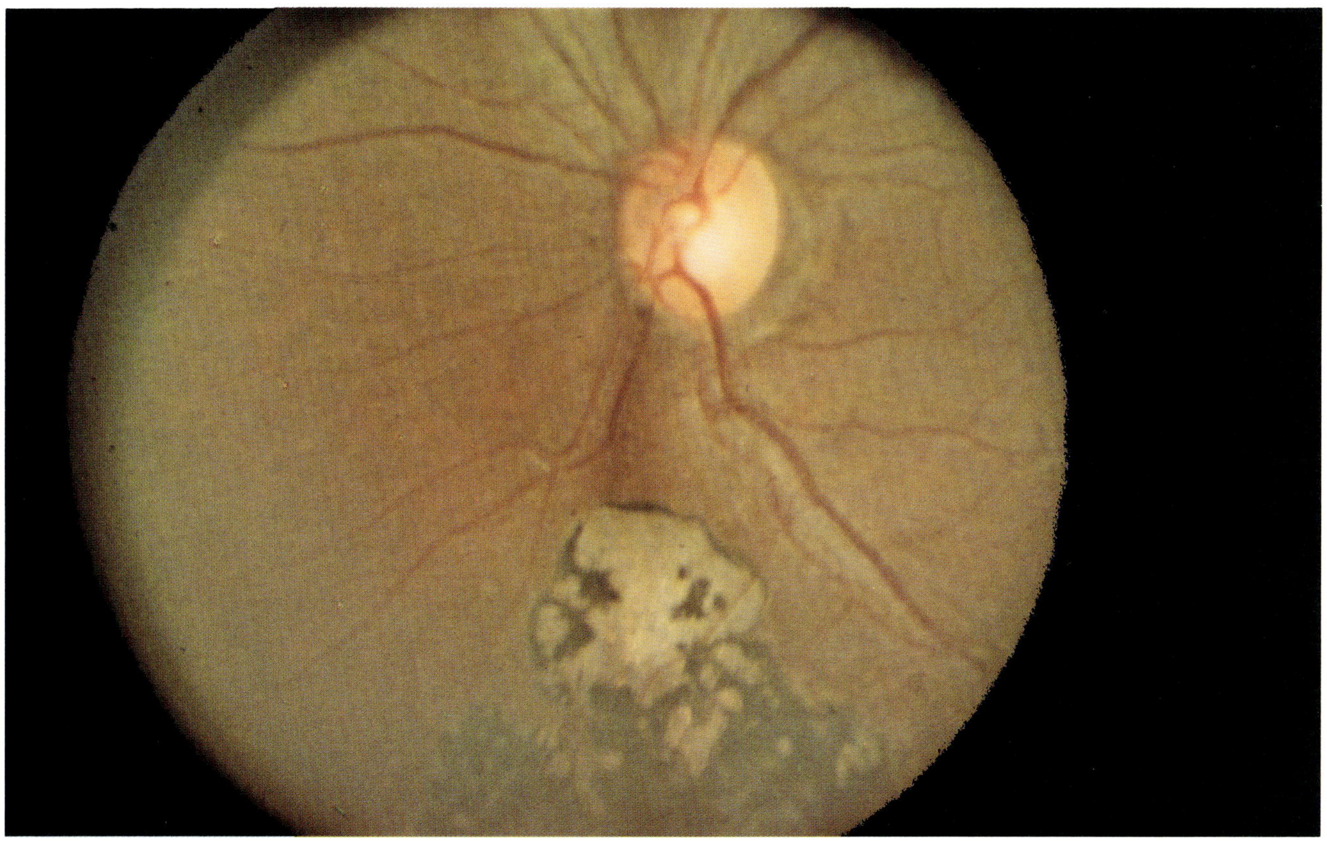

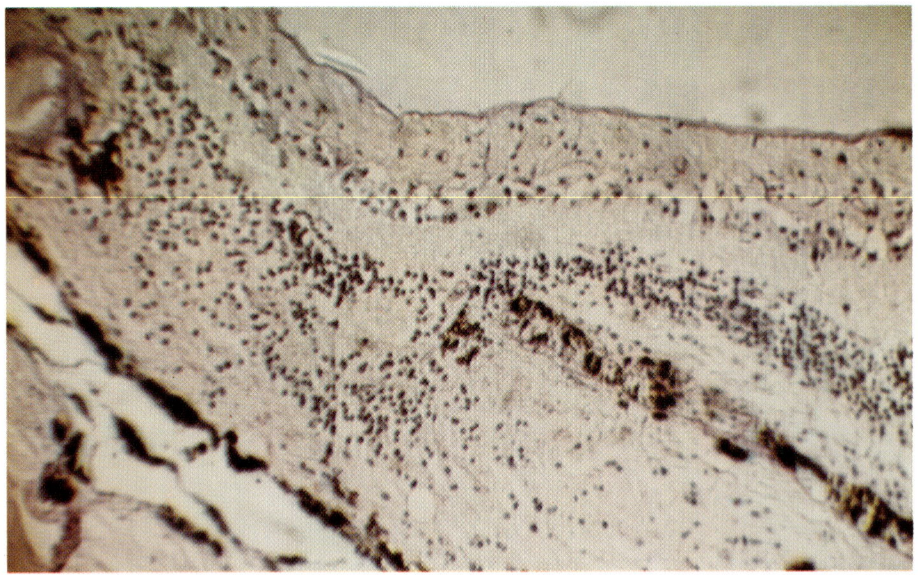

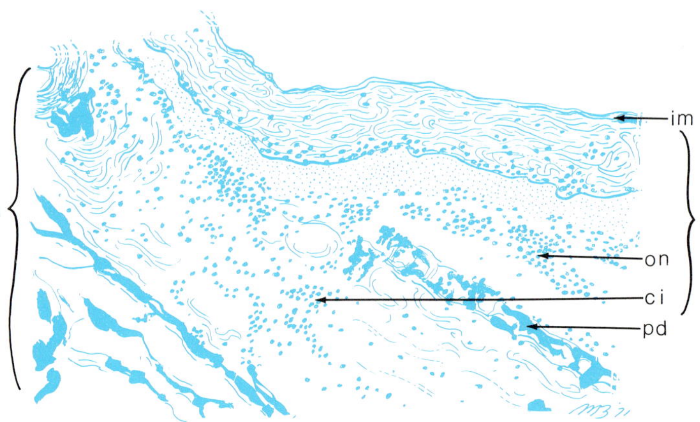

Drawing 91. Plate 91 (im, internal limiting membrane; ci, cellular infiltrate; on, outer nuclear layer; pd, pigment deposit; ch, choroid; r, retina).

Pathology

The response to inflammation, varying degrees of tissue destruction, and scar tissue formation are the typical histologic findings (Plates 91 and 92 and Drawings 91 and 92). Acutely, these consist of exudation of fluid, vascular engorgement, and cellular infiltration, chiefly of mononuclear cells. In some instances, granulomata form. Obliteration of choroidal vessels follows cellular infiltration in and about these structures. Pigment cells are distorted, displaced, and tend to clump about the inflammatory lesion. Ultimately scar tissue forms and the retina and choroid become adherent in the involved area. Masses of fibrous tissue and clumps of melanin replace the normal structures of both of those layers of the eye.

Pathogenesis and Clinical Disease States

Chorioretinitis may follow accidental or surgical trauma to the eye with resulting invasion of pyogenic organisms. Granulomatous lesions may develop in tuberculosis, syphilis, toxoplasmosis, histoplasmosis, a large number of other fungal and parasitic infestations, inclusion body virus disease, brucellosis, and sarcoidosis.[2 (pp. 391-402)] Measles, chickenpox, and smallpox are other offenders.[4 (p. 555)]

Plates 91 and 92. Note adherence of retina and choroid, infiltration of inflammatory cells, and scar tissue formation at that site. Plate 91 (PAS, × 80). Plate 92 (PTAH, × 80).

Drawing 92. Plate 92 (f, fibrosis; ci, cellular infiltrate; r, retina; ch, choroid; pd, pigment deposit).

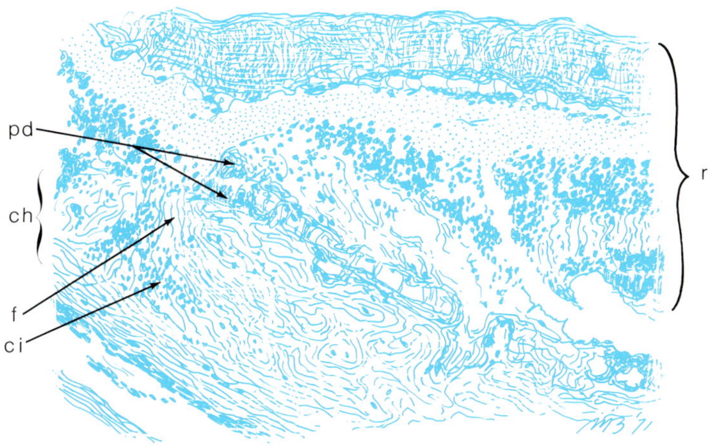

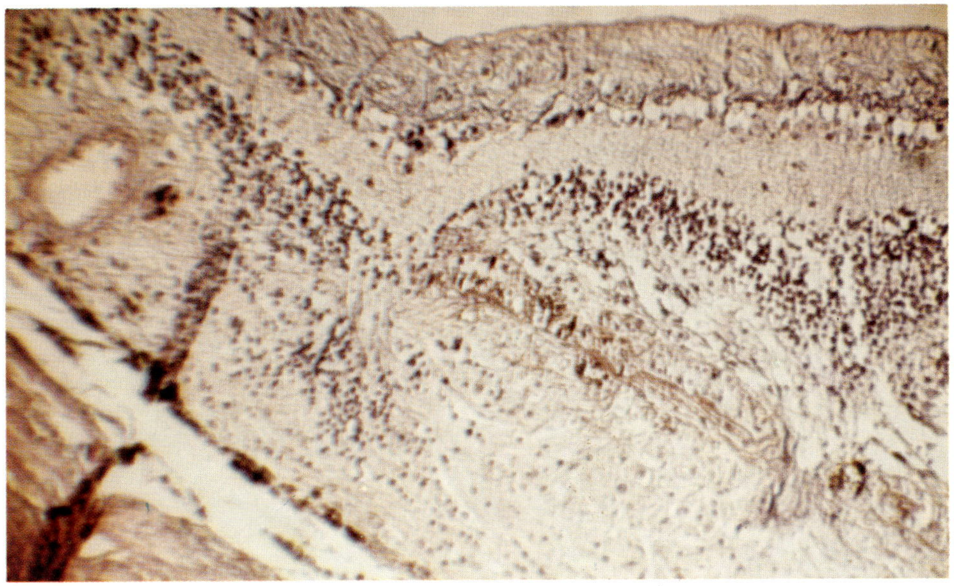

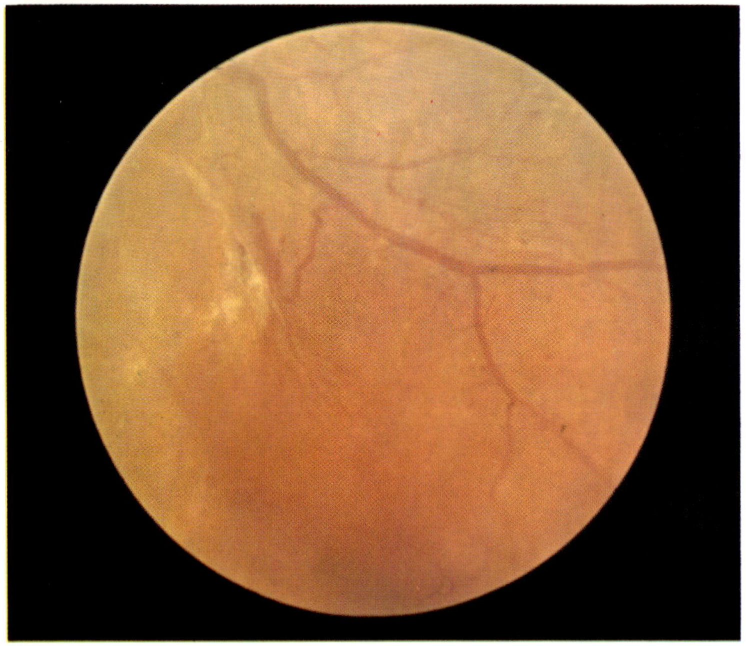

Plate 93. O.D. Inferior temporal. Hemorrhage intermingling with vitreous gel. Hemorrhage has settled inferiorly. Note brown–black color of old blood pigment.

Plate 95. O.D. There is a large vitreous hemorrhage which extends from the inferior portion of the optic disc. Note that the retina underlying that hemorrhage is obscured. The disc is surrounded by another hemorrhage which has diffused into the vitreous gel.

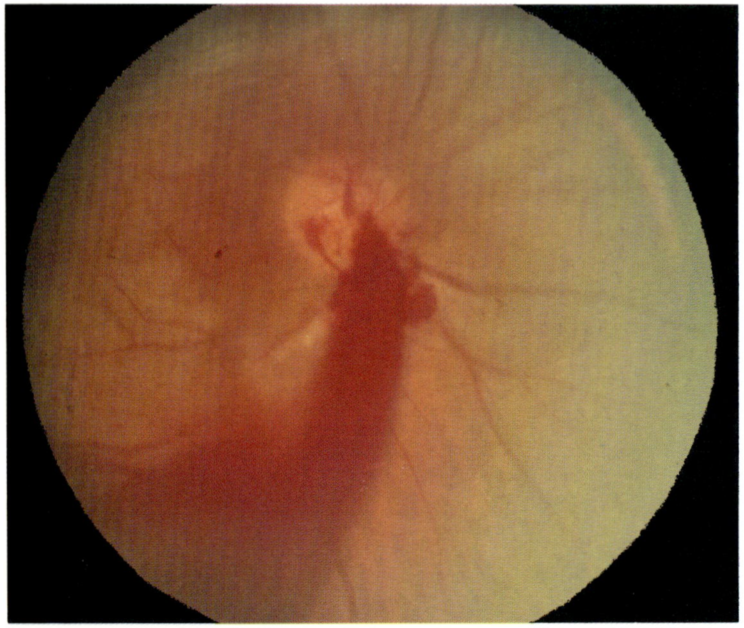

Plate 94. Magnified view of massive vitreous hemorrhage. The normal red reflex is obscured. The glistening white areas represent the fibrosis associated with proliferative retinopathy (see pp. 144–52).

HEMORRHAGE

The form and appearance of ocular hemorrhage are determined by its extent and location. This discussion will deal with three types of hemorrhage:

1. Preretinal — anterior to the retina, including vitreous and subhyaloid hemorrhage.
2. Retinal — within the retina.
3. Choroidal — posterior to the retina and within the choroid.

Preretinal Hemorrhage

VITREOUS HEMORRHAGE

The appearance of hemorrhage within the vitreous depends largely upon its extent. Since the blood tends to disperse within the vitreous gel, it generally does not assume a specific form and with time it tends to settle in the inferior part of that cavity (Plate 93). Over a period of weeks the blood pigment alters and assumes a brown or black color (Plate 93).

When vitreous hemorrhage is massive, it may completely obliterate the normal orange–red fundal reflex (Plate 94). With less blood present, all or part of the vitreous becomes hazy, thus obscuring portions of the retina behind it (Plate 95).

Some vitreous hemorrhages remain as intact masses which displace rather than mix with its gel. As a result, the borders of the hemorrhage are sharply defined (Plates 96 and 97 and Drawing 96).

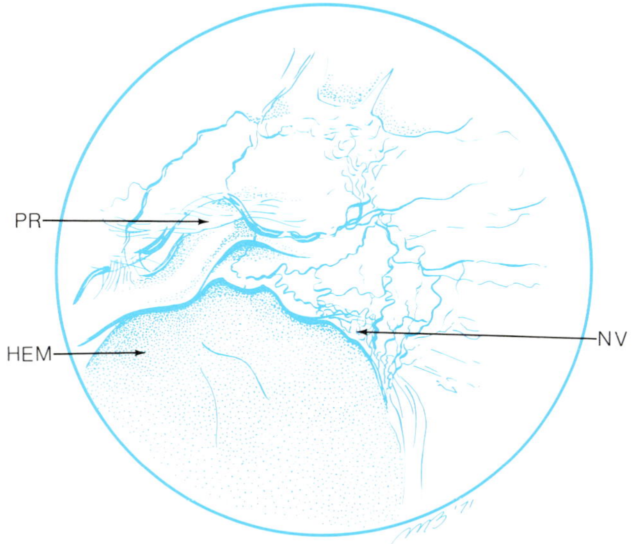

Drawing 96. Plate 96 (HEM, hemorrhage; NV, neovascularization; PR, proliferative retinopathy).

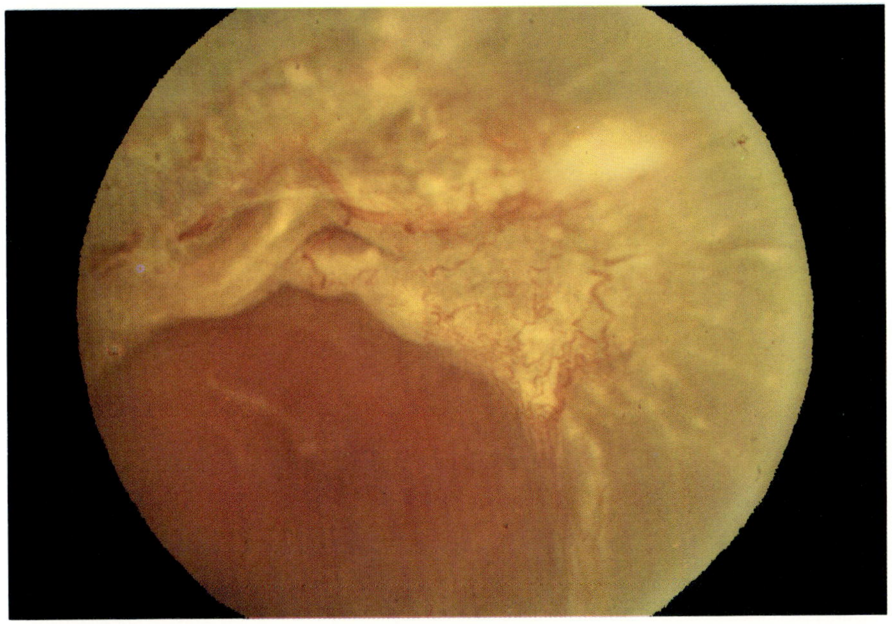

Plate 96. Sharply outlined hemorrhage which displaces vitreous (in patient with proliferative retinopathy). Note new vessel formation and scar tissue (see pp. 137–152).

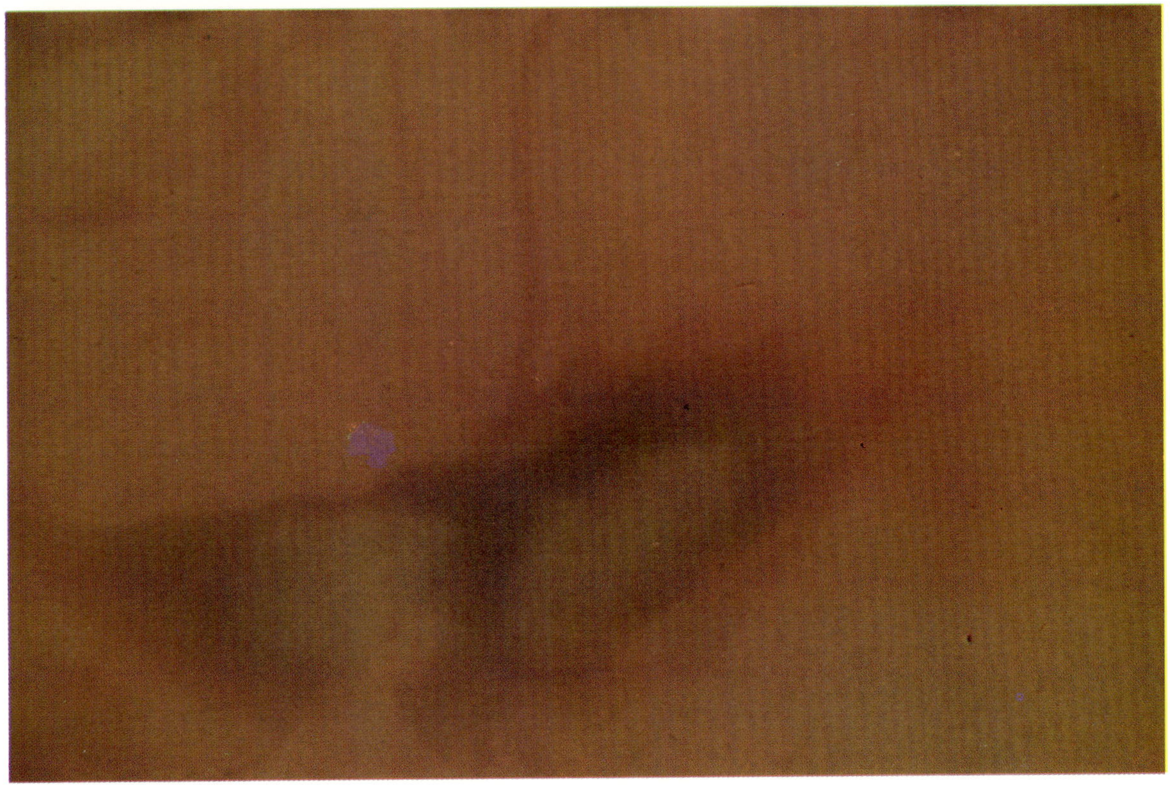

Plate 97. Sharply outlined preretinal hemorrhages, probably in vitreous.

Fate of Vitreous Hemorrhage

The rate of absorption of vitreous hemorrhage is unpredictable. In the majority of patients with no associated ocular disease, the hemorrhage may be absorbed rapidly with little or no lasting damage.[141, 142] With extensive vitreous hemorrhage and/or in the presence of intraocular disease a fibroblastic response may be followed by the development

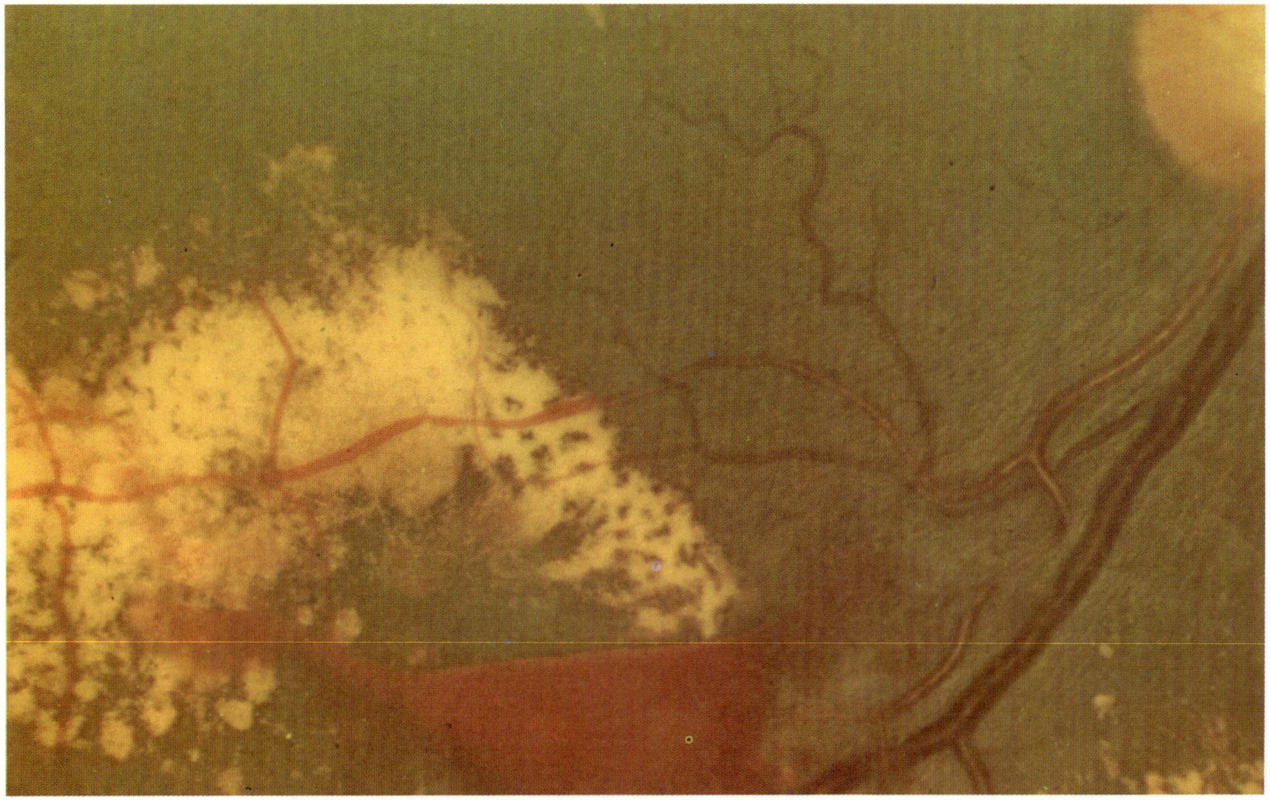

Plate 98. Subhyaloid hemorrhage, crescent–shaped, situated anterior to the retinal vessels. A conglomerate mass of hard exudates is also present.

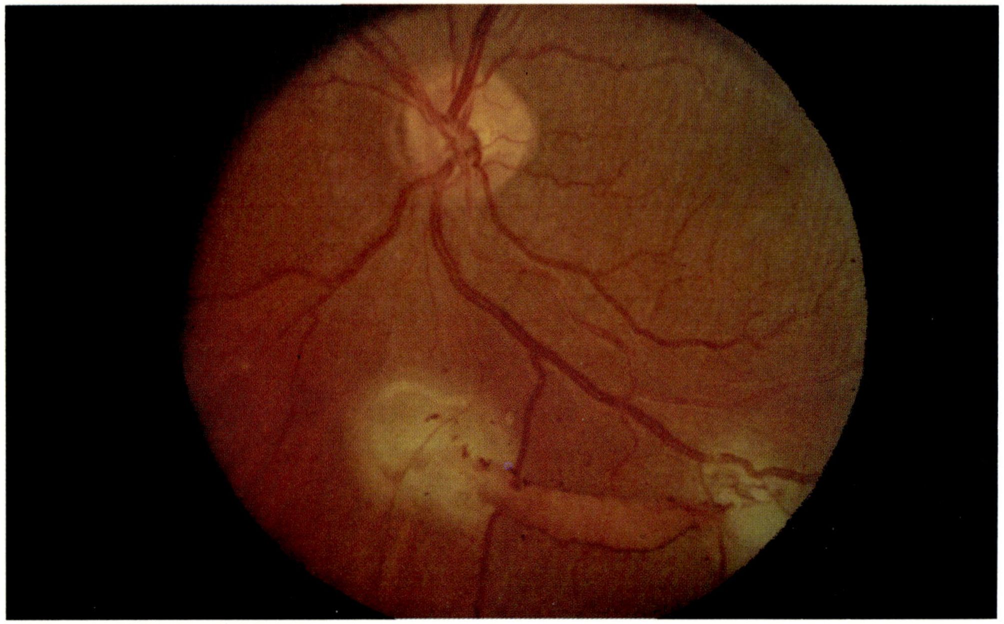

Plate 99. O.S. Inferior central. A crescent–shaped hemorrhage with a straight upper border overlies blood vessels. The hemorrhage was initially observed 1 month before the photograph was taken. Note the two white areas in the region of the hemorrhage. These represent the changes that develop several days after retinal photocoagulation. New vessel formation is present in each of the white patches (see pp. 144–145).

of proliferative retinopathy[143] (see p. 83) and retinal detachment.[143] Ocular hemosiderosis is another serious complication of vitreous hemorrhage.[141, 143] Iron deposits may reach the anterior chamber, produce a fibrotic response, and impede the flow of aqueous humor with glaucoma as the end result.[141, 143].

Pathogenesis and Disease States

Hemorrhage in the vitreous may arise from vessels in the ciliary body, from the newly formed vessels (neovascularization) of proliferative retinopathy (see pp.137–145), or from retinal hemorrhage which breaks through the internal limiting membrane. It may follow trauma, cataract extraction, or a variety of diseases including diabetes mellitus, thrombosis of the central retinal vein, and Eale's disease (retinal vasculitis associated with neovascularization, microaneurysm formation, and retinal hemorrhage).

SUBHYALOID HEMORRHAGE

This form of preretinal hemorrhage appears as a red, round, and sharply outlined mass anterior to the retinal vessels. As the cellular elements of the blood settle, the serum remains above and the upper border becomes a straight line (Plates 98 and 99). The lesion then has a crescentic configuration or may resemble a teardrop, particularly with the patient in the sitting or upright position. With prolonged recumbency the hemorrhage may once again appear to be round. The subhyaloid hemorrhage is believed to be located in the potential space between the coalescing vitreous fibers (hyaloid membrane) and the internal limiting membrane of the retina (Plate 100 and Drawing 100).

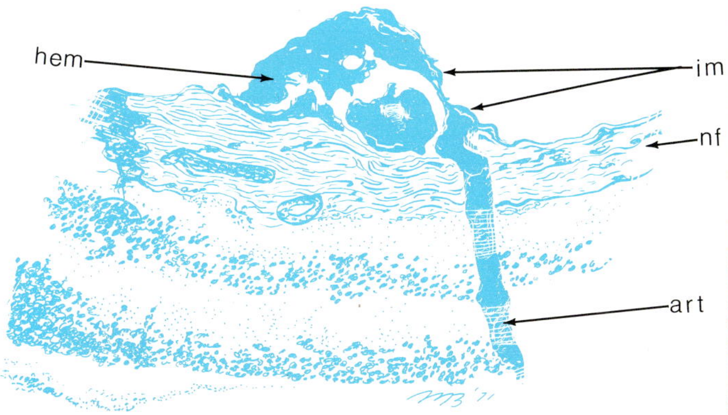

Drawing 100. Plate 100 (im, internal limiting membrane; hem, hemorrhage; nf, nerve fiber layer; art, artefact).

Plate 100. Microscopic section of hemorrhage in anterior part of nerve fiber layer, bound by internal limiting membrane. This hemorrhage clinically appeared to have all the characteristics of a subhyaloid one (PTAH, approx. × 80).

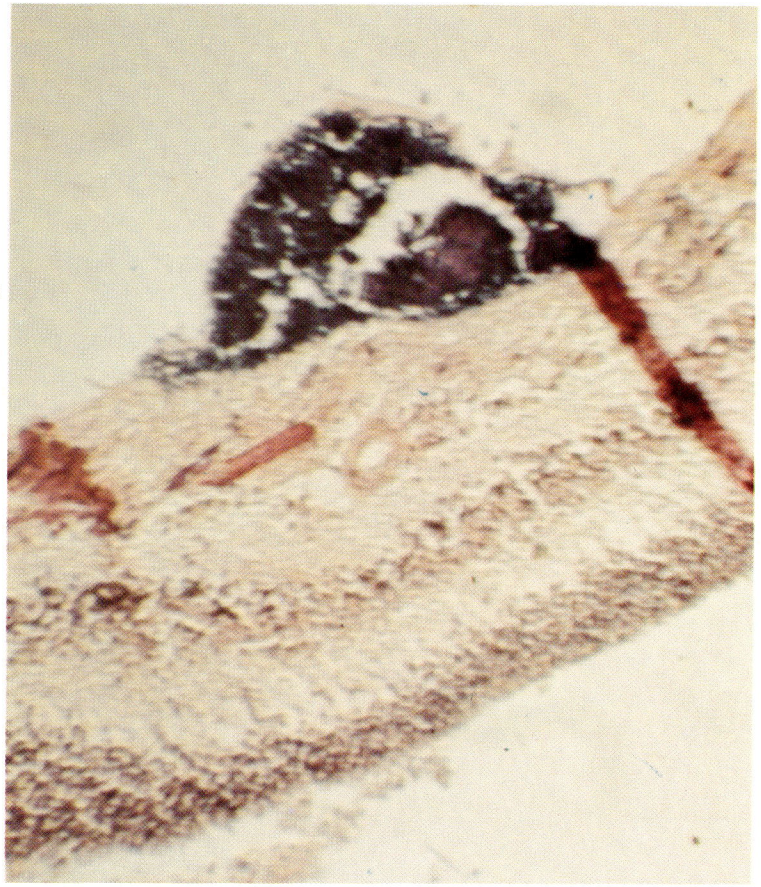

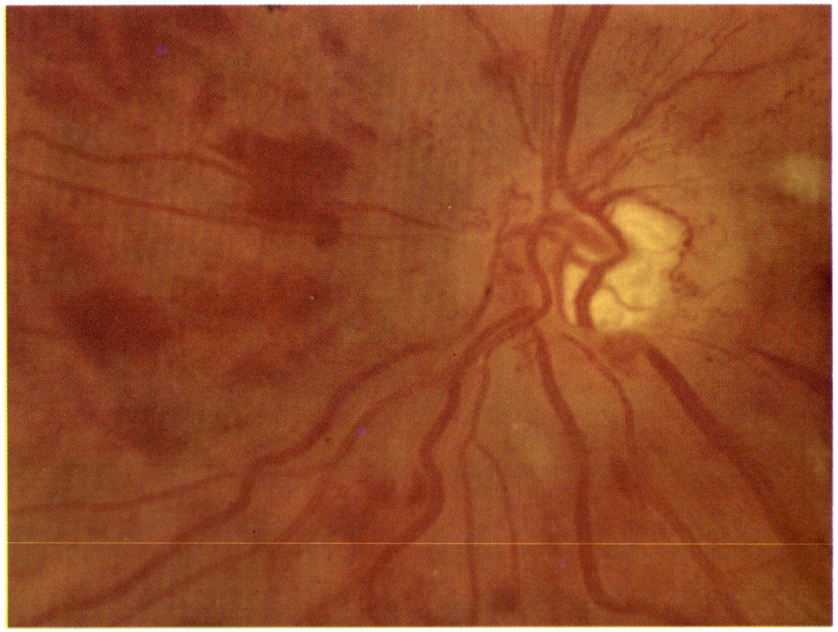

Plate 101

Plates 101 and 102. Note flame–shaped and linear hemorrhages which overlie the retinal vessels. In addition, note that hemorrhages in Plate 102 follow the normally curved nerve fibers as they approach the macula.

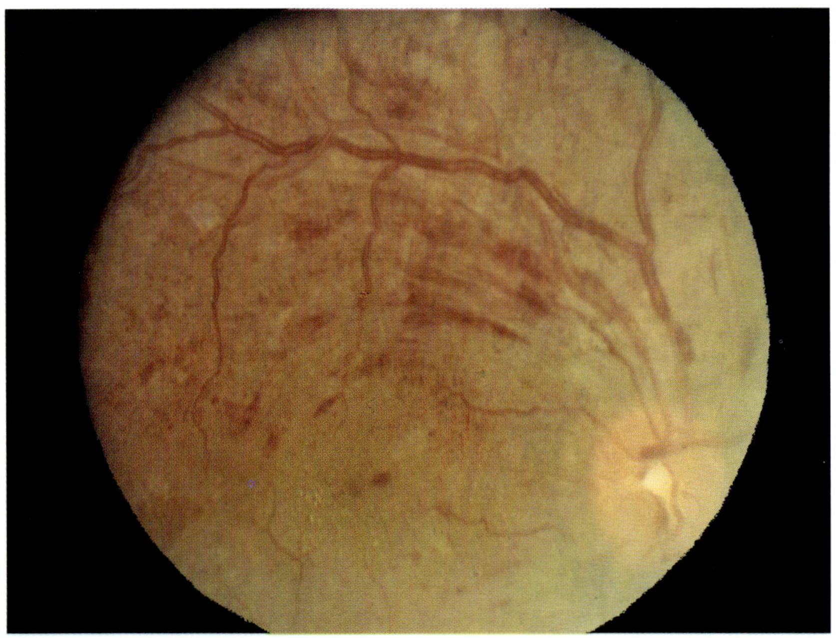

Plate 102

Fate of the Subhyaloid Hemorrhage

Subhyaloid hemorrhage may be absorbed rapidly.[4 (p. 131)] When associated with thrombocytopenia, diabetes mellitus, hypertension, and bacterial endocarditis, such hemorrhage remains unabsorbed for several months.

Pathogenesis and Disease States Associated with Subhyaloid Hemorrhage

Like the vitreous hemorrhage, this lesion follows trauma, and can be associated with retinal hemorrhage in an even greater number of systemic diseases including hypertension, diabetes mellitus, sickle cell disease, and spontaneous subarachnoid hemorrhage.

Retinal Hemorrhage

It will become apparent during this discussion that the ophthalmoscopic appearance of hemorrhage within the retina is largely determined by the architectural arrangement of that structure (see Fig. VII and pp. 6–8).

STRIATE, LINEAR, OR FLAME–SHAPED HEMORRHAGES

These hemorrhages are located in the optic nerve or the nerve fiber layer of the retina. Since the nerve fibers are horizontal in the nerve fiber layer, the shape of the hemorrhage is determined by the direction and force applied by these fibers (Plates 101 and 102). It is important, however, to recognize that as such fibers pass toward the periphery they separate from each other and form a loose network of round or polygonal spaces. Thus the peripheral nerve fiber layer hemorrhage may be round or patchy (Plate 103). Characteristically the nerve fiber layer hemorrhage overlies the retinal vessels which traverse that layer. (See Plate 104 and Drawing 104 for histology of nerve fiber layer hemorrhage.)

Plate 103. Photograph of peripheral portion of fundus. Note several irregular patchy hemorrhages. The dark brown one is probably old. Choroidal vessels are visible.

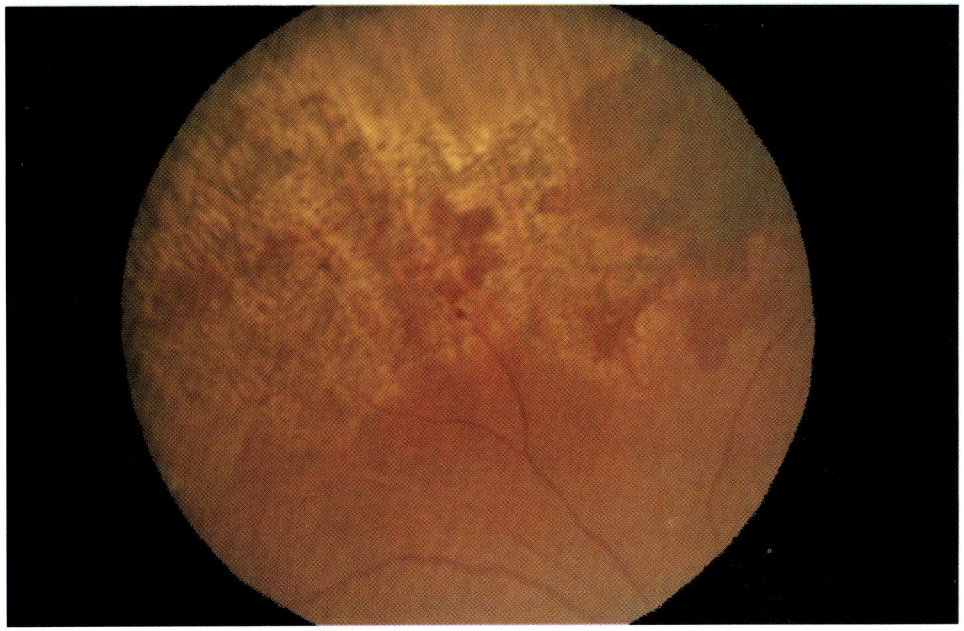

Plate 104. Note hemorrhage in the nerve fiber layer of the retina (PTAH, × 320).

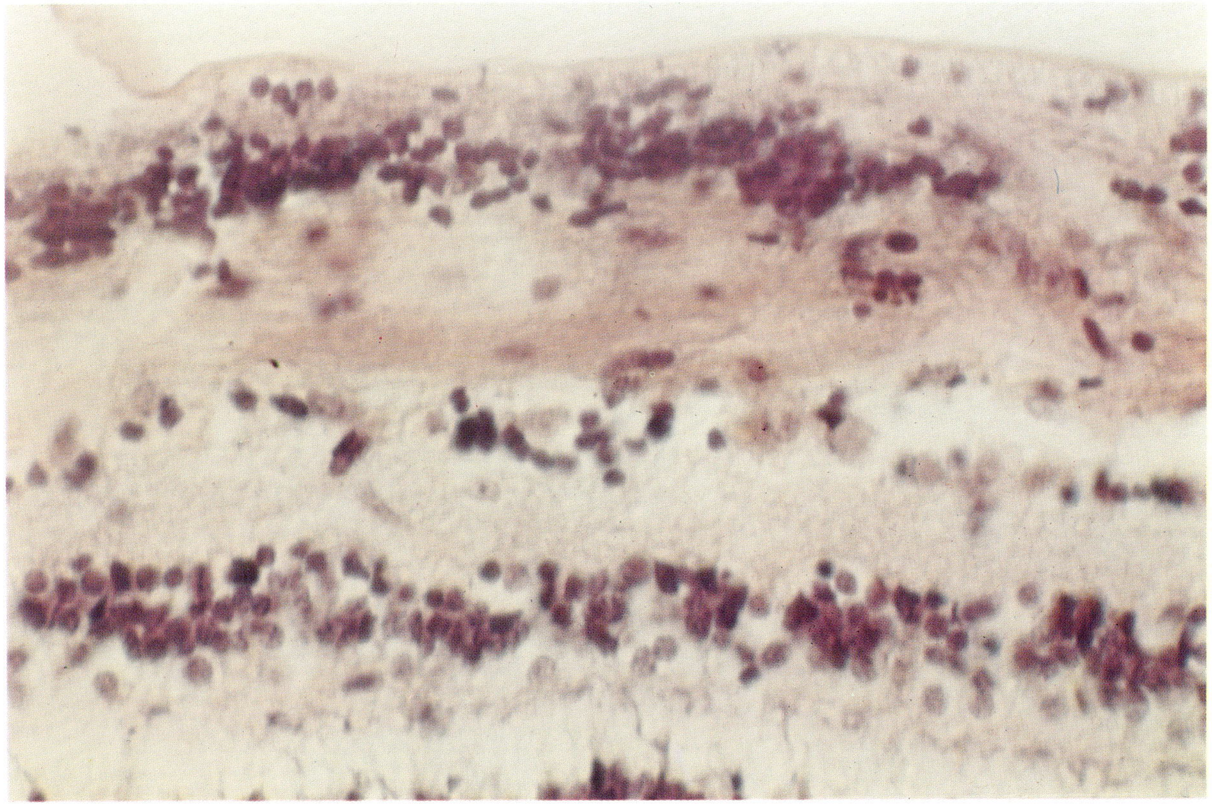

Drawing 104. Plate 104 (hem, hemorrhage; nf, nerve fiber layer).

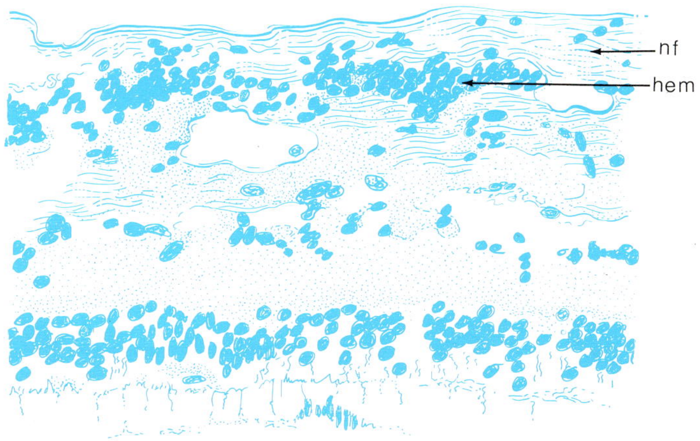

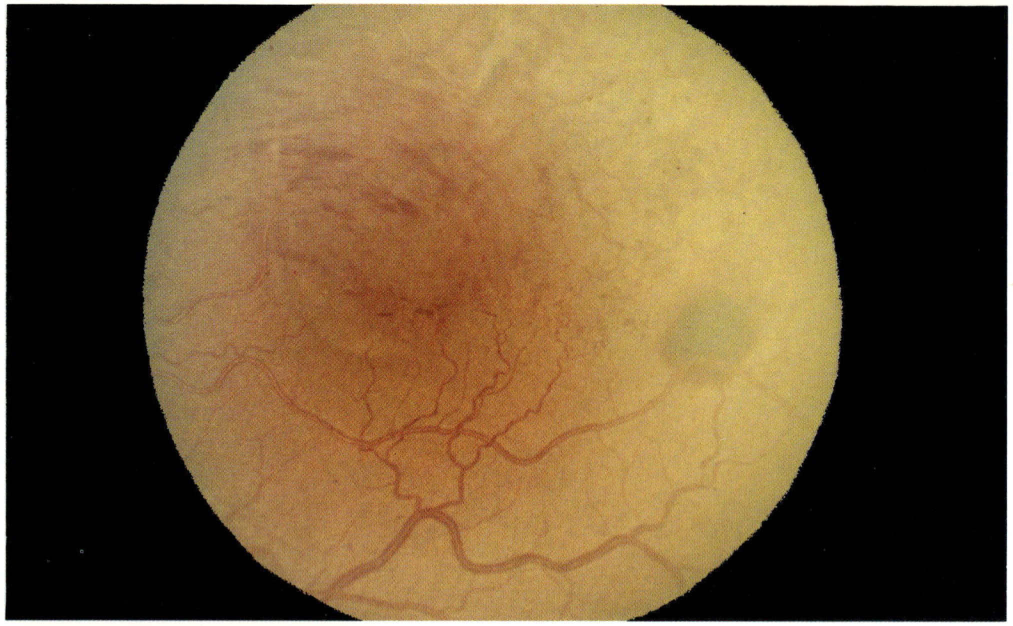

Plate 105. Round, dark brown hemorrhage crossed by arteriole. Numerous linear hemorrhages are also present.

Plate 106. Note large, round hemorrhage posterior to retinal vessels. In addition, there are linear hemorrhages superimposed upon a cotton wool patch.

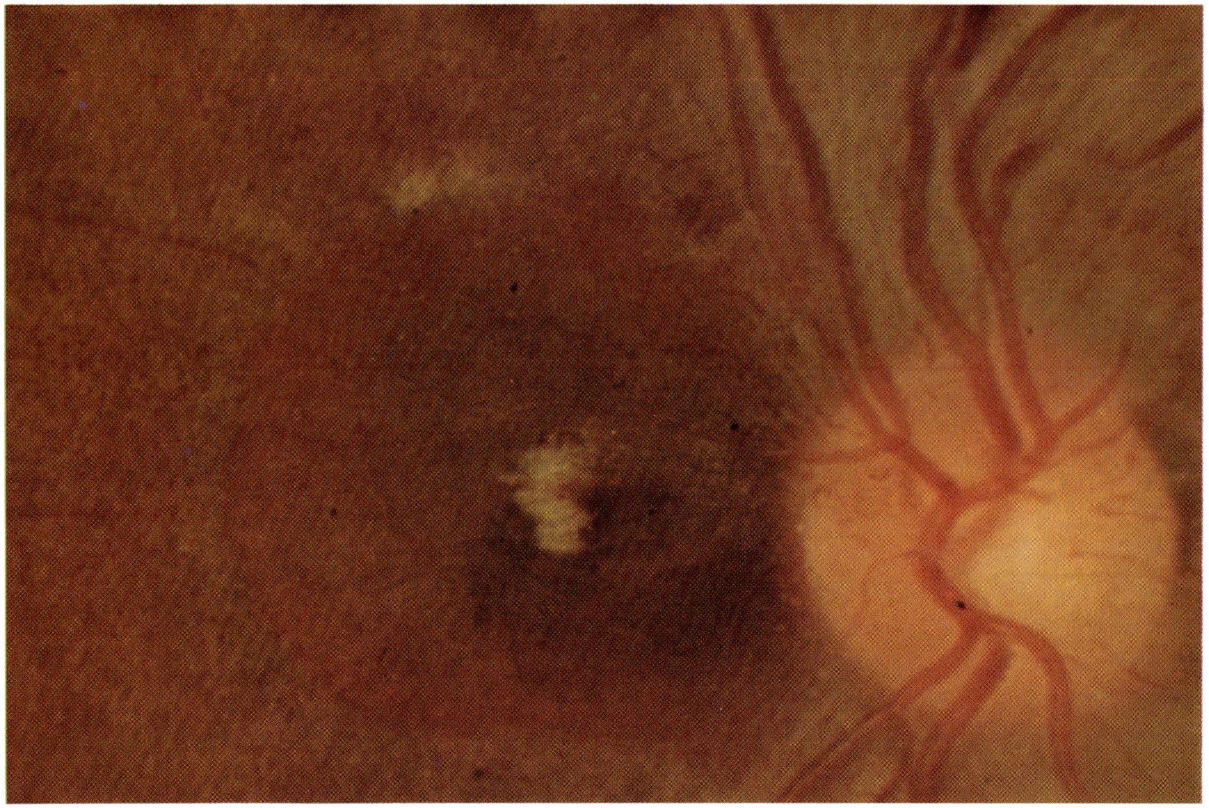

ROUND OR OVAL HEMORRHAGES

These hemorrhages (Plates 105 and 106) are generally situated in the outer plexiform layer. Nerve fibers in that area are arranged in a vertical pattern (see Fig. VII and pp. 6–8). As a result, blood partially confined by these fibers generally accumulates in the form of a cylinder. With the ophthalmoscope one sees the round or oval end of this cylindrical collection of blood. In addition, since the blood vessels end at the junction of the inner nuclear and outer plexiform layers, hemorrhage in the area last mentioned appears behind the retinal vessels. (See Plate 107 and Drawing 107 for histology of hemorrhage in the outer plexiform layer.)

In the macular region, hemorrhage in the deeper layer may assume the starlike arrangement of Henle's fibers.

Plate 107. Hemorrhage in inner nuclear and outer plexiform layers (PTAH, × 300).

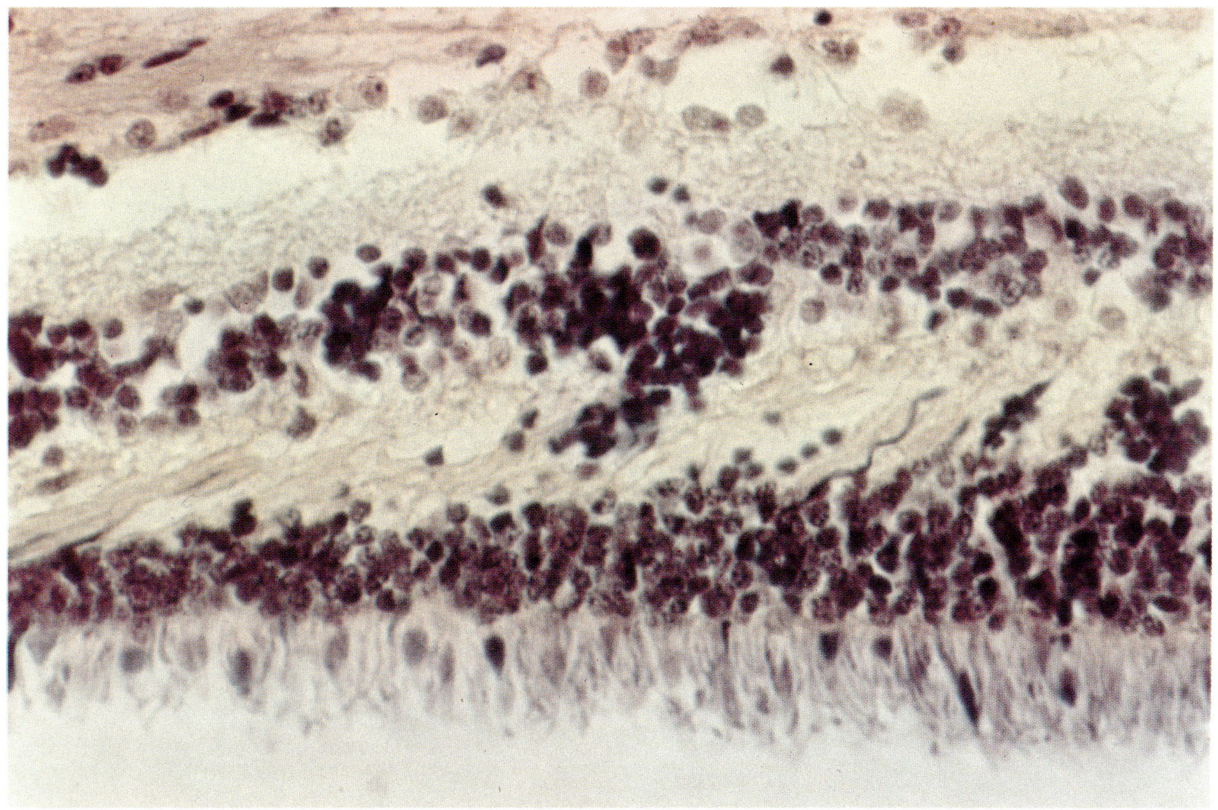

Drawing 107. Plate 107 (hem, hemorrhage; op, outer plexiform layer).

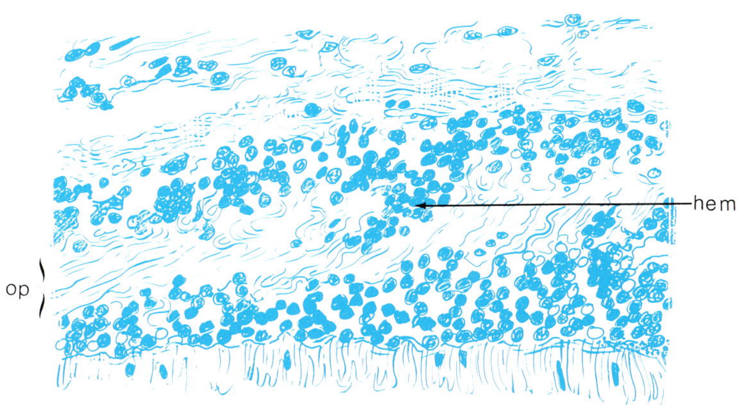

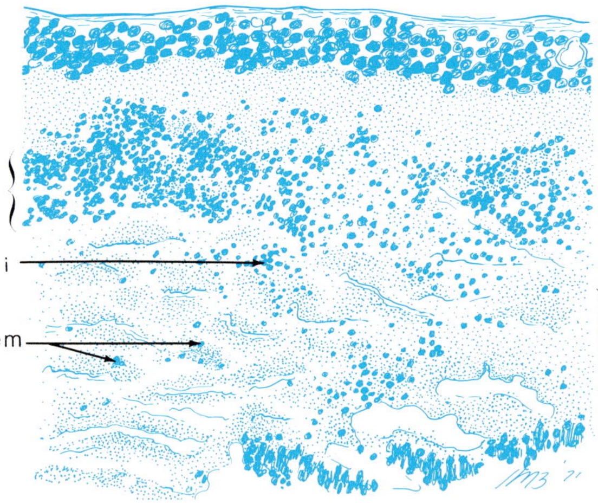

Drawing 109. Plate 109 (hem, hemorrhage; ci, cellular infiltrate; in, inner nuclear layer; op, outer plexiform layer).

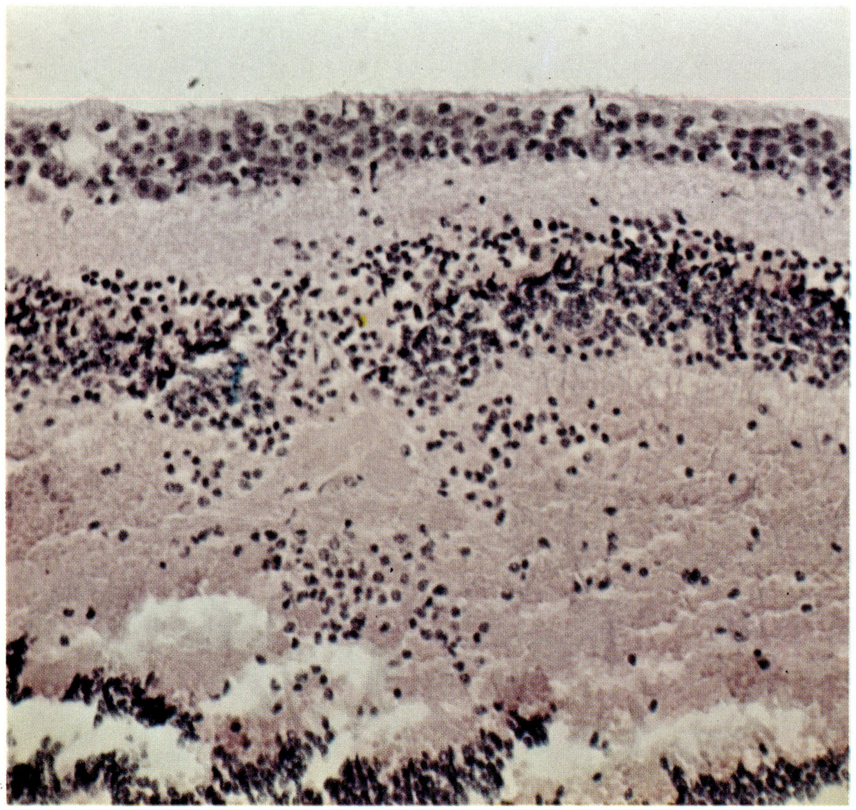

Plate 109. Accumulation of leukocytes in center of hemorrhage within inner and outer plexiform and inner nuclear layers (H&E, × 120).

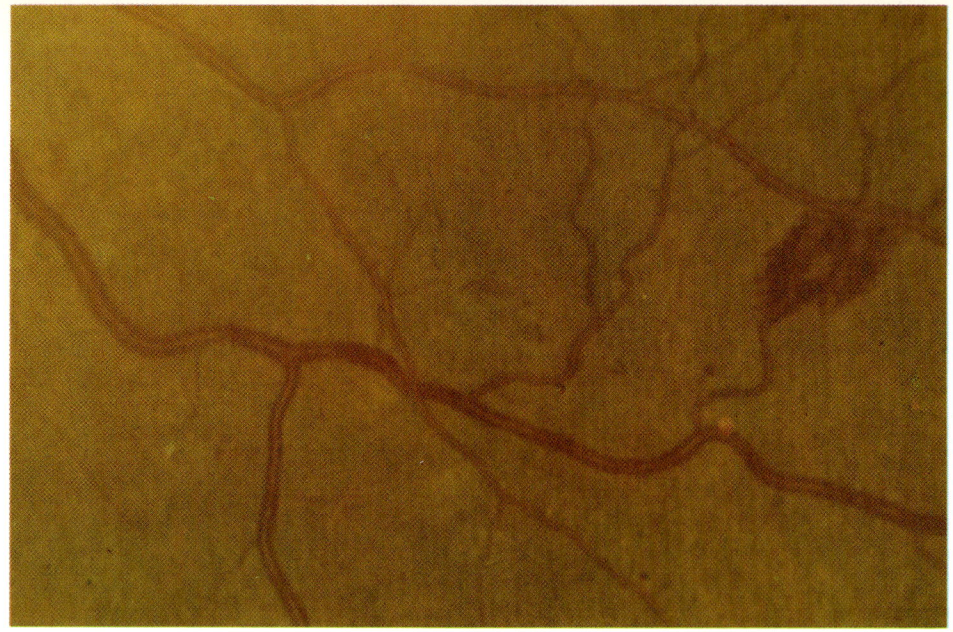

Plate 108. White–centered, flame–shaped hemorrhage (Roth spot). The borders of the hemorrhage are irregular. There are two other small linear hemorrhages. A small red dot (microaneurysm) is present below the Roth spot (see pp. 127–135 for discussion of microaneurysm).

PALE–CENTERED HEMORRHAGE (ROTH SPOT)

Either the superficial flame–shaped or the deep round hemorrhage may develop a central or eccentric white spot (Plate 108). This lesion has been identified as the Roth spot.

Pathology

The histologic counterpart of this lesion can take several forms. A central accumulation of inflammatory cells within the hemorrhage has been demonstrated[144, 145] (Plates 109–111 and Drawings 109–111). "Coagulated albuminous" material,[146] swollen degenerated nerve fibers[145] (Plate 112 and Drawing 112), and fibrin deposits[147] have also been described within the central core of the Roth spot.

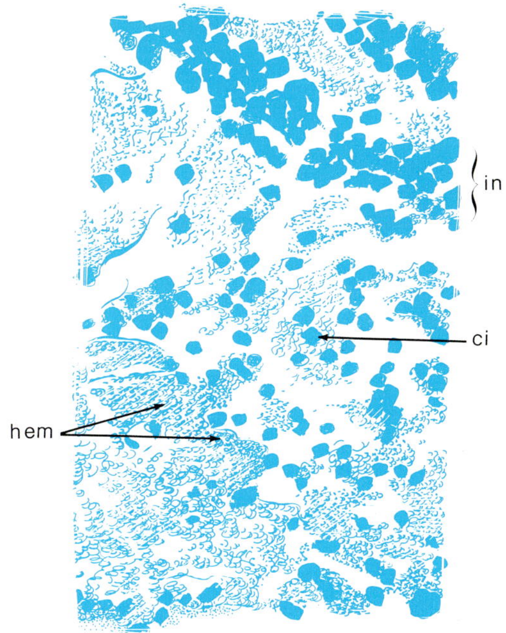

Drawing 110. Plate 110 (hem, hemorrhage; ci, cellular infiltrate; in, inner nuclear layer).

Drawing 111. Plate 111 (hem, hemorrhage; ci, cellular infiltrate; in, inner nuclear layer; on, outer nuclear layer; art, artefact).

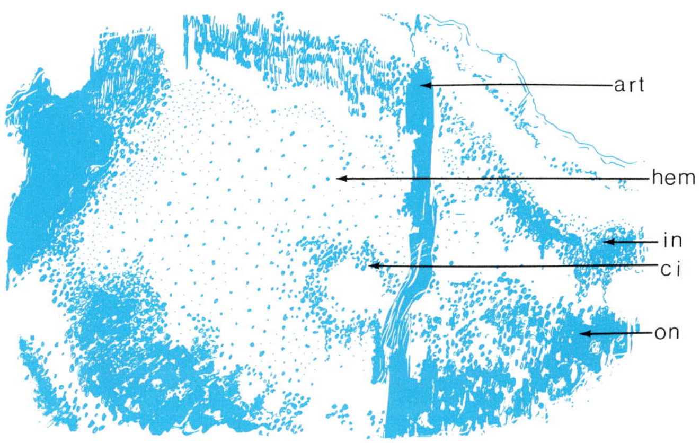

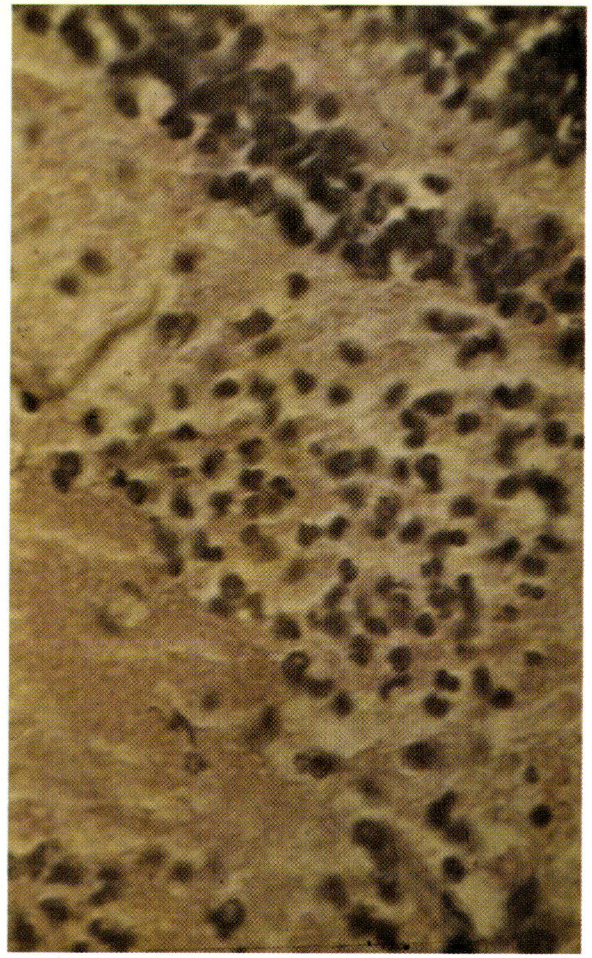

Plate 110. Higher magnification of central accumulation of leukocytes shown in Plate 109 (H&E, approx. × 300).

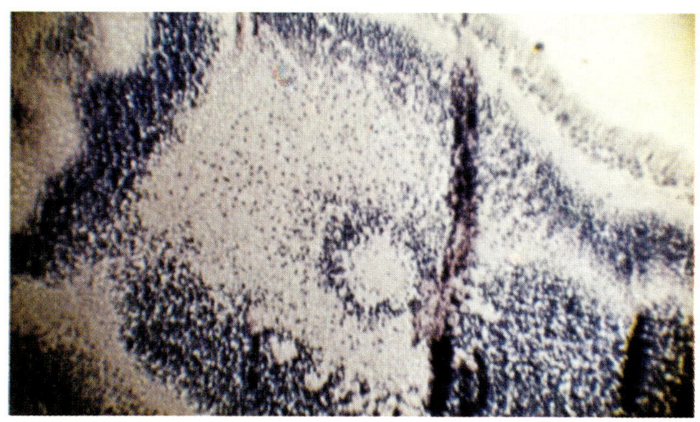

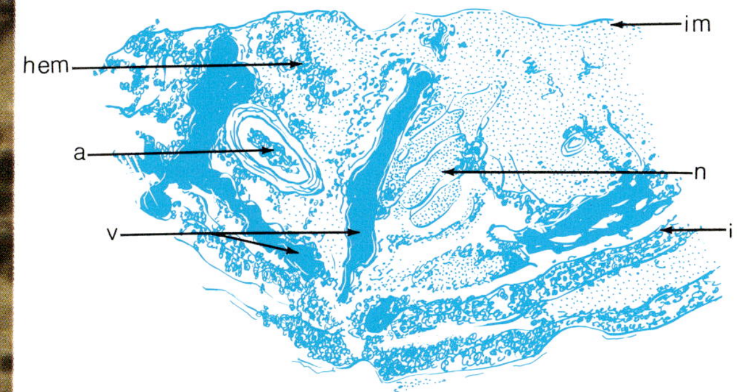

Drawing 112. Plate 112 (im, internal limiting membrane; hem, hemorrhage; a, thick–walled arteriole; n, amorphous material (probably necrotic nervous tissue); v, vein filled with red blood cells; in, inner nuclear layer).

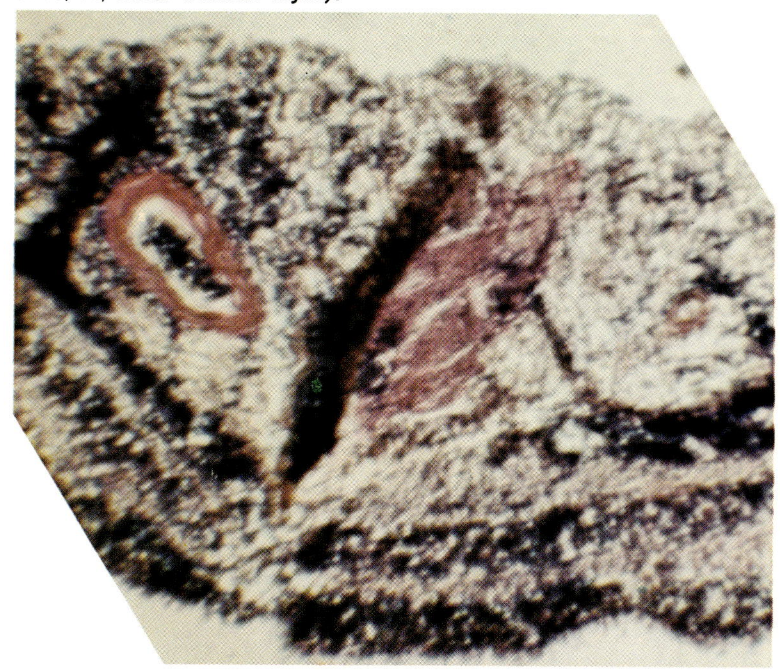

Plate 112. Central area of necrotic nervous tissue of retina surrounded by hemorrhage (PTAH, approx. × 80).

Plate 111. Central area of hemorrhage and cellular debris, surrounded by a ring of inflammatory cells. The latter, in turn, are enveloped by massive hemorrhage (H&E, approx. × 80).

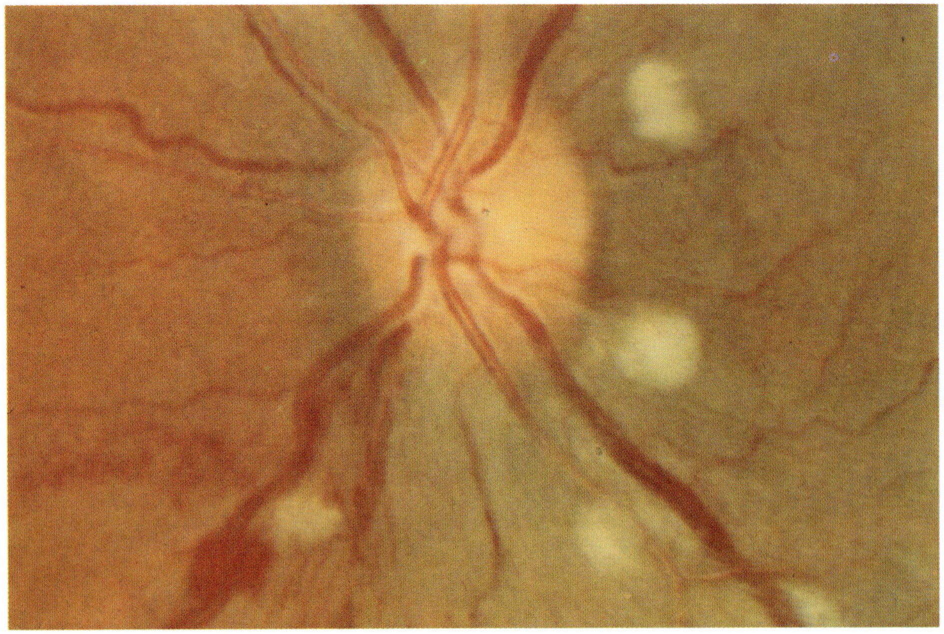

Resolution of hemorrhage in a patient with malignant hypertension.

Plate 113. Magnified view. Note several flame–shaped and irregular hemorrhages at 7 o'clock below the disc. Did you notice the cotton wool patches and "copper wire" arterioles?

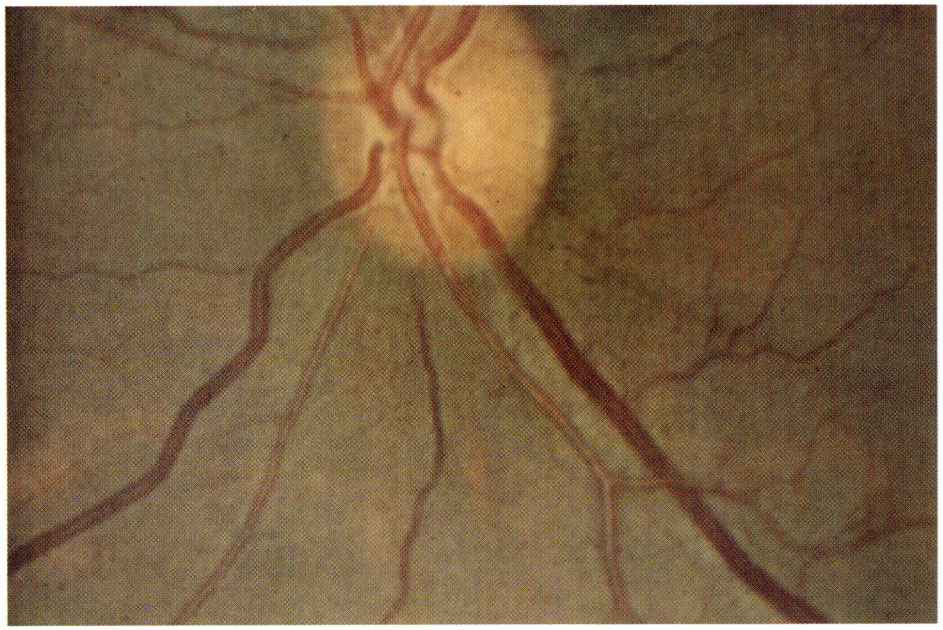

Plate 114. Same patient 1 year later. Note resolution of hemorrhages and cotton wool patches. Background color difference is a photographic aberration.

Clinical Significance

Originally believed to be specific for bacterial endocarditis, the Roth spot has also been described in the hemorrhages associated with a variety of other abnormalities. These include hematologic disorders such as severe anemia, leukemia, and multiple myeloma. The white–centered hemorrhage is also known to occur in patients with hypertension and diabetes mellitus.

Fate of the Retinal Hemorrhage

Hemorrhage in the nerve fiber layer may regress rapidly in patients with anemia and in successfully treated accelerated hypertension (Plates 113 and 114). The rate of disappearance of the deep hemorrhage is much slower. Although deep and superficial hemorrhages may disappear and leave no clinical residua, microscopic foci of gliosis and deposited hemosiderin often remain (Plate 115 and Drawing 115).

Pathogenesis and Disease States

Retinal hemorrhage occurs in a wide variety of disease including hematologic disorders associated with severe anemia, i.e., thrombocytopenia, leukemia, multiple myeloma, malnutrition, and blood loss. Rubenstein *et al.*[132] found that retinal hemorrhages occur most commonly when severe anemia and thrombocytopenia coexist. In the same study, thrombocytopenia alone could not be associated with retinal hemorrhage. On the other hand, hemorrhage and severe anemia rarely occurred together in the absence of thrombocytopenia. In contrast, Merin and Freund[148] found a high incidence of retinal hemorrhage in patients with severe microcytic anemia associated with intestinal parasitic infestation and malnutrition.

Retinal hemorrhage occurs frequently in accelerated hypertension and diabetes mellitus. In the former, it is reasonable to postulate that both the high levels of blood pressure and the severe arteriolar and capillary disease (fibrinoid necrosis and occlusion) may be causative factors. In diabetes mellitus, the microaneurysm may be a source of bleeding (see pp. 127, 129). Chester and Banker[104] suggest that lipid vascular occlusion may produce retinal hemorrhage. It is of interest that other diseases associated with vascular occlusion such as polycythemia vera, sickle cell disease, multiple myeloma, and macroglobulinemia are also frequently associated with retinal hemorrhage.

Hemorrhage occurs as a dominant finding with both venous branch or central retinal vein occlusion, presumably related to venous

Drawing 115. Plate 115 (h, hemosiderin; a, arteriole; in, inner nuclear layer; g, gliosis).

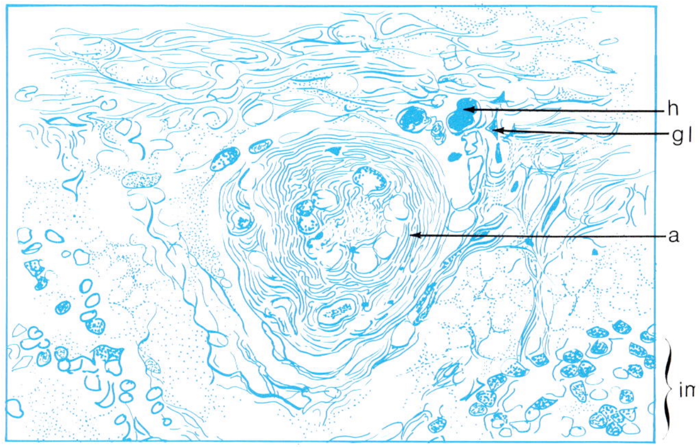

Plate 115. Microscopic section demonstrating residua of hemorrhage. Note distortion of architecture, gliosis, and hemosiderin deposits in the nerve fiber layer above the blood vessel (Turnbull blue, × 300).

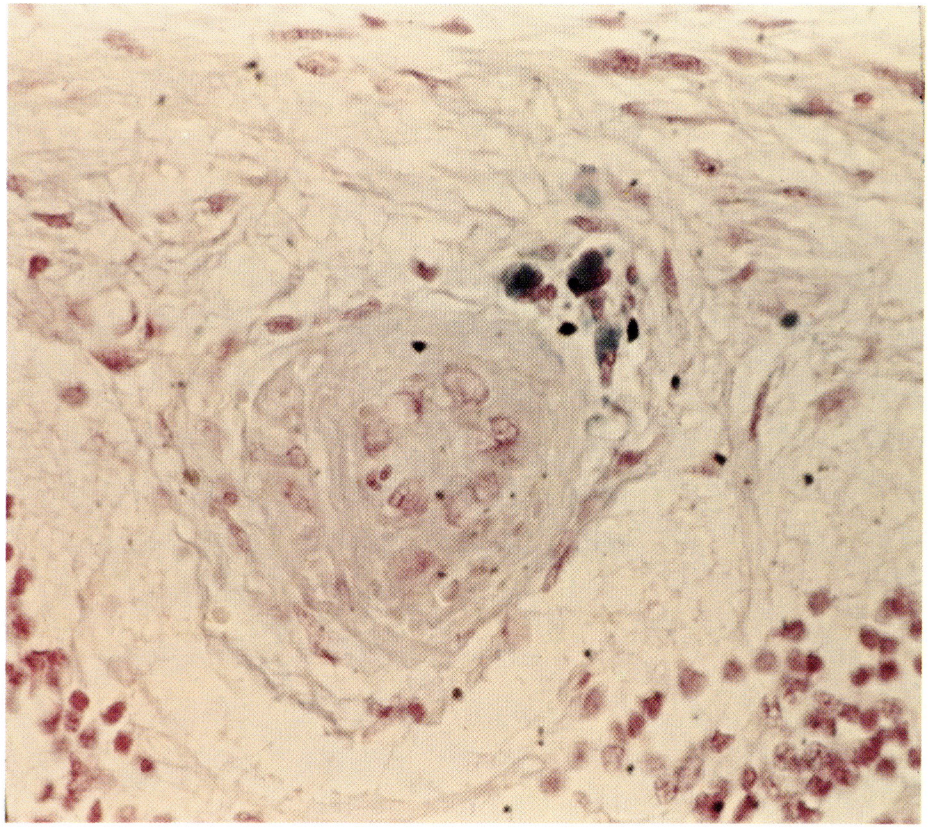

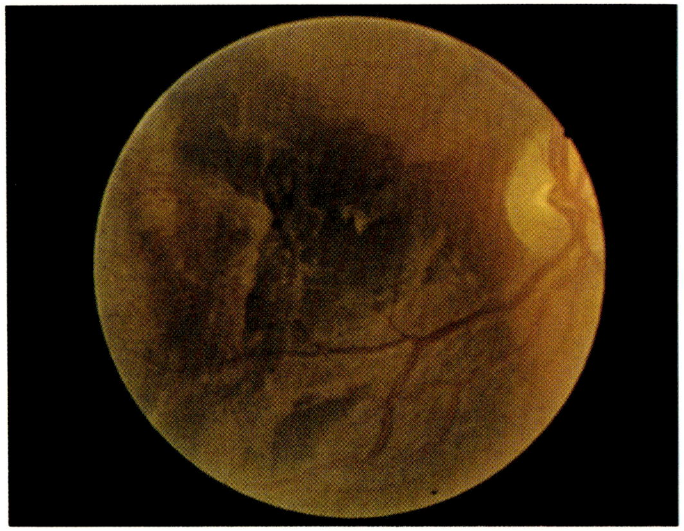

Plate 116. Note irregular red–black mass posterior to the retinal vessels (choroidal hemorrhage).

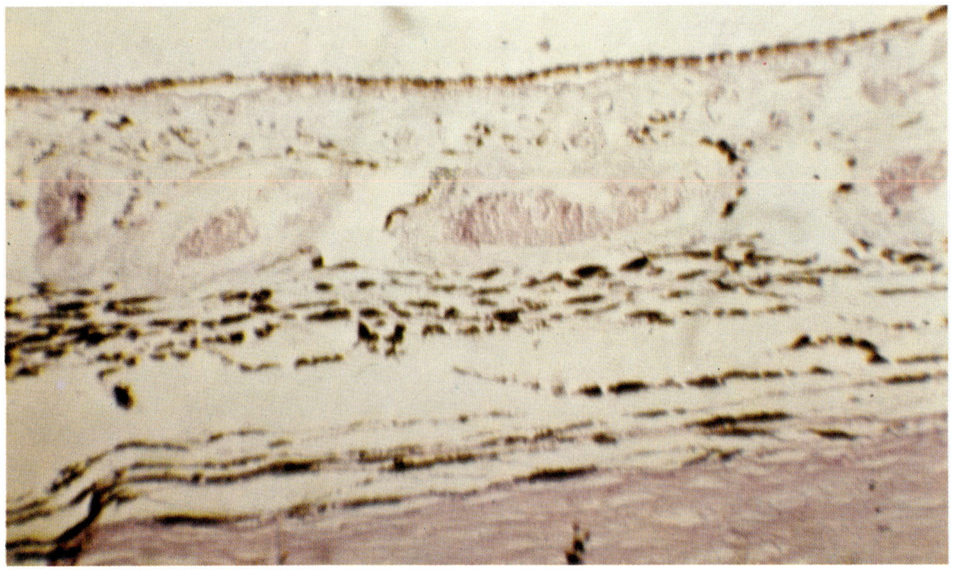

Plate 117. Normal choroid. Note pigment cell layer of retina anterior to Bruch's membrane; many blood vessels and melanin–filled cells bound inferiorly by the sclera (PAS, × 20).

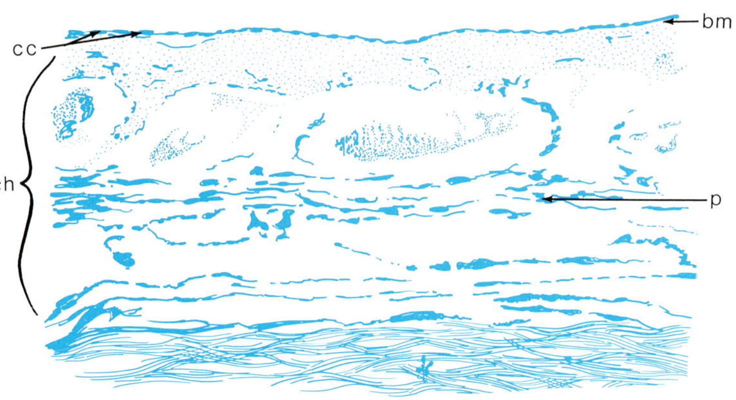

Drawing 117. Plate 117 (ch, choroid; bm, Bruch's membrane; cc, choriocapillaris; p, pigment cells).

engorgement and diapedesis of red cells through the damaged vessel walls. The impaired venous return and engorgement in papilledema may produce hemorrhage by the same mechanism.

Choroidal Hemorrhage

Hemorrhage in the choroid can be recognized by its irregular form, its gray, black, or red color, and its location behind the retinal vessels (Plate 116). Because of these characteristics, it may closely resemble a melanoma of the choroid.

PATHOLOGY

The most posterior portion of the choroid and Bruch's membrane anteriorly provide more resistance than the intervening loose connective tissue, blood vessels, and pigment cells (Plate 117 and Drawing 117). As a result, hemorrhage in the choroid disrupts the less resistant tissue and spreads laterally where it intermingles with liberated pigment and forms an irregular mass of blood and melanin. Very extensive choroidal hemorrhage may disrupt Bruch's membrane, the pigment cell layer of the retina, and the external limiting membrane.[4 (p. 585)] More massive hemorrhage may extend through the retina, markedly raise intraocular pressure, and perforate the cornea (expulsive hemorrhage).[149]

PATHOGENESIS AND DISEASE STATES

Choroidal hemorrhage may be associated with severe myopia or it may follow head and orbital trauma.[4 (p. 585)] Expulsive choroidal hemorrhage may follow cataract extraction. [4 (p. 585)] It is a rare spontaneous event in the eyes of the elderly patient known to have chronic glaucoma.[149]

ANNOTATED BIBLIOGRAPHY

The Cotton Wool Patch

Chester, E. M. and Banker, B. Q.: *The Role of Lipid Thrombi in the Pathogenesis of Diabetic Retinopathy,* Arch. Intern. Med., **120:** 397, 1967. An attempt to relate lipid occlusion of retinal arterioles and capillaries to the formation of the cytoid body.

Dollery, C. T., Henkind, P., Patterson, J. W., Ramolho, P. S., and Hill, D. W.: *Focal Retinal Ischaemia. Part I, Ophthalmoscopic and Circulatory Changes in Focal Retinal Ischaemia,* Br. J. Ophthalmol., **50:** 285, 1966. An excellent presentation of the experimentally induced cotton wool patch and its clinical course.

Friedenwald, J. S.: *A New Approach to Some Problems of Retinal Vascular Disease,* the Jackson Memorial Lecture, Amer. J. Ophthalmol., **32:** 487, 1949. A good presentation of the extravascular lesions of the retina.

Hodge, J. V. and Dollery, C. T.: *Retinal Soft Exudates. A Clinical Study by Colour and Fluorescence Photography,* Q. J. Med., **33:** 117, 1964. A good study of the clinical course of the cotton wool patch and the information gained by the use of fluorescein angiography.

Klien, B. A.: *Comments on the Cotton-Wool Lesion of the Retina,* Amer. J. Ophthalmol., **59:** 17, 1965. A good presentation of the pathogenesis of the cytoid bodies and their correlation with the cotton wool patch.

Shakib, M. and Ashton, N.: *Focal Retinal Ischaemia. Part II, Ultrastructural Changes in Focal Retinal Ischaemia,* Br. J. Ophthalmol., **50:** 325, 1966. An illuminating discussion of the histologic findings in the experimental study by Dollery *et al.*

Wolter, J. R.: *Pathology of a Cotton-Wool Spot,* Amer. J. Ophthalmol., **48:** 473, 1959. An excellent demonstration of the nature of the cytoid body.

The Hard Exudate

Ballantyne, A. J. and Michaelson, I. C.: *Textbook of the Fundus of the Eye,* 2nd ed., pp. 145–151, Williams & Wilkins, Baltimore, 1970. A good discussion of the pathogenesis of a poorly understood group of lesions.

Drusen Bodies

Ballantyne, A. J. and Michaelson, I. C.: *Textbook of the Fundus of the Eye,* 2nd ed., pp. 592–595, Williams & Wilkins, Baltimore, 1970. A concise presentation of the subject. A good picture of the clinical findings outlined on page 593.

Duke-Elder, W. S. and Dobree, J. H.: *Diseases of the Retina,* in: Duke–Elder, W. S. (ed.): *System of Ophthalmology,* Vol. X: pp. 645–652, Mosby, St. Louis, 1967. A good discussion of the colloid bodies.

Chorioretinitis

Ballantyne, A. J. and Michaelson, I. C.: *Textbook of the Fundus of the Eye,* 2nd ed., pp. 552–575, Williams & Wilkins, Baltimore, 1970. A clear and concise presentation.

Hogan, M. J. and Zimmerman, L. E. (eds.): *Ophthalmic Pathology. An Atlas and Textbook,* 2nd ed., pp. 344–468, Saunders, Philadelphia, 1962. An excellent detailed description of the uveal tract including the normal histology and the various pathological changes.

Hemorrhage

Ballantyne, A. J. and Michaelson, I. C.: *Textbook of the Fundus of the Eye,* 2nd ed., pp. 122–139, Williams & Wilkins, Baltimore, 1970. A good clinical pathological correlation of hemorrhage in the vitreous, retina, and choroid. Discussion of the pathogenesis illustrates how little is understood about the actual production of hemorrhage.

Test Plates (unlabeled retinal photographs and unlabeled retinal photomicrographs)

Questions and Answers B1–B10

Plate B1

Clinical findings: A 50–year–old male with known hypertension for 6 years and insulin–dependent diabetes mellitus for 8 years. Plate B1 — O.D. — temporal.

QUESTIONS — B1

Question 1. List abnormalities (see answer, p. 97).

Question 2. What is the histologic counterpart of the cotton wool patch?

Question 3. What is known about its pathogenesis?

Question 4. Can the concept of vascular occlusion be used to explain all cotton wool patches?

Question 5. In what diseases may one find the cotton wool patch?

PLATE B1

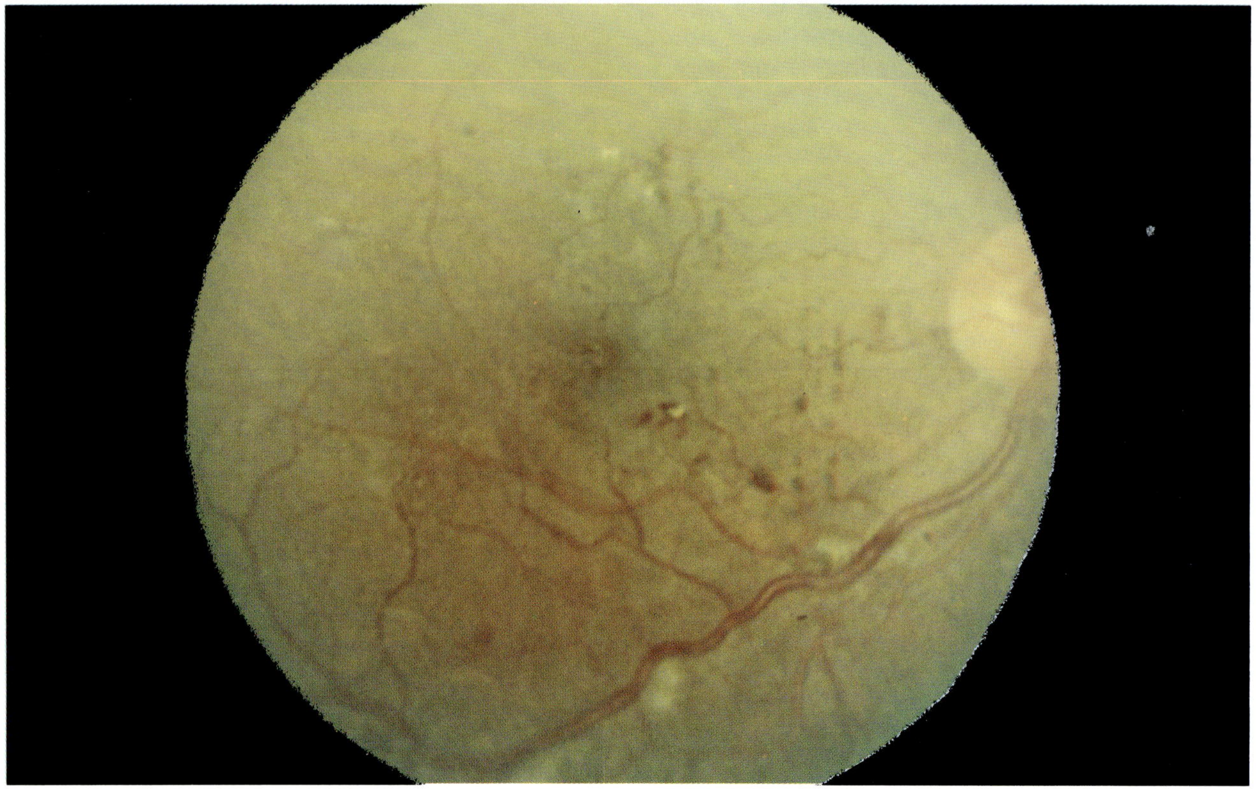

ANSWERS — B1

Answer 1. Normal disc. The right inferior temporal arteriole is tortuous and shows "copper wire" change. The corresponding venule is engorged and tortuous. Cotton wool patches are present along the course of the venule. Small, discrete, white areas of degeneration are visible at 11 o'clock, 2–4 disc diameters temporal to the disc. There are two small hemorrhages and an area of degeneration below and medial to the macula.

Answer 2. Microinfarcts of the nerve fiber layer of the retina form the cotton wool patch. The areas of infarction contain swollen and degenerated axons and the nodes of Cajal, the cytoid bodies (see p. 61).

Answer 3. Impairment of the nutrition of the ganglion cells and their axons in the nerve fiber layer appears to be major cause of the pathologic changes. The ischemic infarct is the result of either vascular occlusion of retinal arterioles and/or capillaries or carotid artery (see pp. 62–64).

Answer 4. No. There is no adequate explanation for the cotton wool patch in severe anemia.

Answer 5. See p. 66.

Reference

Ashton, N., *Pathophysiology of Retinal Cotton–Wool Spots*, Br. Med. Bull., **26:** 143, 1970.

Plate B2

Clinical findings: A 50–year–old male who has had hypertension for 13 years. Bl. P. 290/198 mmHg, BUN 100 mg./100 ml, creatinine 10.8 mg./100 ml. Adult onset diabetes mellitus which developed 1 year ago has been controlled by dietary restriction. Hct. 40%, Hb 13.6 gms/100 ml. Plate B2 — O.D. — temporal and inferior.

PLATE B2

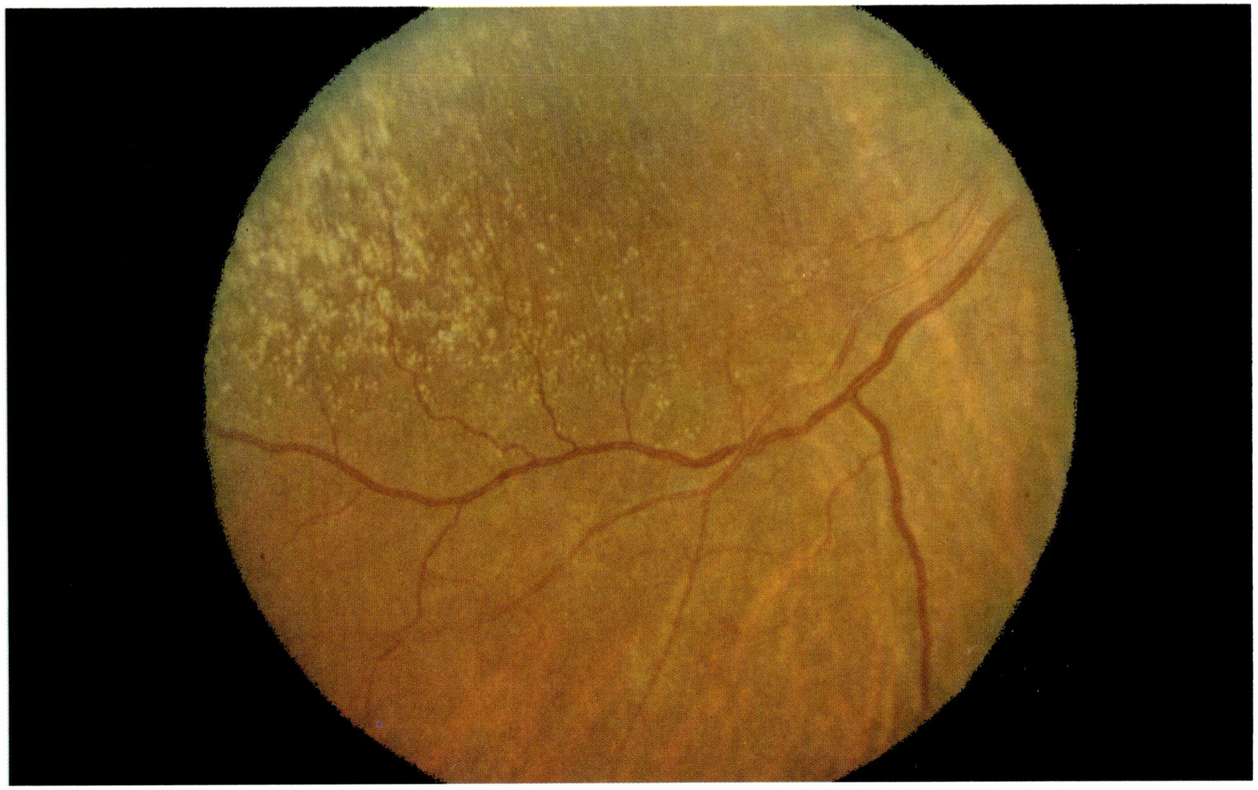

QUESTIONS — B2

Question 1. List abnormalities (see answer, p. 99).

Question 2. In what layer of the retina are the extravascular lesions noted in Plate B2 located?

Question 3. Why do blood vessels cross over the hard exudates?

Question 4. Are there usually differences in the clinical appearance of the hard exudate in hypertension and diabetes mellitus?

Question 5. In the two diseases noted above may there be histochemical differences in the outer plexiform lesions?

ANSWERS — B2

Answer 1. Temporal portion of disc appears to be normal. Arterioles show segmental "copper wire" change. Arteriovenous displacement is present at 7 o'clock, 3 disc diameters inferior and temporal to disc. Venular tortuosity is present. There are numerous hard exudates (note vessels crossing over them) surrounding the macula above, below, and temporal to it. Several similar lesions are present at 7 o'clock, 2–3 disc diameters below the nerve head.

Answer 2. Outer plexiform layer.

Answer 3. The branches of the central retinal artery do not reach the outer plexiform layer.

Answer 4. No. However, at times, the hard exudate appears to be yellow and "waxy" in diabetes mellitus.

Answer 5. In diabetes the lesions are more likely to contain lipid; in accelerated hypertension, fibrin deposits are more likely. Since the two diseases often coexist, there is considerable overlap in the histochemical findings.

Reference

Hogan, M. J. and Zimmerman, L. E. (eds.): *Ophthalmic Pathology. An Atlas and Textbook,* 2nd ed., pp. 500–510, Saunders, Philadelphia, 1962.

Plate B3

Clinical findings: A 64–year–old male with insulin dependent diabetes mellitus for 15 years. Bl. P. 200/100 mmHg, BUN 72 mgs/100 ml, creatinine 3.9 mgs/100 ml. Enlarged heart with myocardial insufficiency. Hb 8 gms/100 ml, Hct. 24%. Plate B3 — O.D. — central and nasal (magnified view).

PLATE B3

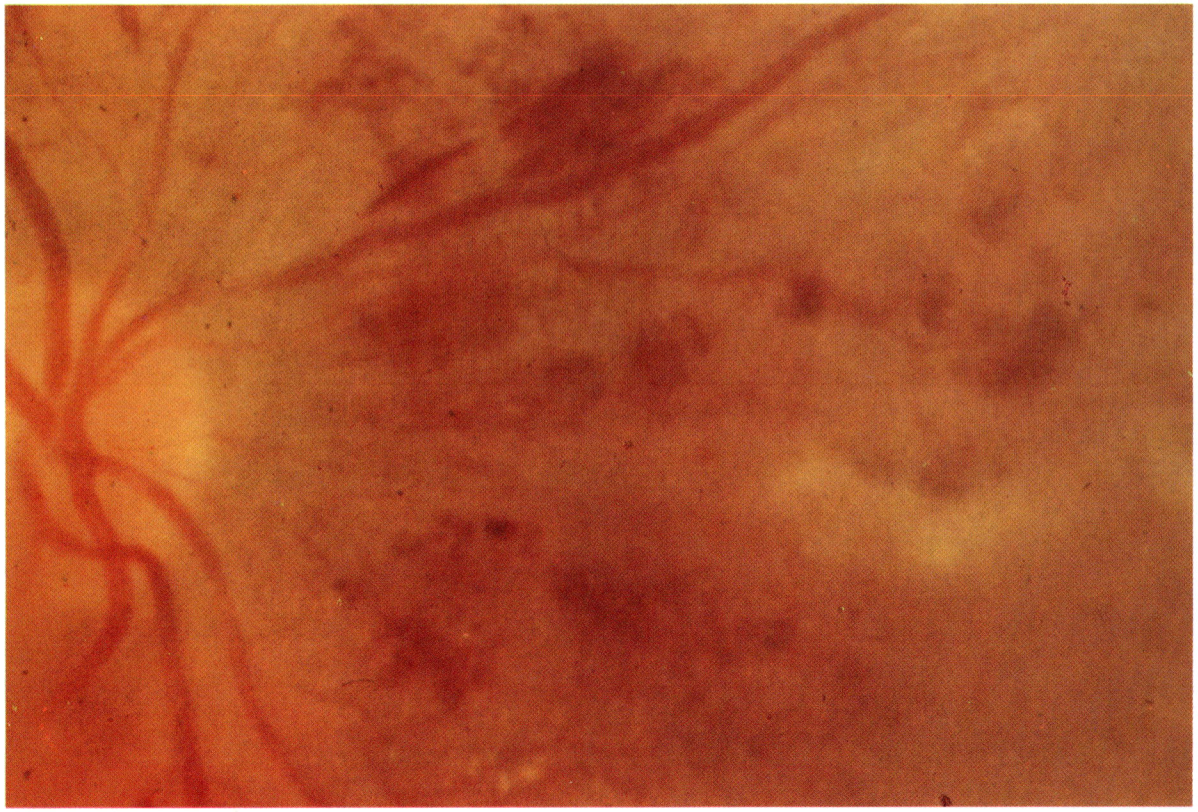

QUESTIONS — B3

Question 1. List abnormalities (see answer p. 101).

Question 2. In general, what criteria are used to distinguish hemorrhage in the nerve fiber layer from that in the outer plexiform layer?

Question 3. Is the location of hemorrhage in the retina specific for any one disease?

Question 4. Does the location of the hemorrhage influence its rate of absorption?

Question 5. Can histologic residua of hemorrhage be found in the retina? If so, what are the findings?

Question 6. Would you expect to see clinical evidence of such residua with the ophthalmoscope?

ANSWERS — B3

Answer 1. This patient's fundus appeared to be hazy because of a cloudy vitreous. Disc is normal. Arterioles are narrow. The venules are somewhat tortuous. There is a cotton wool patch at 4 o'clock, 2 disc diameters from disc. Multiple linear, flame–shaped, irregular striate, round, and oval hemorrhages are visible. Microaneurysms and hard exudates are present between 4 and 6 o'clock.

Answer 2. Nerve fiber layer hemorrhages are linear or flame–shaped. They often have striate borders and generally overlie blood vessels. The deep hemorrhage (generally in the outer plexiform layer) is round or oval. Blood vessels cross over it.

Answer 3. No.

Answer 4. Yes. Hemorrhage in the nerve fiber layer may be absorbed rapidly. Large vitreous hemorrhages are often poorly absorbed in patients with severe retinopathy. A similar hemorrhage following trauma in a normal, young individual may be completely and rapidly absorbed. Subhyaloid, outer plexiform, and choroidal hemorrhages are absorbed slowly.

Answer 5. Yes. Hemosiderin deposits and gliosis.

Answer 6. Rarely, since the residual lesions are small and the magnification of the ophthalmoscope is not sufficient to make them visible.

Reference

Ballantyne, A. J. and Michaelson, I. C.: *Textbook of the Fundus of the Eye,* 2nd ed., pp. 122–139, Williams & Wilkins, Baltimore, 1970.

Plate B4

Clinical findings: A 21–year–old female who has had severe headache and blurred vision for 2 weeks. Bl. P. 240/150 mmHg, BUN 22 mgs/100 ml, creatinine 1.8 mgs/100 ml, Hct. 47%, Hb 15.2 gms/100 ml. Sickle cell preparation — negative. Normal intravenous pyelograms and renal arteriograms. Plate B4 — O.D. — nasal.

QUESTIONS — B4

Question 1. List abnormalities (see answer, p. 103).

Question 2. If antihypertensive therapy were instituted would you expect regression of the patient's symptoms and retinal changes? If the answer is yes, what would be the order of regression?

PLATE B4

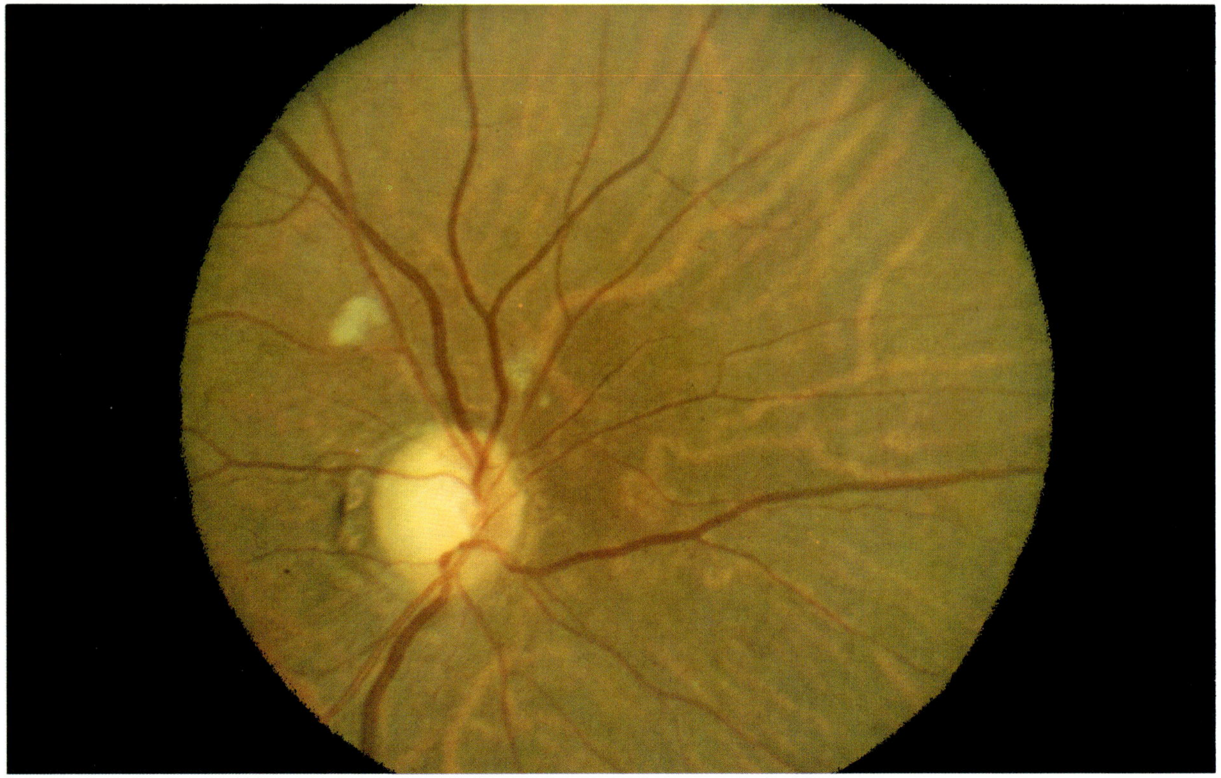

ANSWERS — B4

Plate B4

Answer 1. Disc is flat and its margins are distinct. Arterioles are narrow and show "copper wire" change. Cotton wool patches are present at 11 and 1 o'clock. A–V compression is observed above the disc. Choroidal blood vessels are visible.

Answer 2. Headache would probably be the first symptom to respond favorably. Since the macula was not involved the visual impairment would probably disappear within several days. The cotton wool patches would decrease in size within several weeks. Complete regression of the changes noted, with the exception of the arteriolar abnormalities, could be expected in 2 or 3 months. The arteriolar changes are not likely to regress.

References

Ellis, P. P. and Fonken, H. A.: *Retinopathies of Chronic Glomerulonephritis. A Study of Cases Treated with Renal Transplantation,* Arch. Ophthalmol., **75:** 36, 1966.

Kirkendall, W. M. and Armstrong, M. L.: *Effect of Blood Pressure Reduction on Vascular Changes in the Eye,* in: Moyer, J. H. (ed.): *Hypertension, the First Hahnemann Symposium on Hypertensive Disease,* Saunders, Philadelphia, 1959.

Lockhart, G., von Noorden, G., Duston, H. P., Corcoran, A. C., and Page, I. H.: *The Course of Retinopathy in Treated Malignant Hypertension,* Arch. Intern. Med., **106:** 205, 1960.

Plate B5

Clinical findings: A 55–year–old female. Bl. P. 170/110 mmHg, Hct. 45%, Hb. 14 gms/100 ml, Fasting bl. sugar 94 mgs/100 ml, BUN 15 mgs/100 ml. The patient has no visual complaints. Plate B5 — O.D.

QUESTIONS — B5

Question 1. Describe (see answer, p. 105).

Question 2. What is the lesion?

Question 3. How would you distinguish this lesion from the cotton wool patch?

PLATE B5

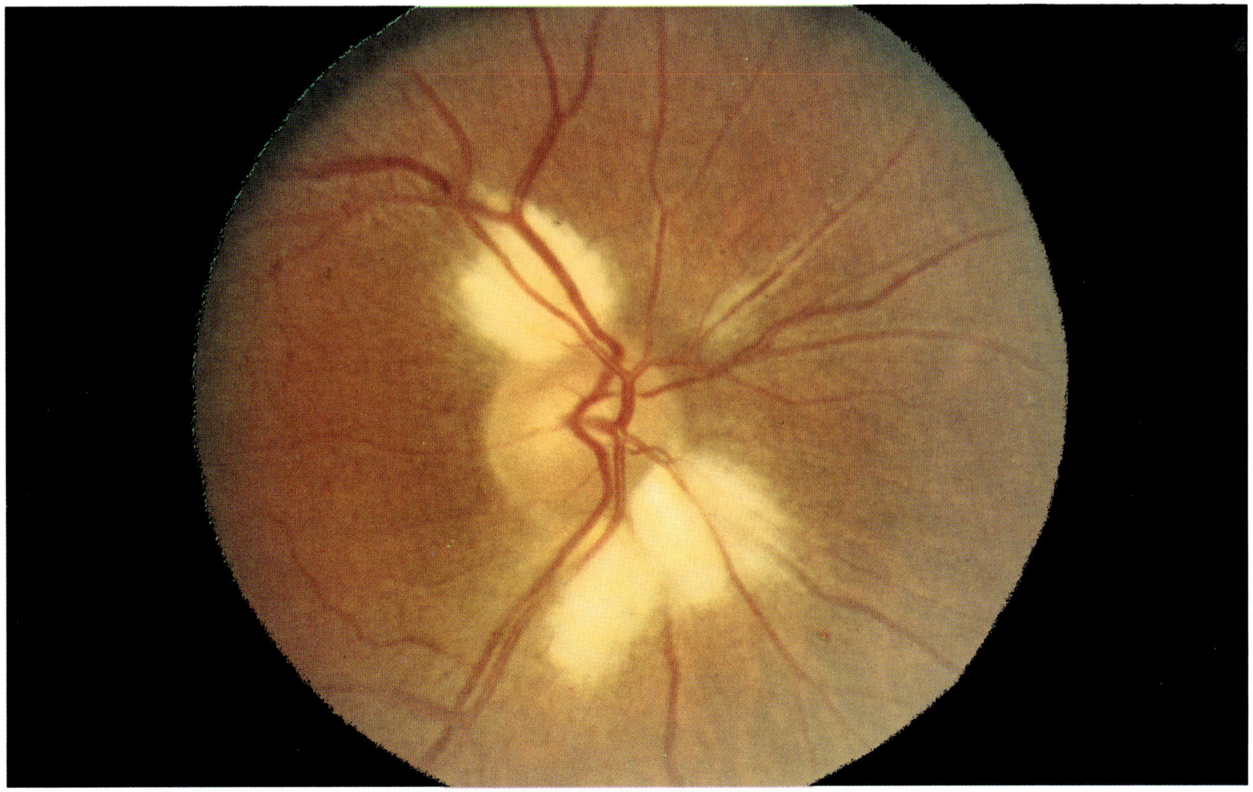

ANSWERS — B5

Answer 1. The disc, arterioles, and venules are normal. Glistening white patches with striate borders extend over and away from the disc at 11 and 4 o'clock. Vessels overlie the lesion at 11 o'clock; the reverse is true at 4 and 6 o'clock. There are similar changes along the superior nasal arteriole.

Answer 2. Myelinated (medullated) nerve fibers (see pp. 20, 21).

Answer 3. Its location, color, and striate borders resemble the findings of the cotton wool patch. To distinguish the two, one must examine the other structures of the retina carefully. The cotton wool patch would be an unlikely finding in the absence of arteriolar or venular disease. In addition, other extravascular lesions such as hemorrhage, hard exudates, and/or microaneurysms are often present. As noted above, the arterioles and venules are normal in Plate B5 and there are no lesions other than the myelinated nerve fibers.

Reference

Duke–Elder, W. S.: *Normal and Abnormal Development. Part II, Congenital Deformities,* in: Duke–Elder, W. S. (ed.): *System of Ophthalmology,* Vol. III: pp. 646–652, Mosby, St. Louis, 1963.

Plate B6

Microscopic section of retina — PAS × 80 (approx). Note PAS positive deposits in outer plexiform layer (see Drawing B6).

QUESTION — B6

Question 1. What would you expect to see on funduscopic examination of a patient with the above lesions? (See answer, p. 107.)

PLATE B6

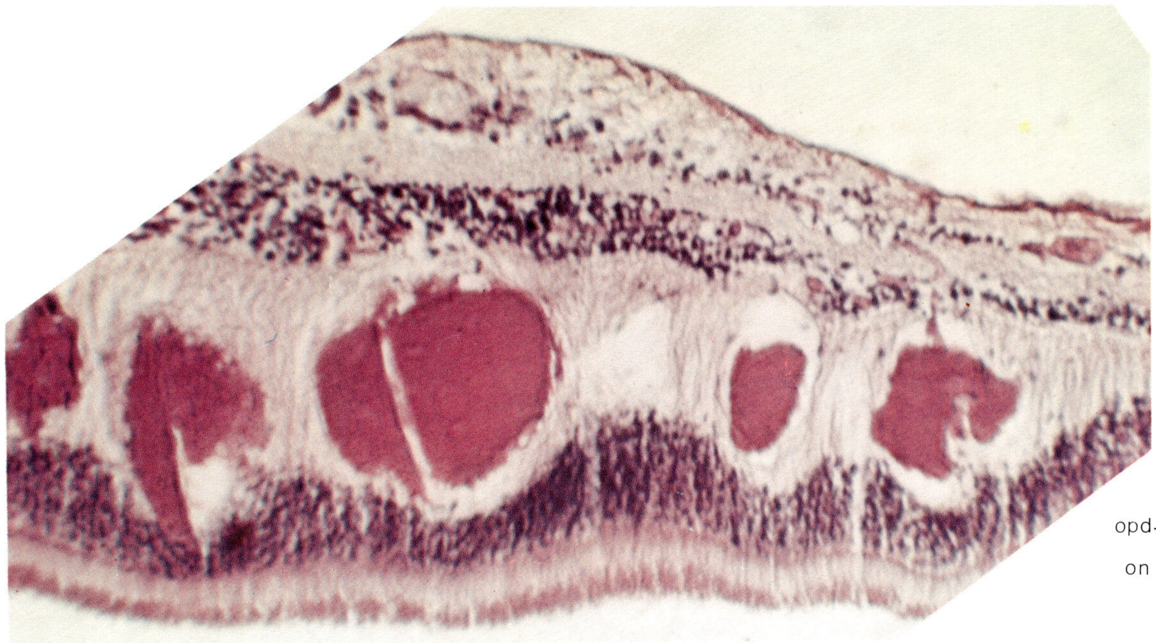

Drawing B6. Plate B6 (opd, outer plexiform deposit; in, inner nuclear layer; on, outer nuclear layer).

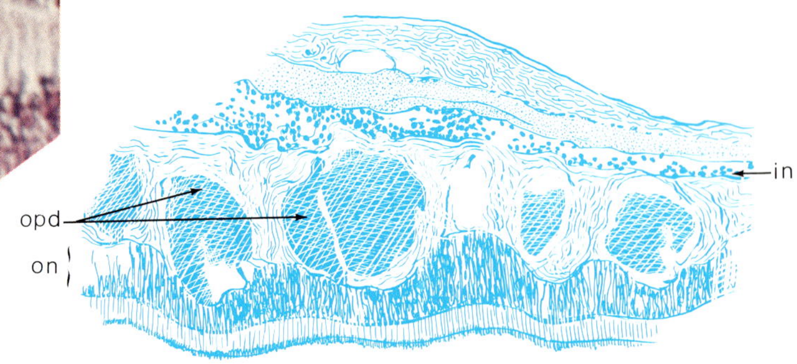

ANSWER — B6

Answer 1. Hard exudates. Discrete yellow or white lesions, perhaps in clusters, would be present. Blood vessels would cross over the lesions.

Plate B7

Microscopic section of retina — LFB × 80 (approx.) Note the cluster of cell–like, oval bodies in the nerve fiber layer of the retina (see Drawing B7).

QUESTIONS — B7

Question 1. What are these structures? (See answer, p. 109.)

Question 2. What clinical abnormality would be present in the retina?

PLATE B7

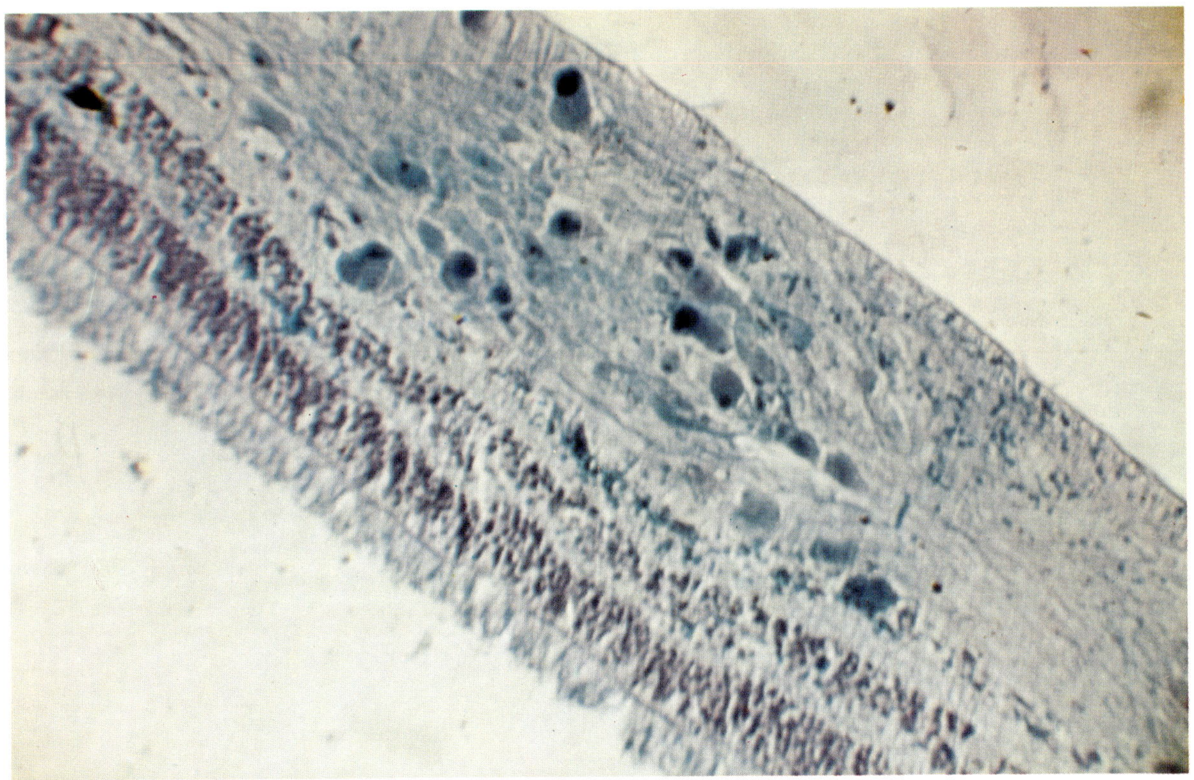

ANSWER — B7

Answer 1. Cytoid bodies.

Answer 2. Cotton wool patch. White or gray lesions which overlie blood vessels and have irregular borders.

Drawing B7. Plate B7 (cb, cytoid bodies; nf, nerve fiber layer; ip, inner plexiform layer).

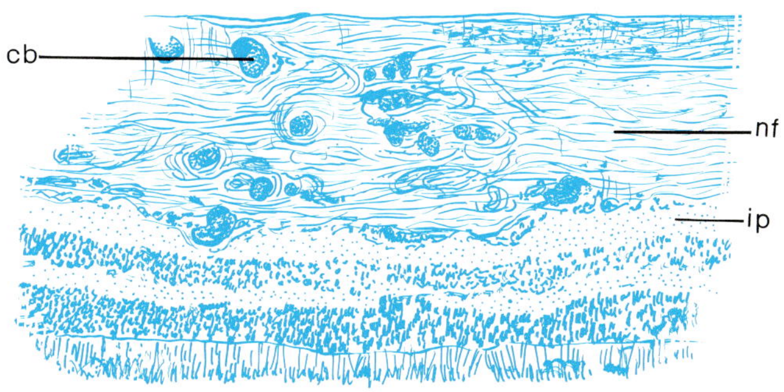

Plate B8

Clinical findings: A 26–year–old female with insulin–dependent diabetes mellitus for 12 years. Bl. P. 160/120 mmHg. Peripheral neuropathy and postural hypotension were prominent findings. Plate B8 — O.D. — central.

QUESTIONS — B8

Question 1. List abnormalities (see answer, p. 111).

Question 2. What is a subhyaloid hemorrhage? Where is it located and what are its clinical characteristics?

PLATE B8

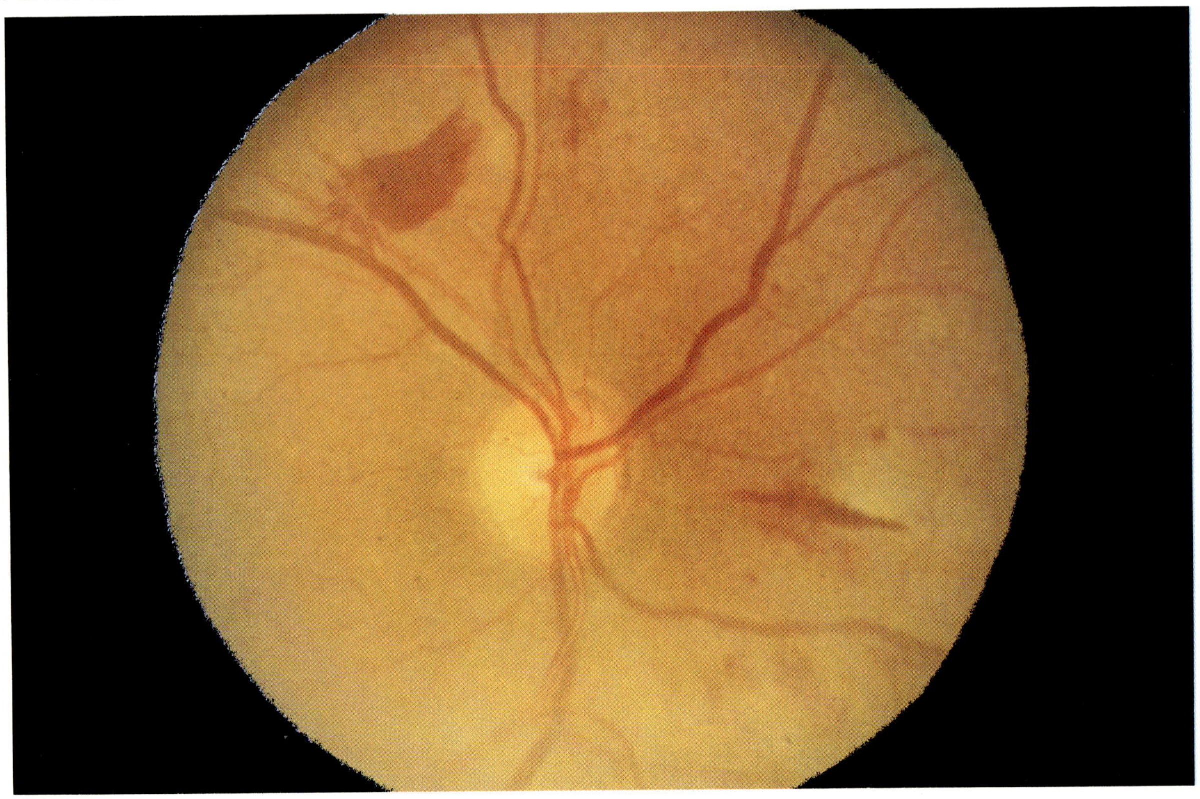

ANSWERS — B8

Answer 1. Normal disc. Increased central light streak of arterioles. Engorged, tortuous, and segmented venules. Linear hemorrhage at 12, 3, and 5 o'clock. Round hemorrhage near macula. A large subhyaloid hemorrhage which seems to extend from spoke–like hemorrhages at 11 o'clock, above the disc. Arteriovenous compression below the disc at first and second crossings. Microaneurysm above linear hemorrhage and cotton wool patch at 3 o'clock (see Chapter V for a discussion of the microaneurysm).

Answer 2. The subhyaloid hemorrhage is round or oval and has distinct borders. It overlies the retinal blood vessels. With the patient upright, a hematocrit effect develops and the hemorrhage has a straight upper border. It is believed to be the result of retinal hemorrhage which penetrates the internal limiting membrane. The blood is then confined between that structure and the hyaloid membrane.

Plate B9

Clinical findings: A 20–year–old female who at age 6 was told that she had an "infection" of her left eye. Since that illness she has had poor vision in that eye. She lived in Kentucky until 2 years ago. Plate B9 — O.S. — temporal.

QUESTIONS — B9

Question 1. Describe findings (see answer, p. 113).

Question 2. What is your diagnosis?

Question 3. What are the pathologic changes in that disorder?

Question 4. What diagnostic procedures may help find the cause of chorioretinitis?

PLATE B9

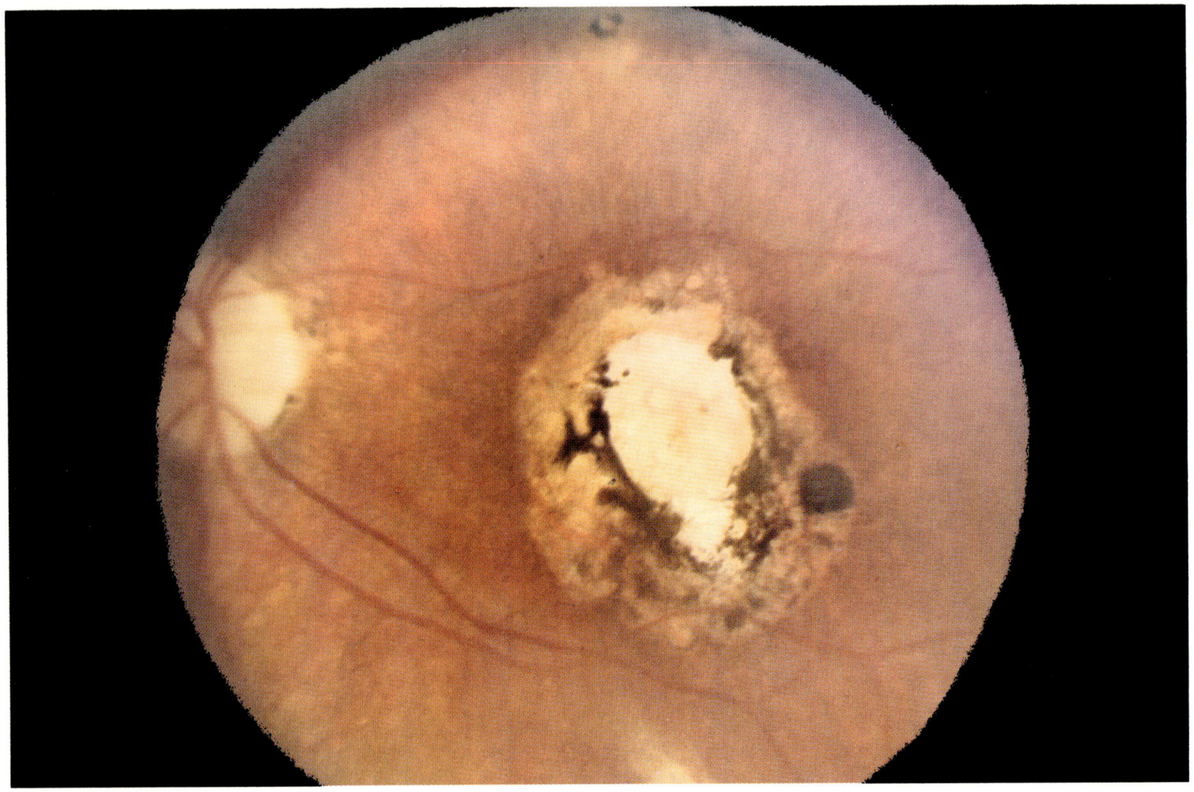

ANSWERS — B9

Answer 1. The disc has an irregular, temporal border. A pigmented crescent is present. Choroidal vessels are visible at the disc border. There is a large white patch in the macular area. It is surrounded by clumps of brown–black pigment. In turn, there is another band outside of the pigmented area. Choroidal vessels are visible in the outer band. The latter is crossed, at its edge, by the inferior temporal venule. No blood vessels are visible in the white central patch.

Answer 2. Chorioretinitis.

Answer 3. Chorioretinitis is generally the result of infection. The ensuing inflammatory response consists of tissue destruction, fibrosis, occasionally granulomata, and pigment migration (see p. 80).

Answer 4.

a. chest x-ray
b. skin tests
   1. tuberculin (P.P.D.)
   2. toxoplasmosis
   3. histoplasmosis
c. serologic tests
   1. toxoplasmosis
   2. histoplasmosis
   3. syphilis

Although there are many other diseases associated with chorioretinitis, tuberculosis, syphilis, and toxoplasmosis are believed to be the most common offenders.

Reference

Hogan, M. J. and Zimmerman, L. E. (eds.): *Ophthalmic Pathology. An Atlas and Textbook*, 2nd ed., pp. 373–403, Saunders, Philadelphia, 1962.

Plate B10

Clinical findings: A 38–year–old male. BUN 150 mgs/100 ml; creatinine 8.0 mgs/100 ml; Bl. P. 230/150 mmHg; cardiac enlargement; 2 hour p.c. blood sugar 194 mgs/100 ml; Hct. 20%, Hb, 6.5 mgs/100 ml. Plate B10 — O.S. — temporal.

PLATE B10

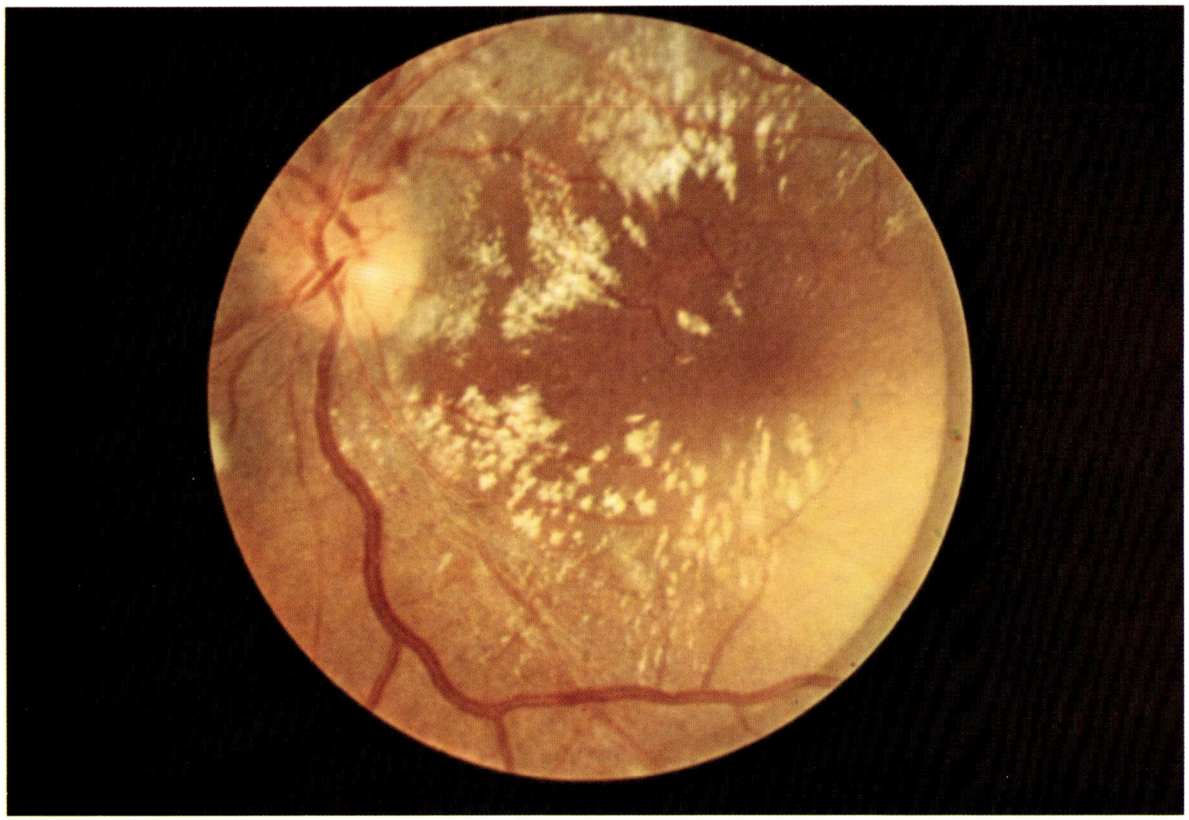

QUESTIONS — B10

Question 1. List abnormalities (see answer, p. 115).

Question 2. What term is applied to the pattern of hard exudates which extend from the macula?

Question 3. Is the macular star specific for any one disease?

Question 4. In what layer of the retina would you expect to find the lesion of the macular star?

Question 5. Why does the outer plexiform lesion in the macular area assume the star-like pattern?

Question 6. Where in the retina is the hemorrhage noted?

ANSWERS — B10

Answer 1. The optic disc is hyperemic and its margins are indistinct. A small cilioretinal artery is present on temporal side of the disc. The arterioles are narrow. The venules are engorged and tortuous. Numerous discrete and conglomerate yellow areas of degeneration extend from the macular area. They are arranged in a starlike pattern. Blood vessels cross over some of these lesions. There is a hemorrhage which overlies a blood vessel at 1 o'clock, close to the disc.

Answer 2. Macular star.

Answer 3. No. It is, however, most commonly found in patients with accelerated or malignant hypertension.

Answer 4. Outer plexiform layer.

Answer 5. The outer plexiform layer (Henle's fibers) radiates into the hub-like fovea like the spokes of a wheel. Lesions in that layer of the macula assume the same anatomical pattern.

Answer 6. Nerve fiber layer.

Reference

Duke–Elder, W. S. and Dobree, J. H.: *Diseases of the Retina,* in: Duke–Elder, W. S. (ed.): *System of Ophthalmology,* Vol. X: pp. 30–32, Mosby, St. Louis, 1967.

Drawing 118. Plate 118 (O, indistinct disc margins; HEM, hemorrhage; CWP, cotton wool patch; V, venous engorgement; NV, neovascularization).

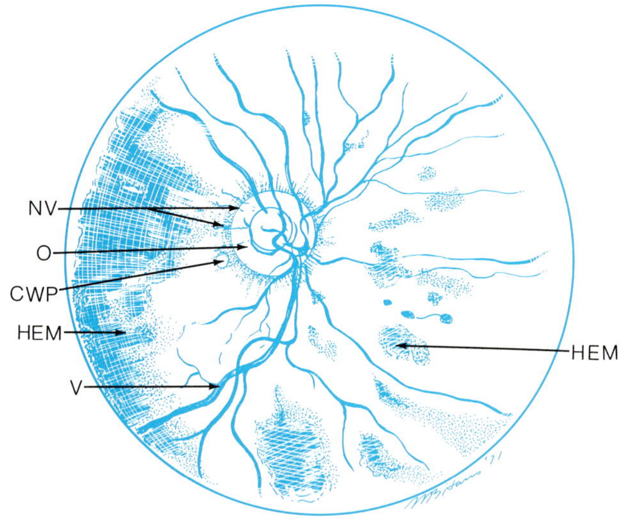

Plate 118. O.D. Multiple retinal hemorrhages extend from the disc. The disc margins are indistinct; new vessel formation of the disc (see Chapter VI) and venous engorgement are present. A cotton wool patch is present at 10 o'clock close to the disc.

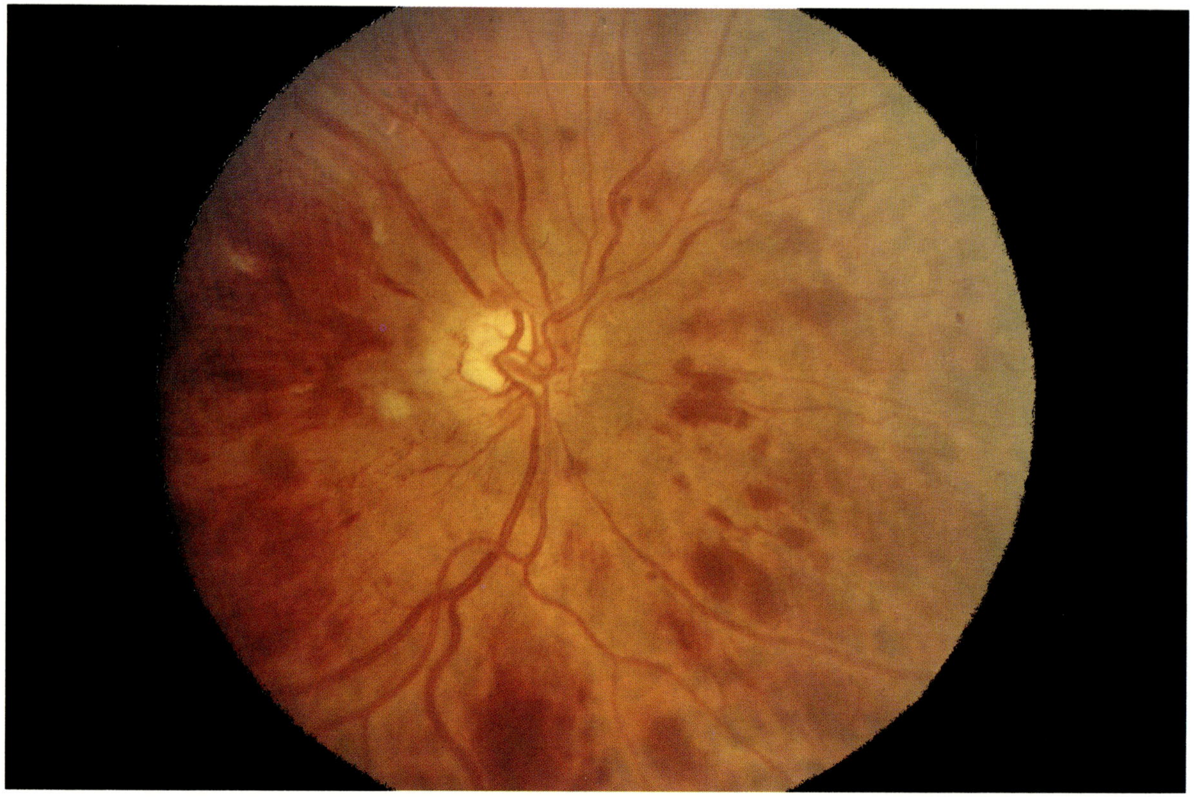

Chapter IV
RETINAL VENOUS DISEASE

VENOUS DISEASE

The clinically recognizable retinal venous alterations include:

1. Central retinal vein occlusion
2. Venous branch occlusion
3. Alteration of venous caliber
   a. widening (engorgement, dilatation)
   b. segmentation
   c. tortuosity
4. Venous sheathing

Central Retinal Vein Occlusion

CLINICAL FINDINGS

Generally central retinal vein occlusion is heralded by a painless and sudden loss of vision in one eye. Less commonly, there is a gradual visual loss; and occasionally, both eyes are affected. Unless there is associated central retinal artery occlusion, the visual loss is not complete and light perception persists.[4 (p. 204)] Multiple flame–shaped, linear, and round hemorrhages extend from the optic disc (Plate 118 and Drawing 118). Blood may also be observed in the vitreous. Venous engorgement and tortuosity are marked. The central retinal vein does not pulsate and papilledema may be present. Cotton wool patches and hard exudates may also be present. Within several weeks, neovascularization of the disc and microaneurysms are often observed. Venous sheathing (see p. 123) develops later. Glaucoma may develop within a period of several months.

PATHOLOGY AND PATHOGENESIS

Extensive hemorrhage is observed in all retinal layers. The blood may penetrate the internal limiting membrane and enter the vitreous or extend posteriorly and separate the rods and cones from the pigment cells.[2 (p. 499)] Cystic spaces and deposits of fibrin may be observed in internuclear layers. Scattered areas of necrosis may also be present. The hemorrhage and necrosis may leave such residua as hemosiderin deposits and gliosis. Neovascularization[150] and microaneurysms[151, 152] are other documented histologic abnormalities.

The obstruction of the central retinal vein is generally found in the region of the lamina cribrosa. At that site the caliber of the vein normally decreases and the artery and vein are often enveloped by a single sheath, and may share a common wall. It is reasonable to postulate that such an anatomic arrangement offers a mechanism for compression of the vein by a sclerotic central retinal artery. Retardation of venous flow could then be followed by thrombosis. Venous sclerosis[4 (p. 207)] and inflammation[151] are less common causes of central retinal vein thrombosis. Subendothelial and endothelial proliferation, without thrombus formation, may also produce complete obstruction of the central retinal vein.[153] In the absence of venous disease, thrombus formation results from the increased viscosity of blood in macroglobulinemia[154] and polycythemia vera.[4 (p. 207)]

Based upon clinical evidence Paton *et al.*[155] offer the idea that central and branch retinal vein occlusion may be the result of disease of the central retinal artery and its branches. They observed that injected fluorescein passed promptly through the venous system during the acute phase of the disease. There were, however, demonstrable constrictions and occlusions in the arterial system. In central retinal vein occlusion all the branches of the retinal artery were narrowed. In venous branch occlusion, the arterioles in the involved quadrant were narrowed. Visual field changes were those expected with involvement of the retinal segment supplied by the involved arteriole rather than that of the observed retinal hemorrhage. When ophthaldynamometry was performed in 73 patients, 22 had decreased systolic pressures. That concept is further supported by the clinical observation that unilateral retinopathy consisting of dilatation of retinal veins, hemorrhage, and microaneurysms occurs with ipsilateral carotid artery occlusion.[156] In the monkey, experimentally produced occlusion of the central retinal vein did not lead to the anticipated funduscopic changes unless the central retinal artery was also obstructed.[157] These observations lend support to the concept that retinal ischemia produced by arterial insufficiency plays an important role in occlusion of the central retinal vein.

Plate 119. O.S. Marked A–V compression of the superior temporal vein. A white sheath is visible at the crossing site. Hemorrhage is present along the engorged portion of the vein. The white patches between 1 and 2 o'clock, 2 disc diameters temporal to the disc, are cotton wool patches.

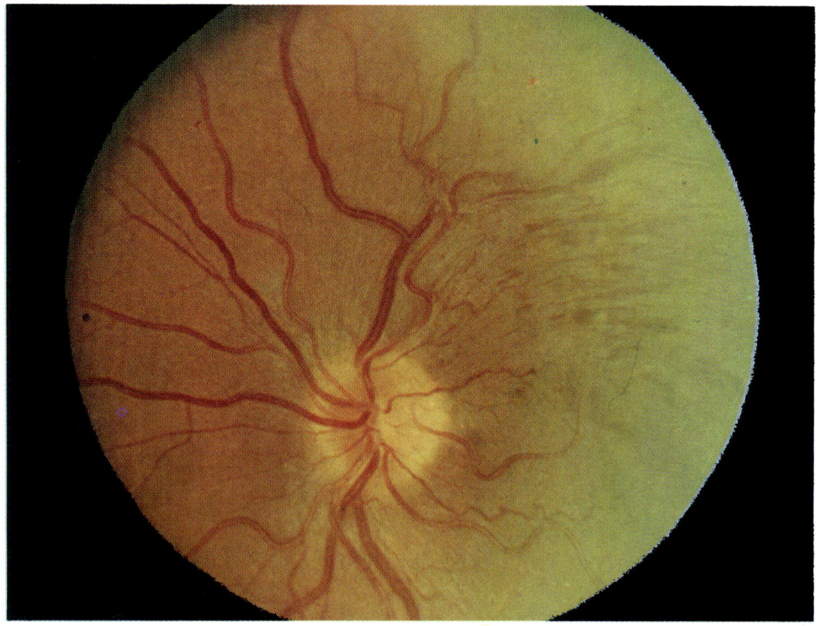

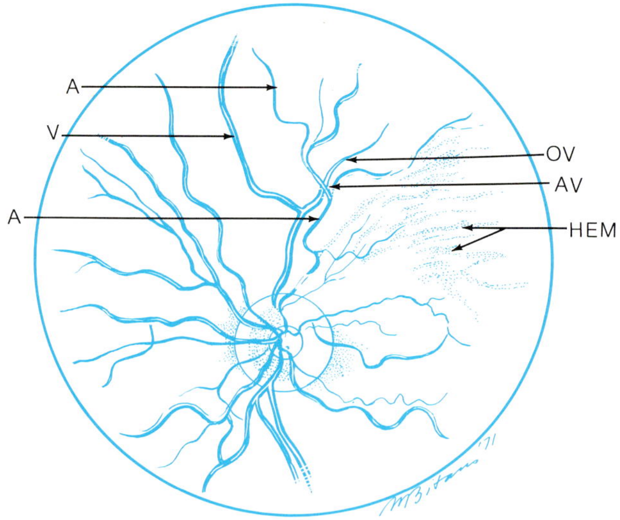

Drawing 119. Plate 119 (V, vein; AV, arteriovenous compression; OV, occluded vein; HEM, hemorrhage; A, arteriole).

Plate 120. O.S. The tortuous, superior temporal arteriole crosses the corresponding venule twice. The outline of the venule becomes indistinct distal to the first crossing. After the second crossing it is replaced by a white streak. Did you notice the pigmented crescent at the temporal border of the disc, the fine "silver wire" arterioles, and the hard exudates close to the macula? One microaneurysm is visible in the macular area.

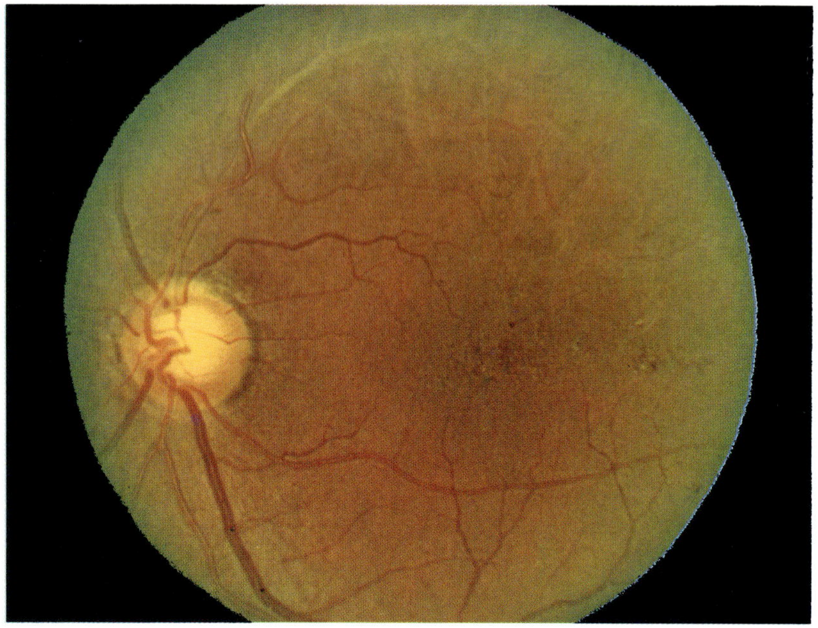

Drawing 120. Plate 120 (V, occluded vein).

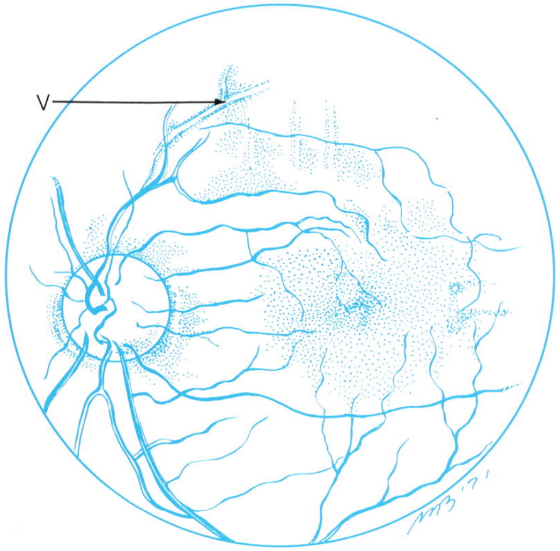

CENTRAL RETINAL VEIN OCCLUSION AND CLINICAL STATES

This abnormality occurs most commonly in middle–aged or elderly patients who have hypertension[155] and/or diabetes mellitus.[151] Polycythemia vera,[4 (p. 207)] lymphoma, leukemia, the dysproteinemias (multiple myeloma and macroglobulinemia), and sickle cell disease are less common causes of central retinal vein occlusion.[158 (pp. 167-168)] This serious ophthalmic disorder occurs uncommonly in young women who use oral contraceptives.[51]

Venous Branch Occlusion

Occlusion of a venous branch commonly occurs at the site of arteriovenous compression. The superior temporal vein is most often involved (Plate 119 and Drawing 119). Hemorrhage is observed along the course of the affected vessel. The vein distal to the site of compression is generally engorged and tortuous. Visual loss generally corresponds with the involved retinal segment and may not be a serious handicap. Involvement of the macula often results in permanent and marked visual loss.

Venous branch and central retinal vein occlusion occur in the same group of diseases above.

The obstructed venous branch becomes a white streak (Plate 120 and Drawing 120).

Fluorescein angiograms demonstrate the site of arteriovenous compression and disclose the presence of new vessels and microaneurysms which arise from the obstructed venule and its branches[159] (Plates 121 and 122 and Drawings 121 and 122). See pp. 137–146 and 127–135 for a discussion of neovascularization and microaneurysms.

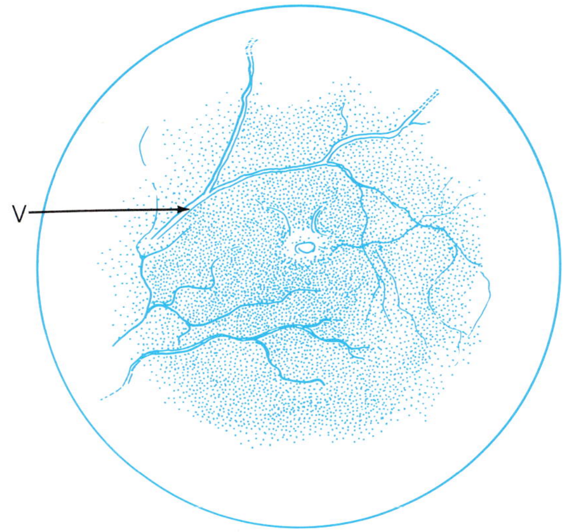

Drawing 121. Plate 121 (V, occluded vein).

Plates 121 and 122. O.S. (Same patient as Plate 120.)

Drawing 122. Plate 122 (V, occluded vein; NV, neovascularization; MA, microaneurysm).

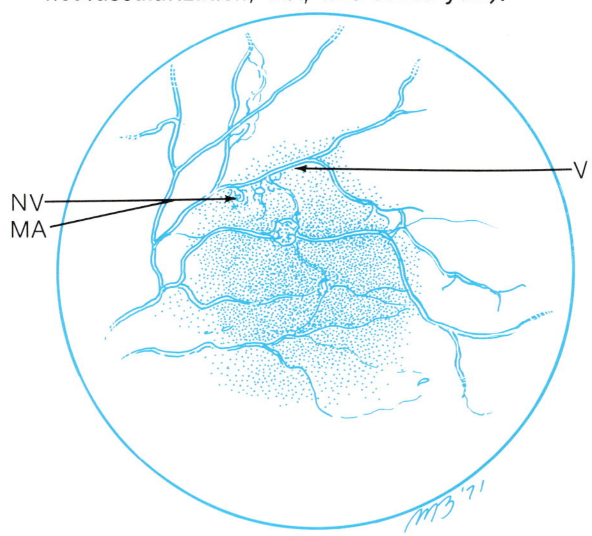

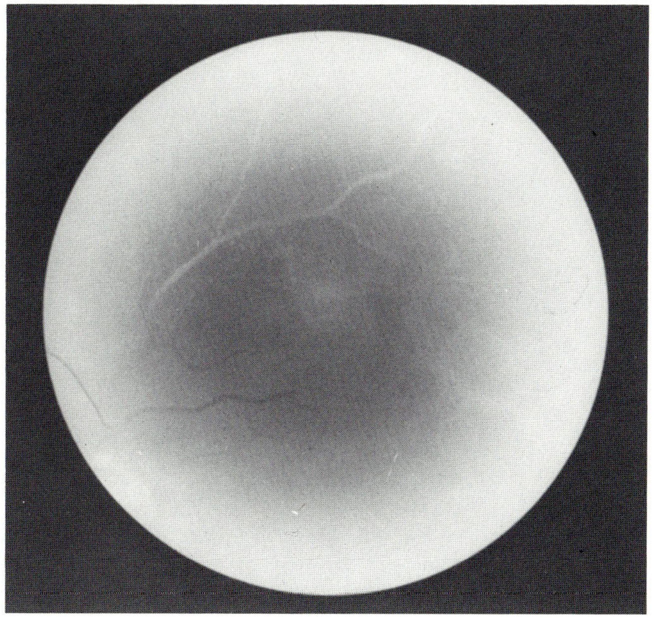

Plate 121. Photograph of O.S. before injection of fluorescein. Note the obliterated venule (portion of it is shown in Plate 120) which appears to be a tortuous white streak. The arteriovenous crossings are visible.

Plate 122. Fluorescein angiogram (arteriovenous phase). The dye–filled, tortuous arteriole compresses the venule twice. New vessels (neovascularization) arise from the venular branches, interconnecting and perhaps serving as collaterals. Numerous microaneurysms are observed to originate from the new vessels.

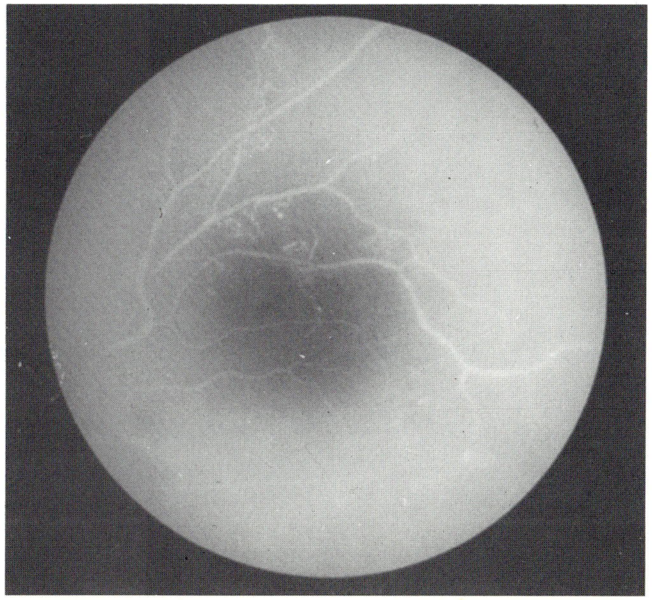

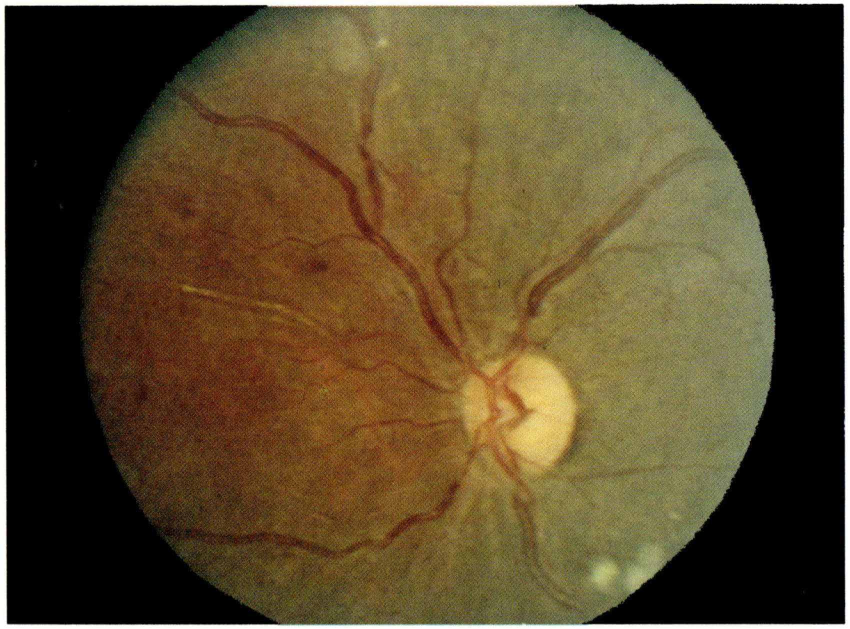

Plate 123. O.S. Central superior. Engorgement and tortuosity of superior nasal and temporal veins. Patient with hypertension and diabetes mellitus. Did you notice a "silver wire" arteriole at 10 o'clock, cotton wool patches at 5 o'clock, and hemorrhages at 11 o'clock?

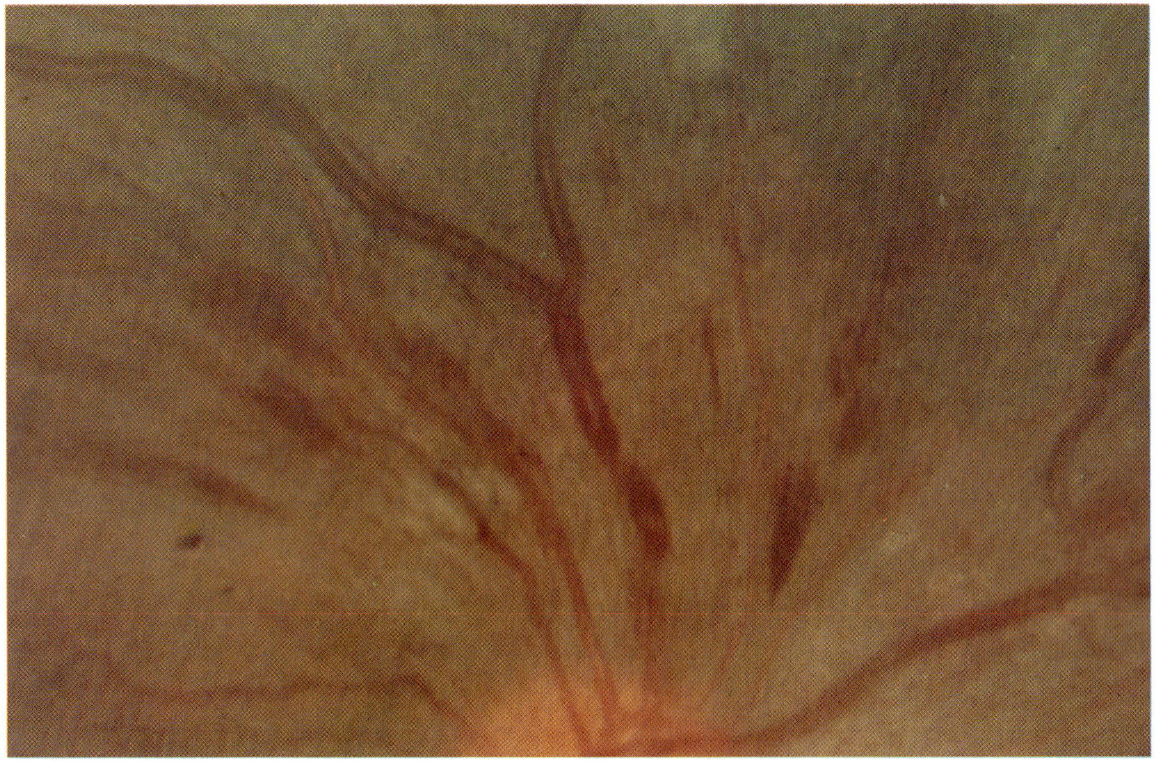

Plate 124. Above the disc (magnified). Venous engorgement, segmentation, tortuosity, and nerve fiber layer hemorrhage in accelerated hypertension.

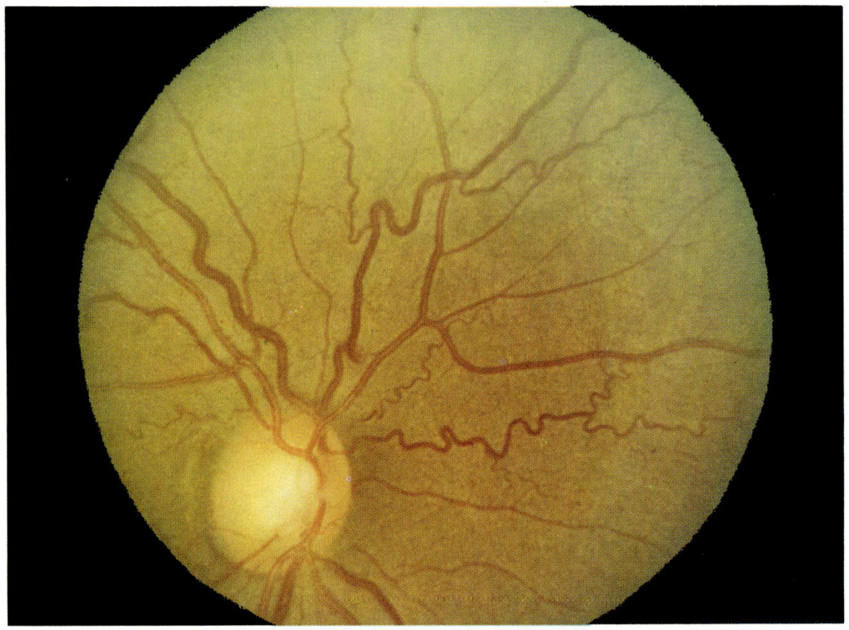

Plate 125. O.D. Superior. Venous tortuosity in patient with diabetes mellitus.

Alteration of Venous Caliber

WIDENING OF THE VEINS

Widening of retinal veins, commonly described as venous engorgement, fullness, or dilatation, may be generalized (Plates 123 and 124), involving the larger veins with extension into smaller branches or affecting only one or few branches. Leukemia, multiple myeloma, macroglobulinemia, polycythemia, central retinal vein occlusion, papilledema, and accelerated hypertension are associated with generalized retinal venous engorgement. In diabetes mellitus the change may involve only one or all of the veins. Arteriovenous compression and venous branch occlusion are associated with engorgement distal to the site of obstruction.

SEGMENTATION

Particularly in diabetes mellitus, a portion of the vein appears to be constricted (Plate 124). This change may be present along the entire vein producing a beaded effect. When multiple areas of constriction are associated with dilatation, the venous abnormality may resemble a chain of sausage links.

TORTUOSITY

This condition frequently accompanies venous engorgement (Plate 125). Bizarre configurations such as loops (Plates 126 and 127), coils, and "cork screw" changes may be observed. Tortuosity, unaccompanied by dilatation, frequently is observed in severe anemia, hypertension, and Fabry's disease. A congenital variety is described as well.

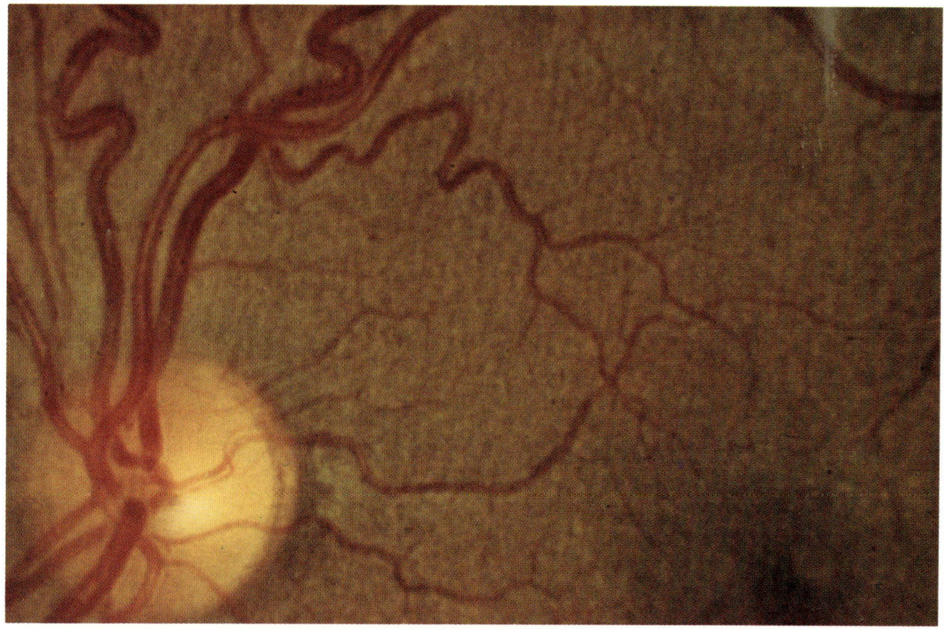

Plate 126. O.D. Superior temporal. Venous tortuosity involving small branch in patient with sickle cell disease.

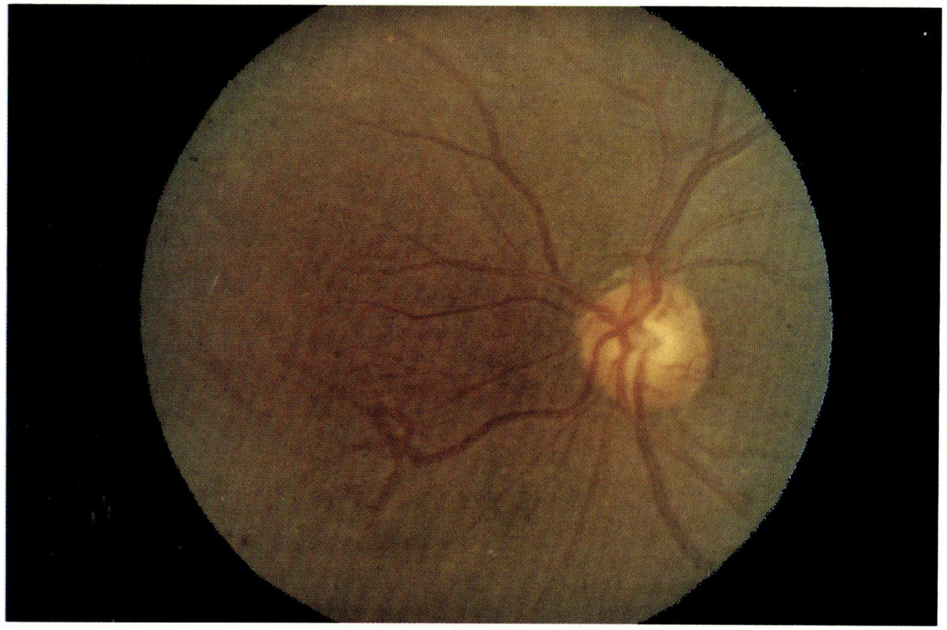

Plate 127. O.S. Venous tortuosity with loop formation in patient with diabetes mellitus.

Plate 128. Venous sheathing, new vessel formation (neovascularization), and hard exudates in patient with diabetes mellitus.

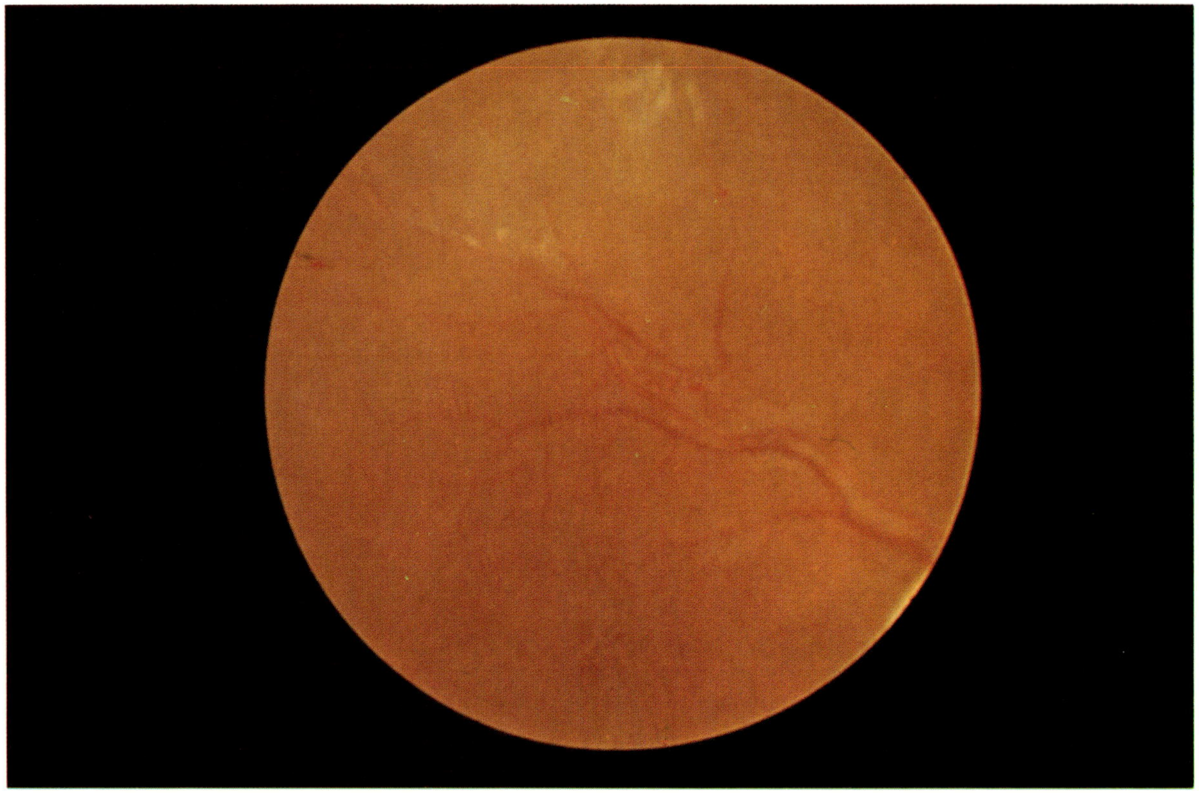

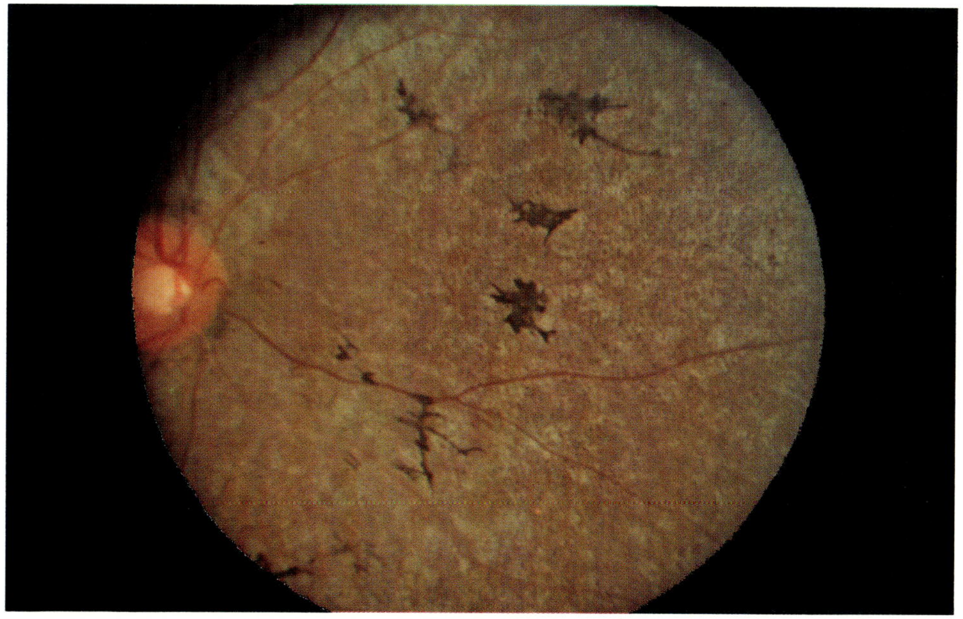

Plate 129. O.D. Nasal. Pigment deposits in the retina, in the wall of a venule (4 o'clock, 2 disc diameters from the disc), and in wall of an arteriole at 1 o'clock in a patient with retinitis pigmentosa (see p. 199).

Venous Sheathing

Venous sheathing may be parallel (Plate 128) or pipe–stem (Plate 130). In the former the white sheath may occur on one or both sides of the involved vein. Venous occlusion, either central or branch, reaction to injury such as photocoagulation, diabetes mellitus, leukemia, and the periphlebitis of Eale's disease (see p. 85) are the most common causes of parallel sheathing. In retinitis pigmentosa sheaths of brown pigment occur along the course of the vein (Plate 129).

Pipe–stem sheathing produces a broad white streak which contains no blood column (Plate 130). It is generally associated with venous branch occlusion, diabetes mellitus, and sickle cell disease.

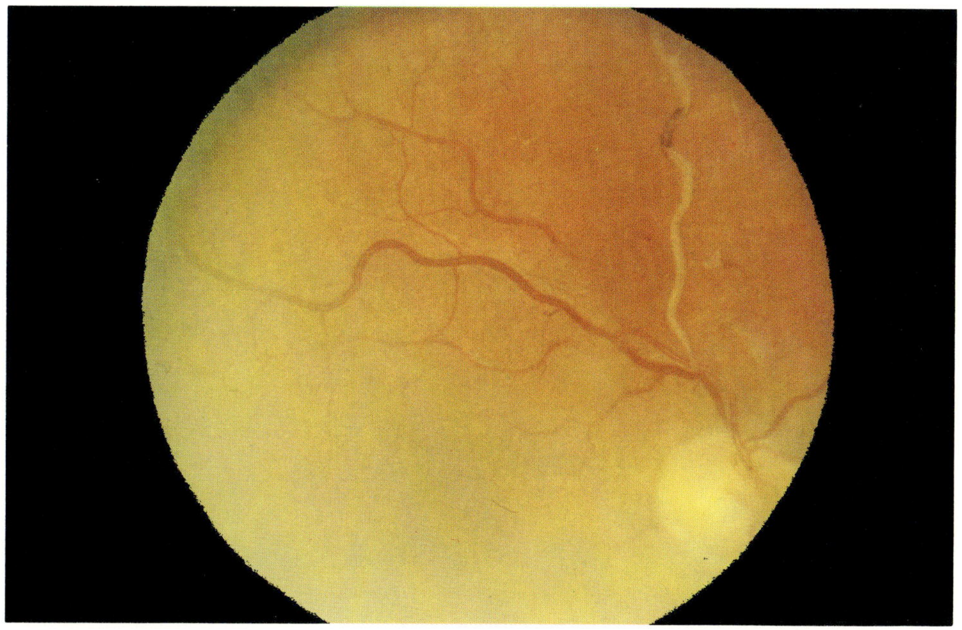

Plate 130. O.D. Superior temporal. Venous wall is a broad white streak. No blood column is visible. Patient with diabetes and hypertension.

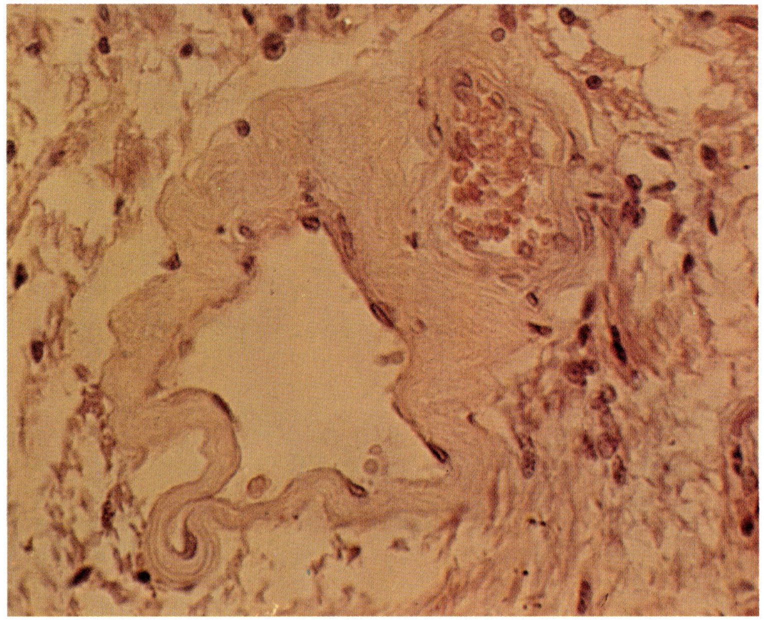

Plate 131. Phlebosclerosis of retinal vein with hyalinization and thickening of media and adventitia. Patient with diabetes mellitus (H&E, × 250).

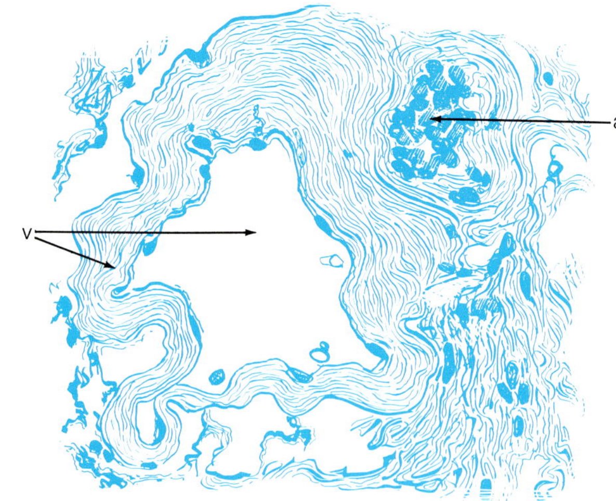

Drawing 131. Plate 131 (v, thick–walled venule; a, arteriole).

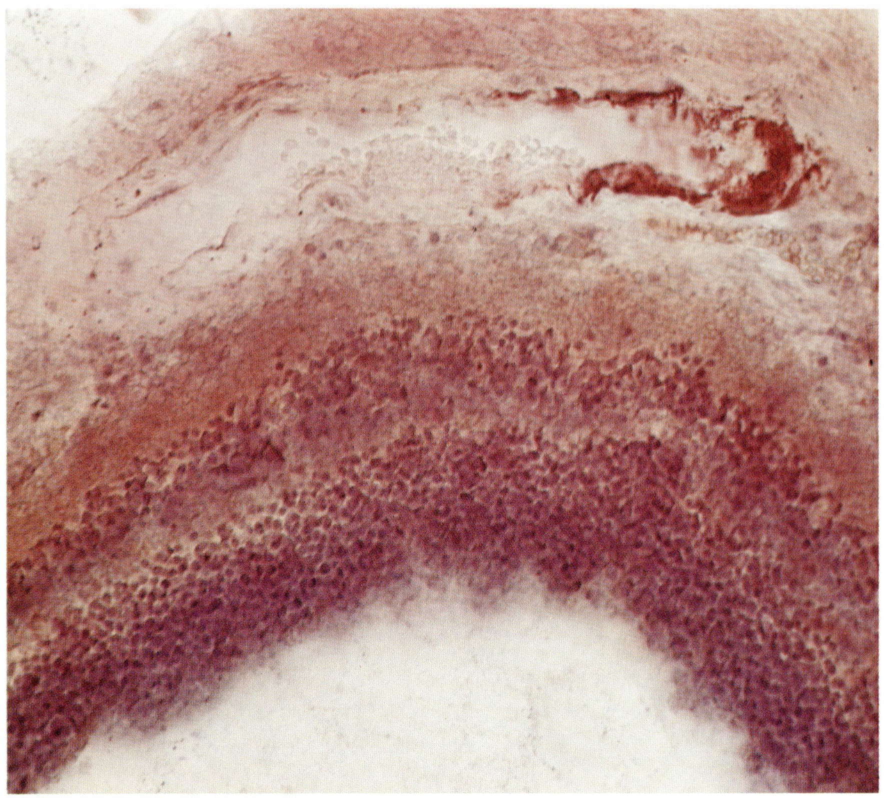

Plate 132. Lipid infiltration of venular wall. Diabetes mellitus (Schar. R, × 120).

Drawing 132. Plate 132 (nf, nerve fiber layer; v, lipid deposit in venous wall; ip, inner plexiform layer).

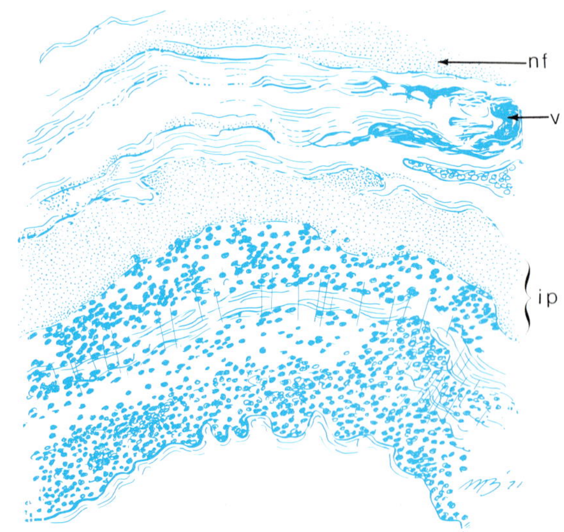

PATHOLOGY AND PATHOGENESIS OF ALTERATION OF VENOUS CALIBER

A number of pathologic changes, such as phlebosclerosis (Plate 131 and Drawing 131), periphlebitis, infiltration of the venous wall with lipid (Plate 132 and Drawing 132), leukemic cells, melanin (Plate 133 and Drawing 133), and occlusive phenomena, have been observed by several authors. However, good clinical pathological correlation has rarely been recorded. Moreover, retinal venous pathology is often not apparent, particularly with reference to correlation with such clinical signs as venous engorgement and tortuosity.

Phlebosclerosis, or venofibrosis, consists of replacement fibrosis of the muscle cells and collagen of the venous wall and subendothelial fibrosis of the intima[160] (Plate 131 and Drawing 131). Comparable changes have been observed in patients with diabetes mellitus.[161, 162] Venous occlusion,[162] lipid infiltration[163] of the intima, sclerosis, and hyalinization[164] have been associated with phlebosclerosis in diabetic retinopathy.

Although it is tempting to try to relate phlebosclerosis and lipid infiltration of the intima to such venous changes as fullness and tortuosity, the pathologic changes do not occur as frequently as one might expect and generally such changes are described only in diabetes mellitus. Venular pathology has not been evident in macroglobulinemia, multiple myeloma, polycythemia vera, and severe anemia of varied causes. Ballantyne[165] has stated that the clinical findings suggest stasis on the venous side of the circulation. This may well apply to central retinal vein occlusion, polycythemia vera, polycythemia associated with cyanotic congenital heart disease such as tricuspid atresia or severe pul-

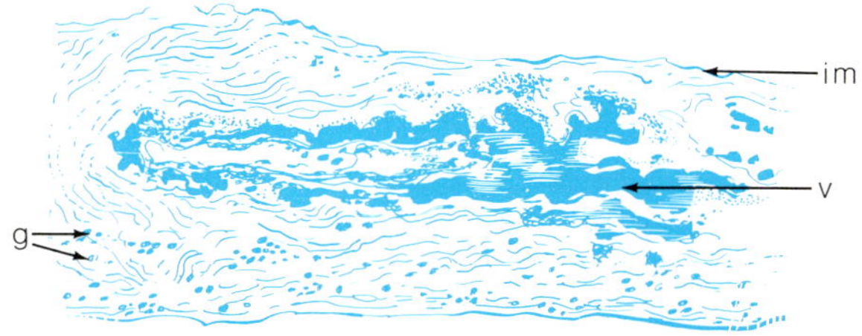

Drawing 133. Plate 133 (v, pigment deposit within and around venous wall; im, internal limiting membrane; g, ganglion cells).

Drawing 134. Plate 134 (v, vein; ci, cellular infiltrate; ip, inner plexiform layer).

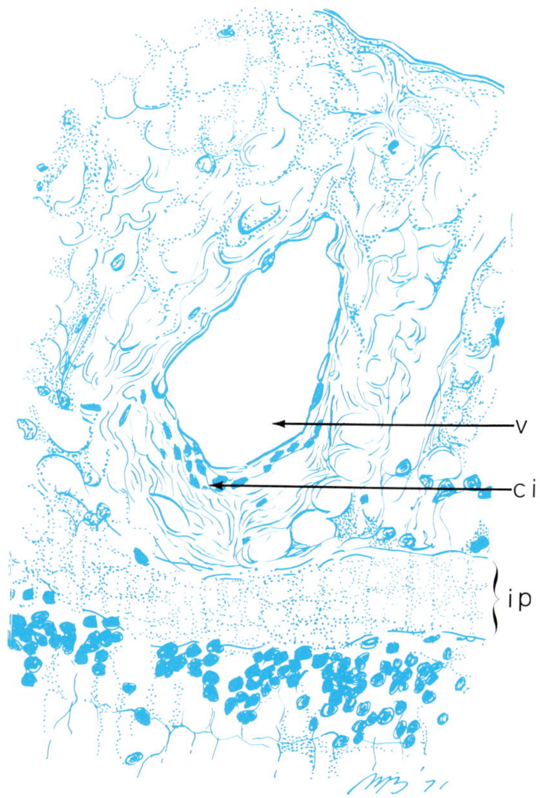

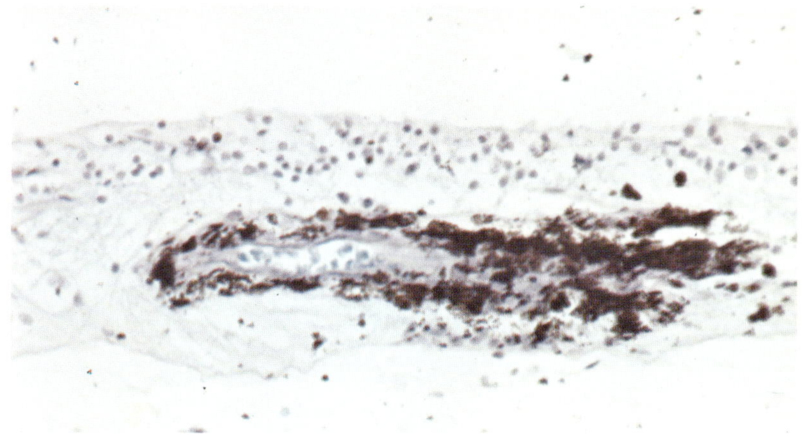

Plate 133. Melanin granules deposited about vein from patient with retinitis pigmentosa (LFB, × 120).

Plate 134. Cellular infiltrate about inferior portion of thickened venular wall. Malignant hypertension (H&E, × 400).

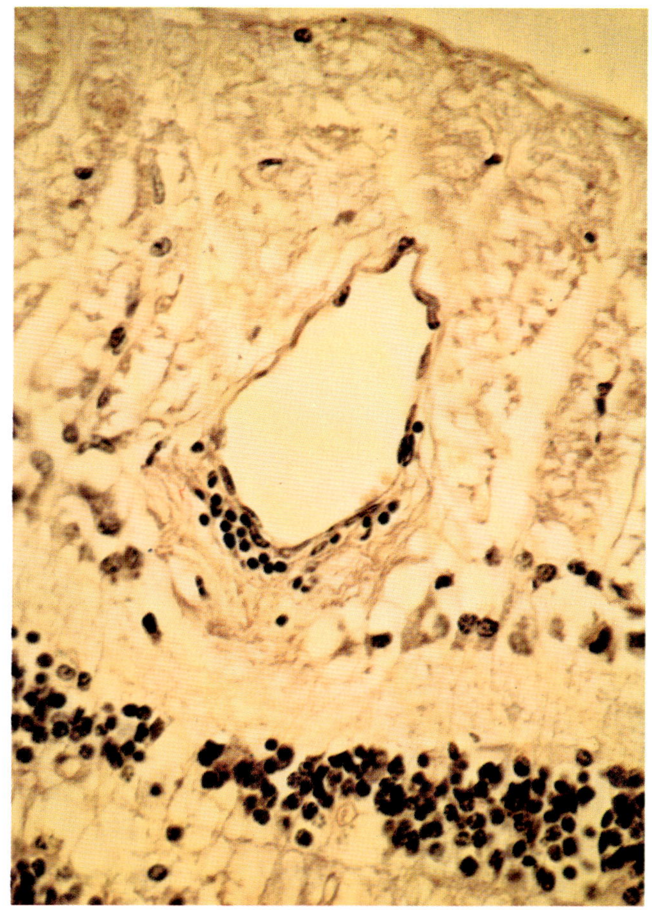

monary disease, macroglobulinemia, and sickle cell disease. That mechanism is not tenable in pernicious and iron deficiency anemias. Yet, clinically recognizable venous abnormalities are frequent in those disorders.

PATHOLOGY AND PATHOGENESIS OF VENOUS SHEATHING

Infiltration of the venous wall, particularly the adventitia, has been described and correlates well with the sheathing observed. In leukemia, the infiltrate consists of leukemic cells;[95] in vasculitis, inflammatory cells (Plate 134 and Drawing 134); in diabetes mellitus, lipid (Plate 132 and Drawing 132); and in retinitis pigmentosa, melanin (Plate 133 and Drawing 133). The explanation for sheathing in central retinal vein occlusion is not obvious.

VENOUS ABNORMALITIES AND CLINICAL STATES

As indicated in the preceding discussion a multiplicity of diseases are associated with venous abnormalities. Generally such changes are accompanied by hemorrhage, particularly in central retinal vein occlusion. Cotton wool patches and hard exudates are frequently associated findings in malignant hypertension, severe anemia, and diabetes mellitus. New vessel formation (neovascularization) and microaneurysms may be present in patients with diabetes.

Diabetes mellitus is the most frequent cause of venous abnormalities. In that disease, venous engorgement, tortuosity, and segmentation may exist without any other evidence of retinopathy and may be present in the absence of overt diabetes. Venous abnormalities are most commonly found in patients under 60 years of age.[166, 167] Retinal venous changes are frequently observed in the presence of proliferative retinopathy[168] (see pp. 147–52). Some observers report that generalized venous dilatation may disappear with improved control of diabetes[133, 169] as well as after pituitary ablation.[170]

Venous abnormalities are commonly found in sickle cell disease as well as in patients with sickle trait.[76] Venous tortuosity was most commonly observed in the (S–S) hemoglobin S and the hemoglobin C (S–C) forms. Retinal venous changes were less commonly observed in the presence of sickle cell trait (SA).

The association of venous engorgement and/or tortuosity with microaneurysms in diabetes mellitus, sickle cell disorders, Waldenström's macroglobulinemia,[171] multiple myeloma,[172, 173] and central retinal vein occlusion is well recognized. Occlusive vascular disease is a common denominator in these disorders. In multiple myeloma and macroglobulinemia, venous stasis resulting from increased viscosity of the blood was also suggested to be the cause of venous abnormalities.[154, 171]

ANNOTATED BIBLIOGRAPHY

Central Retinal Vein Occlusion

Becker, B. and Post, L. T., Jr.: *Retinal Vein Occlusion; Clinical and Experimental Observations*, Am. J. Ophthalmol., **34:** 677, 1951. A good discussion of the clinical findings of retinal vein occlusion in man and in the experimental animal.

Paton, A., Rubinstein, K., and Smith, V. H.: *Arterial Insufficiency in Retinal Venous Occlusion*, Trans. Ophthalmol. Soc. U. K., **84:** 559, 1964. Clinical and experimental data are presented to show the role of arterial insufficiency in the genesis of retinal vein occlusion.

Verhoeff, F. H.: *Obstruction of the Central Retinal Vein*, Arch. Ophthalmol., **36:** 1, 1907. An excellent presentation of the pathological alterations of the central retinal vein.

Venular Disease

Ballantyne, A. J. and Lowenstein, A.: *The Pathology of Diabetic Retinopathy*, Trans. Ophthalmol. Soc. U. K., **63:** 95, 1943. One of the very good early descriptions of the pathology of the retina in diabetes mellitus. The discussion of venous changes is still up to date.

Ballantyne, A. J. and Michaelson, I. C.: *Textbook of the Fundus of the Eye*, 2nd ed., pp. 99–105, Williams & Wilkins, Baltimore, 1970. A good and concise presentation of retinal venous changes.

Chapter V

THE MICROANEURYSM

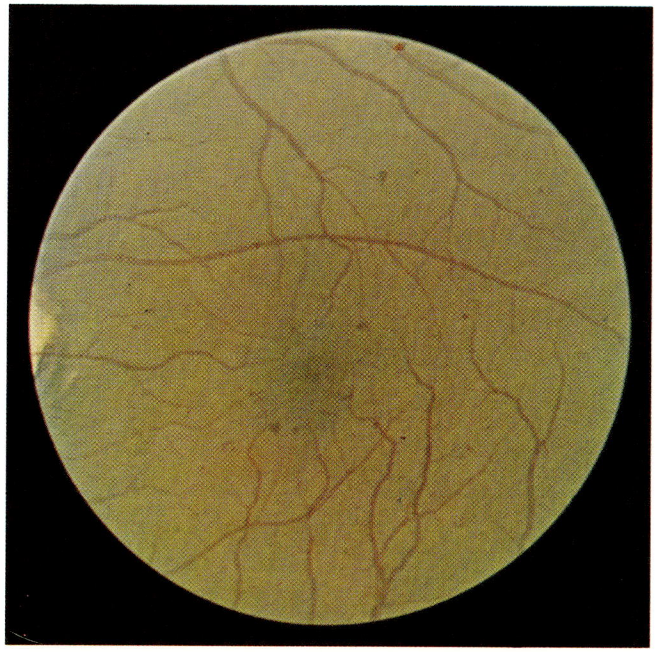

Plate 135. O.S. Two microaneurysms in the region of the macula. Each one appears to be attached to a small blood vessel.

CLINICAL APPEARANCE

The microaneurysm appears as a discrete small red dot (Plate 135); on occasion, it may appear to be attached to a small vascular twig. Although the lesion may occur throughout the retina, it frequently is first observed in the macular region. As a rule the largest number of aneurysms are located in the area between the optic disc and macula. The number of visible microaneurysms is markedly increased with the use of fluorescein angiography[174] (Plates 136 and 137). On occasion, hemorrhage may be noted around the aneu-

Plate 136. O.D. Several microaneurysms are barely visible in the macular region.

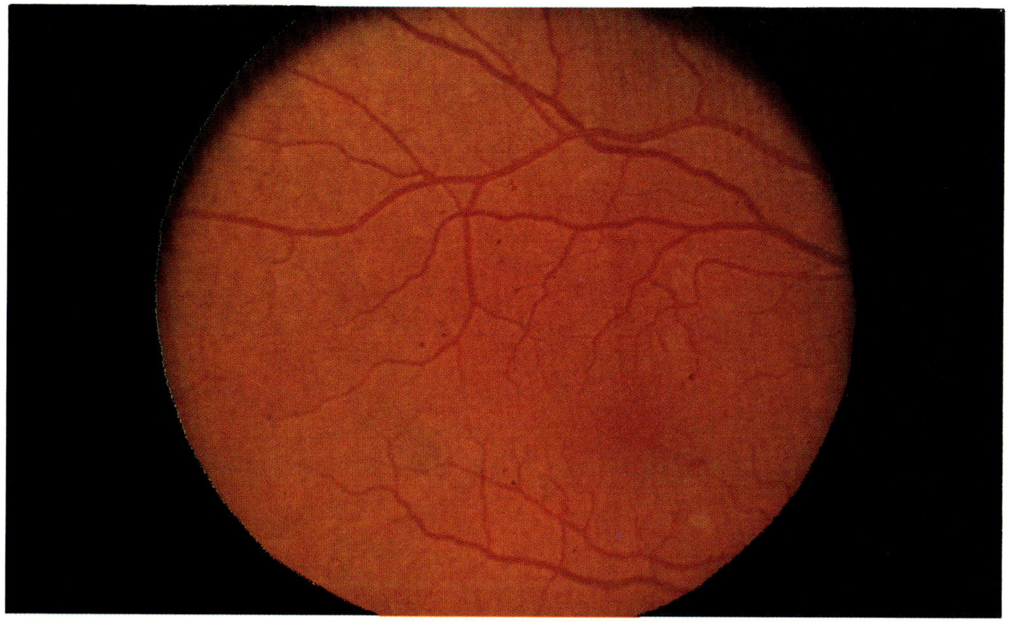

Plate 137. O.D. Fluorescein angiogram of the same patient. Photograph of same area as noted in Plate 136. Note marked increase in number of visible microaneurysms filled with fluorescein.

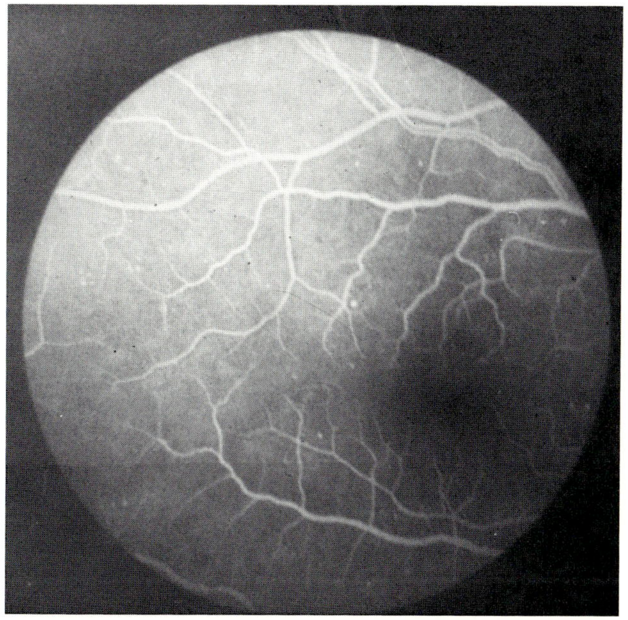

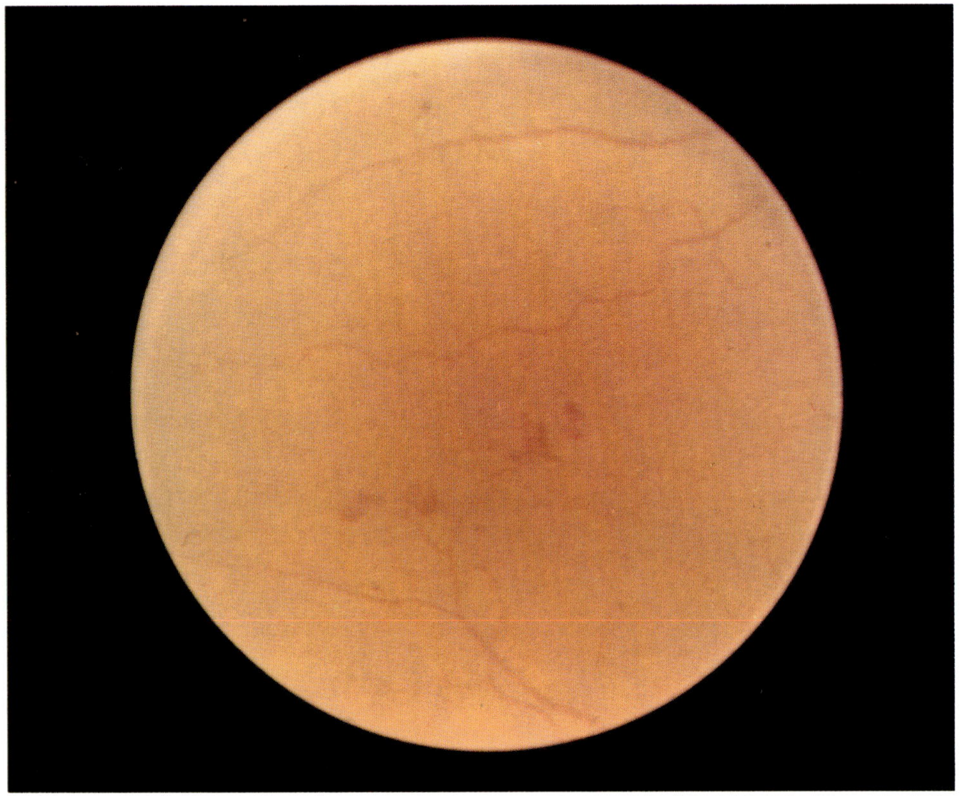

Plate 138. Several areas of hemorrhage which are intermingled with microaneurysms. Did you notice the venous tortuosity?

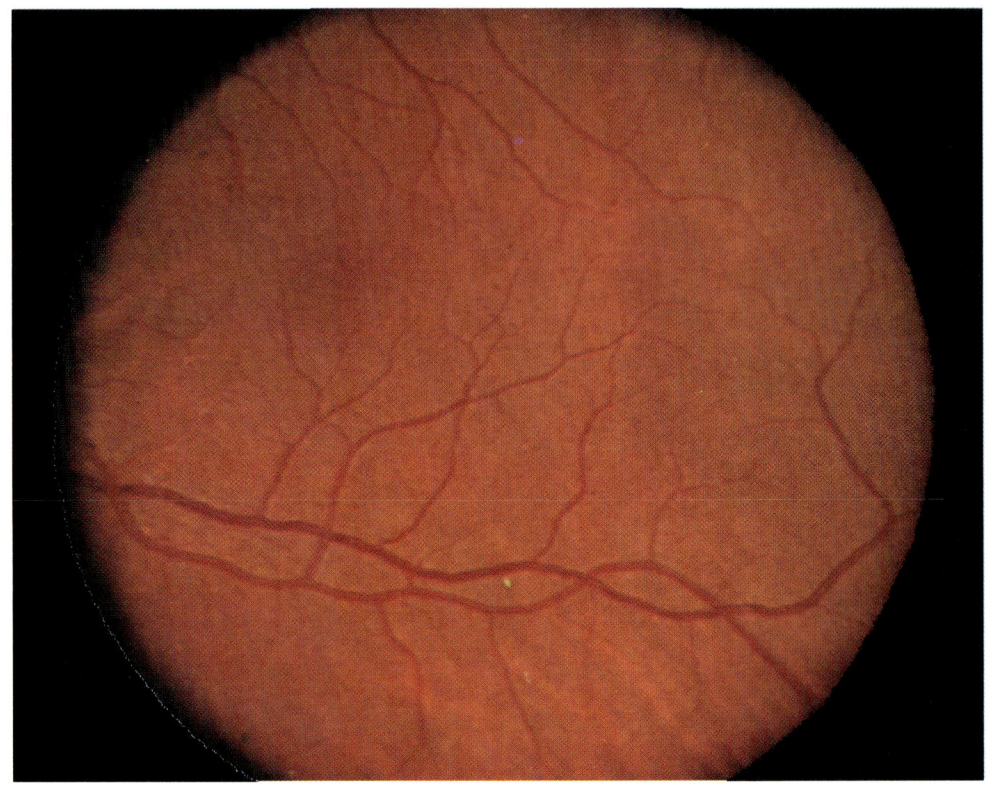

Plate 139. O.S. Temporal. White dot (probably a thrombosed microaneurysm) located below the inferior temporal venule.

rysms, presumably the result of extrusion of blood through their walls (Plate 138). Reference is frequently made to the difficulty of distinguishing the microaneurysm from a small round hemorrhage. The aneurysm is discrete and fluorescein angiograms show it as an outpouching of the vessel wall. Although it will generally persist for several months, it may either disappear completely[75] or develop a white halo and ultimately be replaced by a white dot,[175, 176] presumably the result of hyalinization and cicatricization of the aneurysm[165] (Plate 139). In contrast, the hemorrhage has a hazy and less distinct border and disappears within a period of weeks leaving no clinical residua.[175, 176] In addition, when angiography is performed the hemorrhage will neither fluoresce nor have a vascular attachment. The microaneurysm may occur without any other signs of retinopathy. More likely, however, it is accompanied, and at times preceded, by such venous changes as tortuosity, engorgement, and segmentation. Hemorrhage, cotton wool patches, and hard exudates are frequently associated lesions (Plates 140 and 141). Did you notice the discrete white dots in Plates 140 and 141? They probably represent hyalinized microaneurysms. That microaneurysms may develop rapidly is evident from the observations of clinical and experimental retinal vein occlusion.[152] In clinical observations the microaneurysms are visible within several weeks after the onset of venous occlusion. Generally the other characteristics of that disorder such as venous engorgement, hemorrhage, neovascularization, and hyperemia of the optic disc are evident as well. In the laboratory animal, histologic evidence of microaneurysms was present two to three days after experimental occlusion of retinal veins.

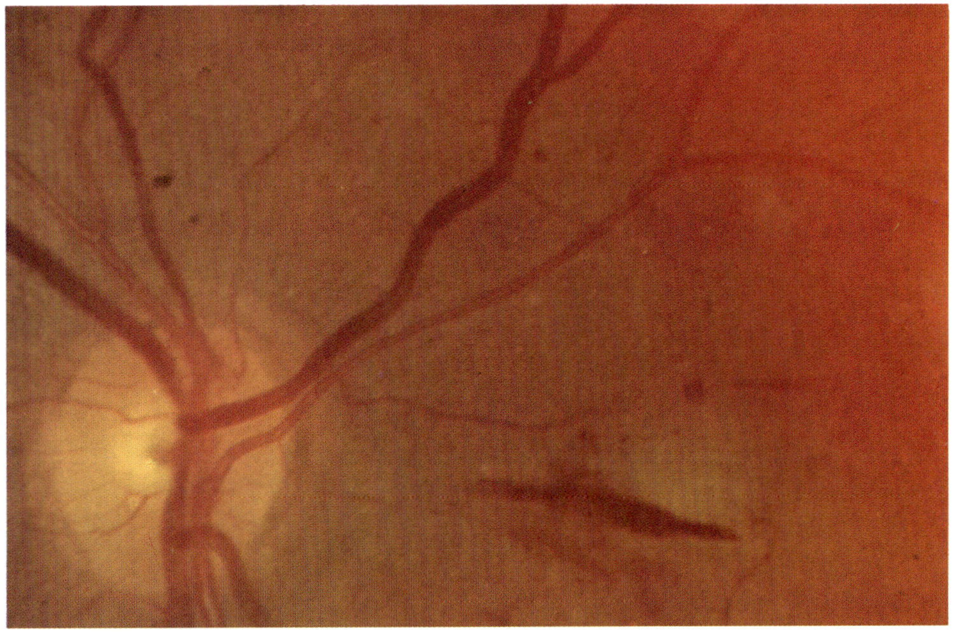

Plate 140. O.D. Nasal area. Microaneurysms, linear hemorrhage, cotton wool patch, and venous tortuosity.

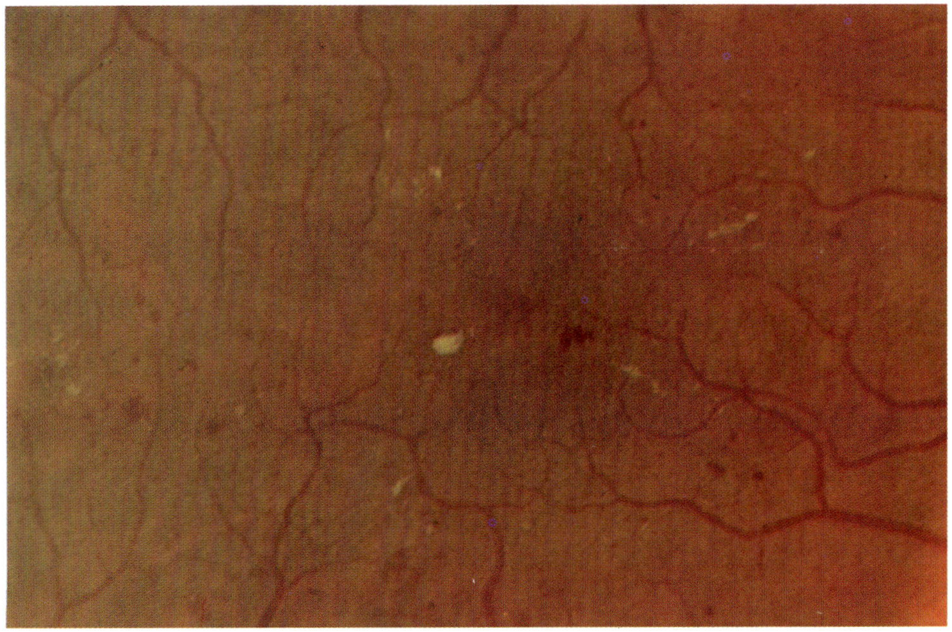

Plate 141. Macular area. Microaneurysms and hard exudates.

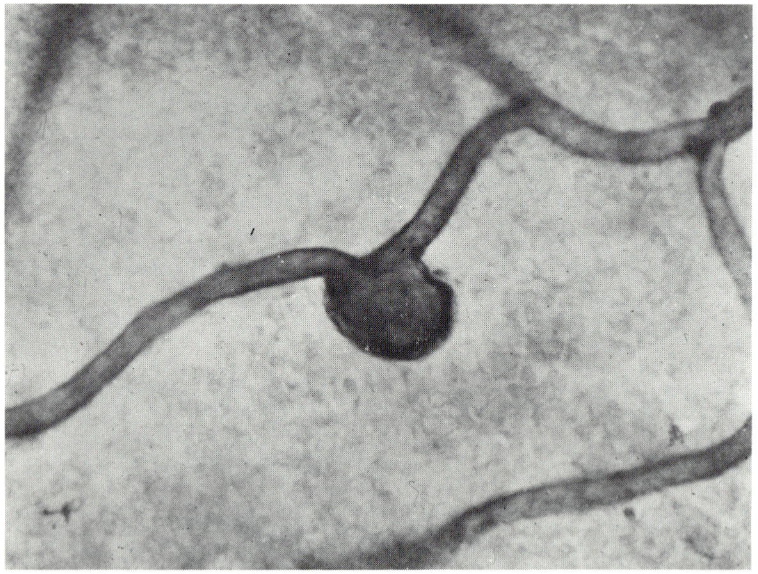

Plate 142. Saccular outpouching arising from one side of a capillary wall. Aneurysm wall appears to be thickened. Whole retinal flat mount, stained by periodic acid–Schiff method (PAS).

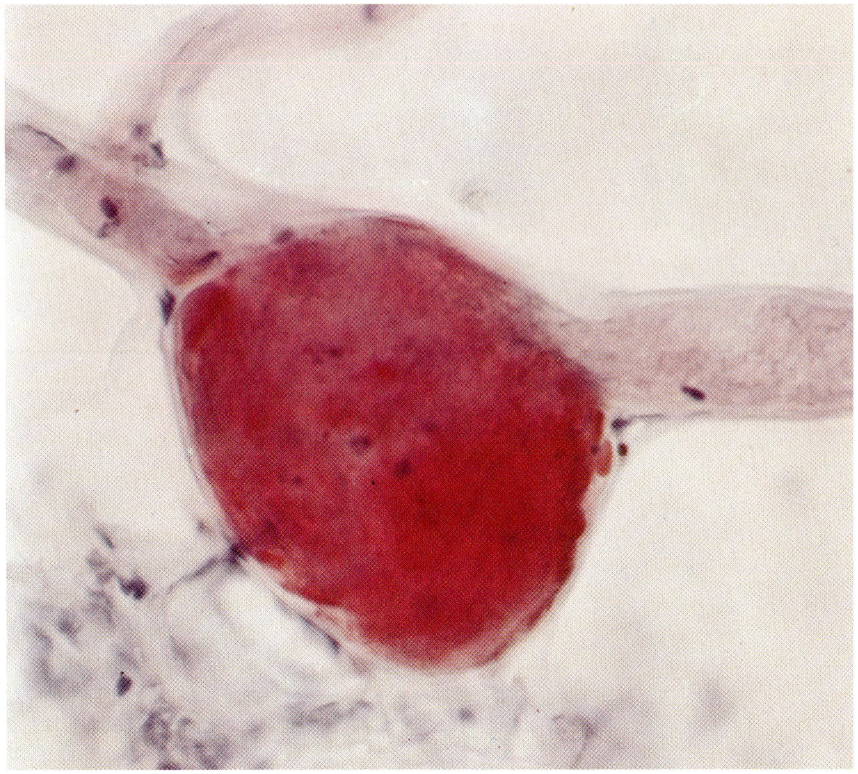

Plate 143. Lipid–containing microaneurysm. Its wall is continuous with that of capillary. Retinal digest (Schar. R stain, approx. × 400).

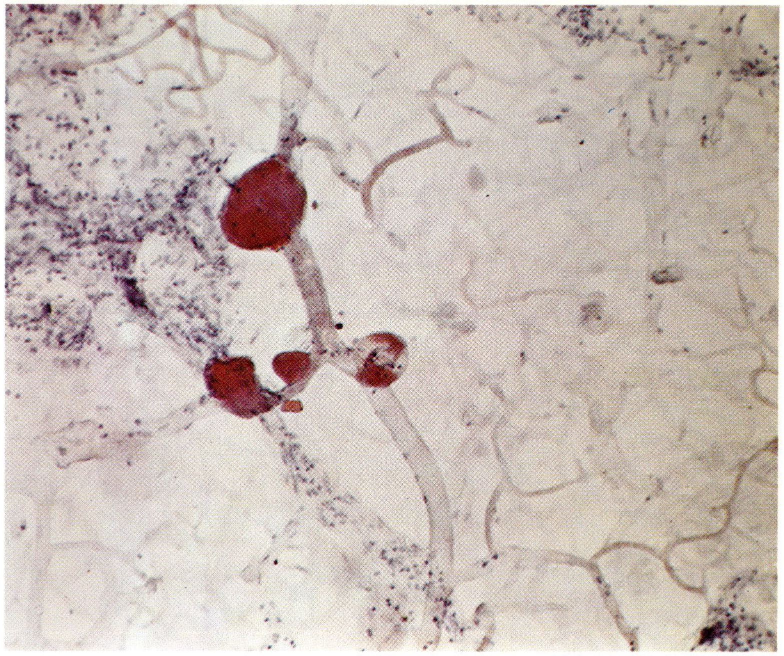

Plate 144. Cluster of lipid–filled microaneurysms arising from acellular vessels. Note lipid-occluded capillaries. Retinal digest (Schar. R, × 80). (Chester, E. M. and Banker, B. Q., *The Role of Lipid Thrombi in Pathogenesis of Diabetic Retinopathy,* Arch. Intern. Med., **120:** 391, 1967.)

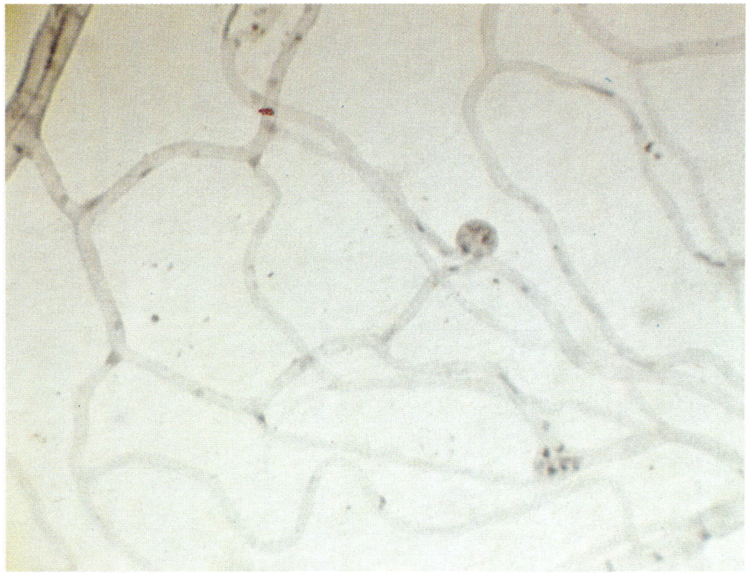

Plate 145. Two microaneurysms containing cellular elements. Retinal digest (Schar. R, approx. × 20).

Plate 146. Microaneurysm connected via a capillary to another microaneurysm which appears to be completely hyalinized with PAS positive material. Did you notice the outer plexiform deposits? (PAS, × 250).

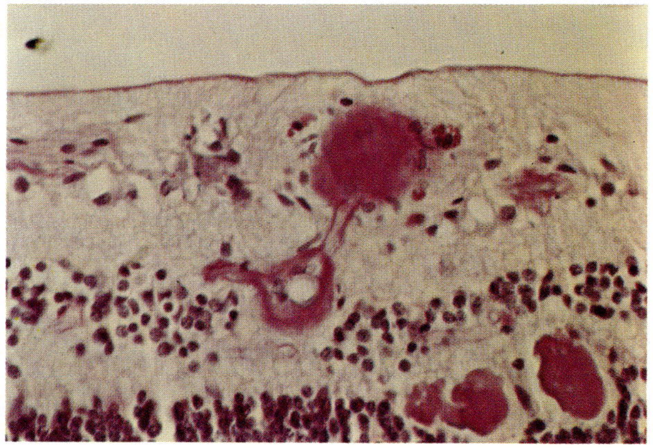

PATHOLOGY

The microaneurysm, a saccular outpouching, 20–90 micra in size, appears on one side of the vessel wall (Plate 142). Although it generally arises from either a venous or arteriolar capillary, it may originate from arterioles, precapillary arterioles, or venules. Its walls are continuous with those of the vessel from which it originates (Plate 143). The aneurysms often occur in clusters, particularly in the central and paracentral regions of the retina (Plate 144). They vary in appearance, ranging from small saccular or fusiform outpouching on one side of the capillary wall, producing a beaded effect, to large globular swellings. Lipid, fibrin, endothelial cells, leukocytes, erythrocytes, and cellular debris are often found within their lumens (Plate 145). The lumen may be completely occluded by a laminated thrombus (Plate 146).

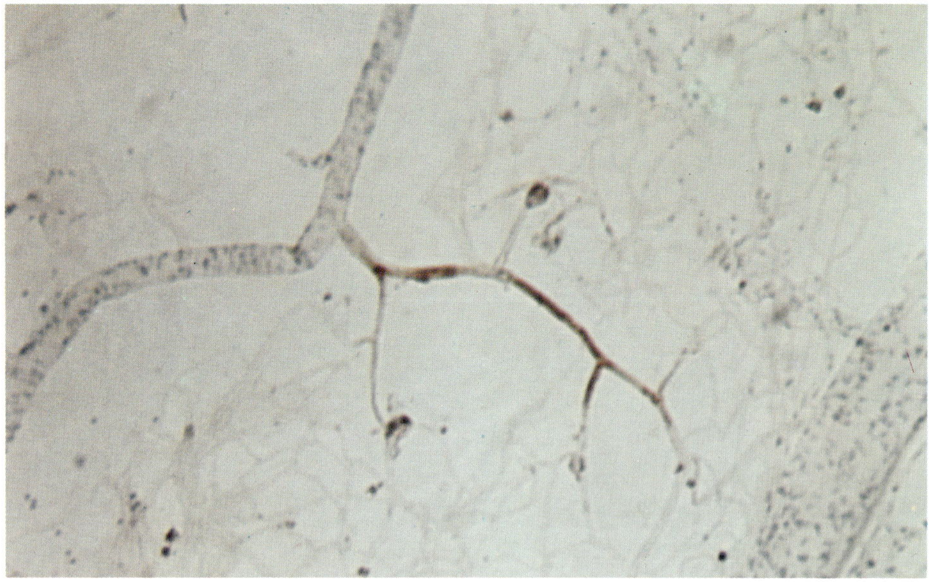

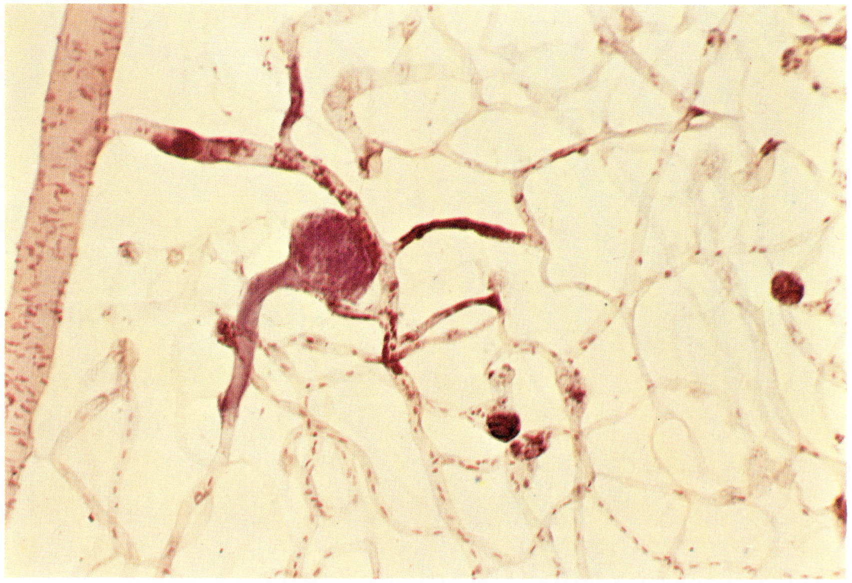

Plates 147 and 148. Microaneurysms arising from lipid–occluded capillaries and precapillary arterioles. Note acellular capillaries connected to lipid–occluded vessels. Retinal digests (Schar. R, approx × 20).

Plate 149 and 150. Microaneurysms arising from acellular or fibrin–occluded capillaries in malignant hypertension. PTAH stain—retinal digests (149 × 80 approx.) (150 × 100 approx.).

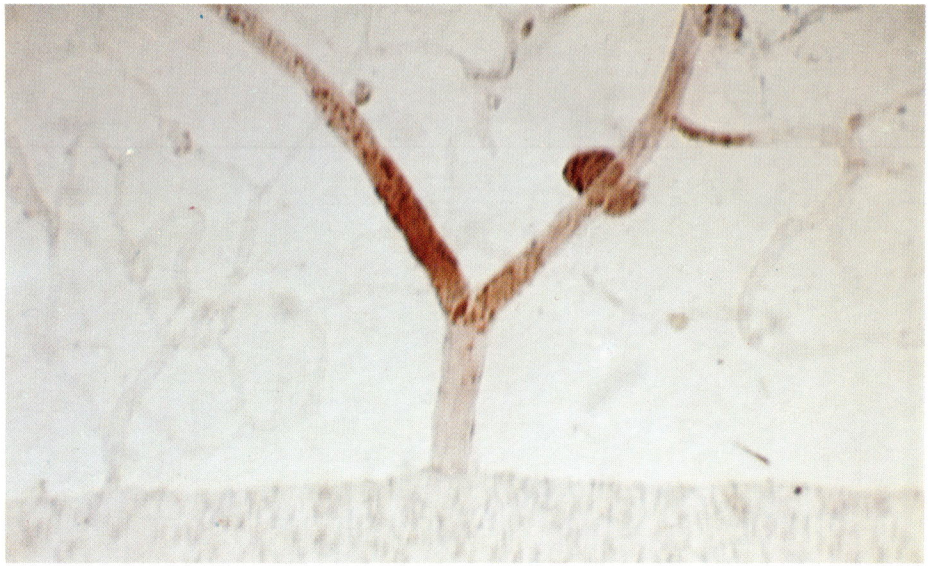

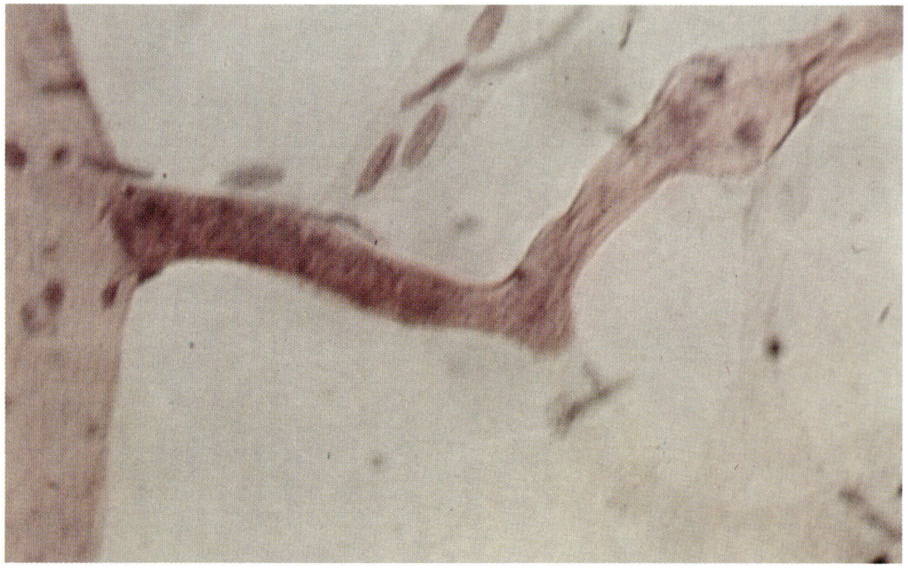

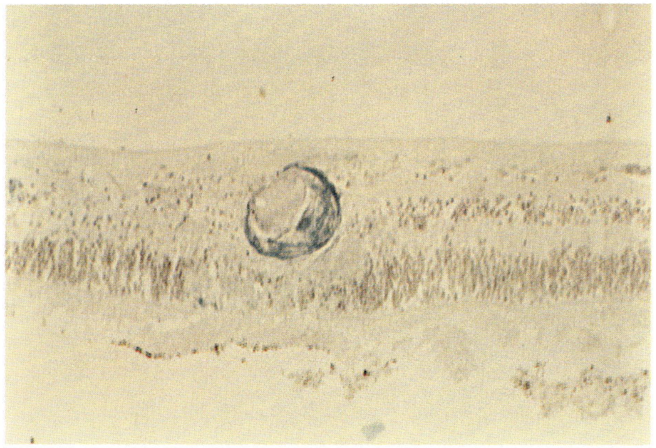

Plate 151. Microaneurysm which extends through inner plexiform and nuclear layers (LFB, × 80).

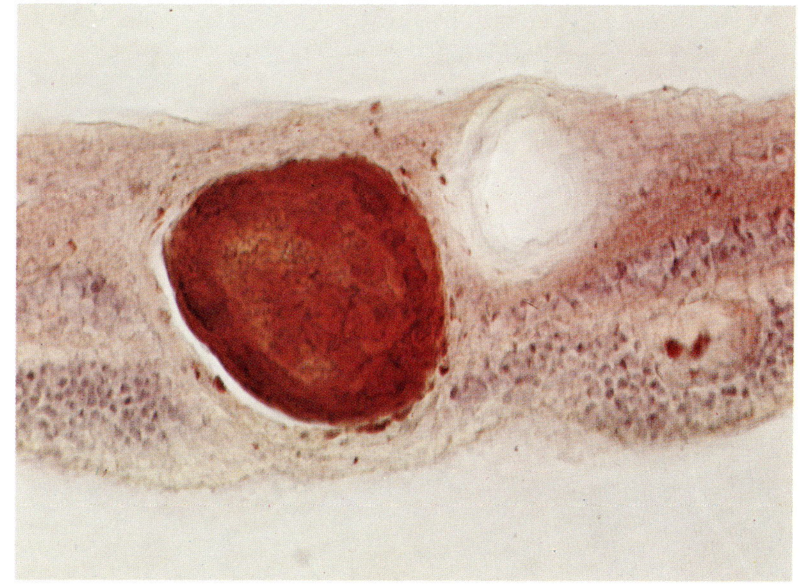

Plate 152. Large lipid-filled microaneurysm extending from nerve fiber layer to outer plexiform layer. Whole retina embedded in gelatin (oil red 0, × 120).

The vessel of origin is invariably abnormal (Plates 143–145). It is either occluded with lipid[104] (Plates 147 and 148) or fibrin[103] (Plates 149 and 150), completely acellular or devoid of mural cells. Cogan, Toussaint, and Kuwabara[177] state that microaneurysms border zones of acellular capillaries and originate from vessels which have normal or hyperplastic endothelial lining without mural cells. In contrast, Chester and Banker[104] found aneurysms arising from capillaries which usually contained neither endothelial nor mural cells.

Although it is difficult to detect in paraffin or gelatin embedded sections of whole retina, the microaneurysm is most frequently observed in the inner nuclear and inner plexiform layers (Plate 151). It may, however, extend throughout the entire thickness of the retinal tissue (Plate 152). Its wall appears thickened in embedded or flat mounted whole retina, as well as in trypsin–digested flat mounts. When stained with periodic acid–Schiff reagent, the wall stains a purple–red color, suggesting the presence of glycoprotein (Plate 153). Bloodworth[15] describes

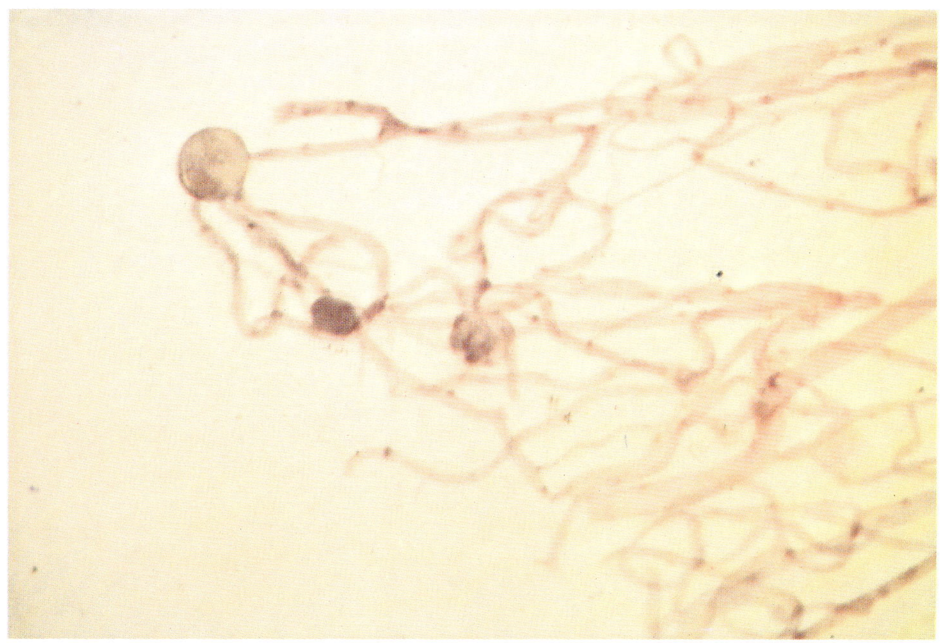

Plate 153. Hyalinized microaneurysm with thickened, purple–red stained walls. Retinal digest (PAS, approx. × 20).

microaneurysms with duplicated basement membranes. He observed pericytes and red blood cells within the split in the wall. He suggests that breaks in the wall of the basement membrane permit blood to separate the layers of that structure and form dissecting aneurysms. A thickened basement membrane of the wall of the microaneurysm has been described in electron microscopic studies of diabetic retinopathy by several investigators.[178-180] In addition, alteration of mural cells and proliferation and loss of endothelial cells were observed.[180]

The concept of a generalized diabetic microangiopathy has developed as a result of the ultramicroscopic evidence of capillary basement membrane thickening in glomerular,[179] retinal,[179] muscle,[181, 182] and dermal tissues.[183] Even prior to the development of such evidence, efforts were made to find the microaneurysm in other tissues of the diabetic; Friedenwald[175] found only one microaneurysm in a study of the brain in ten patients with diabetes. Ashton[184] found no microaneurysms in either cerebral vessels or meninges in patients with diabetes mellitus. His[184] studies of the omentum, peritoneum, pleura, pericardium, bladder wall, liver, and renal capsules were fruitless regardless of whether diabetic retinopathy was present. In addition, he could not find microaneurysms in tissues of the eye other than the retina, including the iris, ciliary body, choroid, or conjunctiva. Contrasting evidence has been presented by other investigators[185, 186] who found microaneurysms in the conjunctiva during a clinical study of patients with diabetes mellitus. In one study conjunctival biopsies provided histologic confirmation of the microaneurysms.[186] Of added interest is the ultramicroscopic evidence of thickened conjunctival capillary basement membranes in diabetic patients.[187]

PATHOGENESIS

Although Mackenzie and Nettleship[188] identified the microaneurysm histologically in 1877, its mechanism of production is still not completely understood. Fusion of kinked capillary loops[189] and traction of mesodermal bridges between capillaries[190] have been offered as mechanisms for the production of localized capillary dilatation. Cogan *et al.*,[74, 191] referring specifically to diabetic retinopathy, offer the loss of the mural cell as the basic lesion responsible for the formation of the microaneurysm. They[191] contend that the mural cells normally maintain retinal capillary tone and thus insure uniform distribution of blood throughout the vascular bed. The loss of mural cells and corresponding loss of vascular tone, according to their concept, leads to rerouting of blood into capillaries which become distended and act as direct shunts between arterioles and venules. The shunt vessels, which have a normal endothelial lining, are subjected to increased hydrostatic pressure by the increased blood flow. As a result, diffuse distention and saccular outpouchings occur in these vessels. The bypassed capillaries, according to this view, undergo secondary occlusion and are not the direct source of microaneurysm.

Disease of the capillary wall as a cause of microaneurysm formation was first suggested by Ballantyne and Loewenstein.[163] They demonstrated the presence of lipid in the vessel wall and suggested that such changes led to distention and fragmentation of the capillary wall. Subsequently, Pope[192] observed that lipid extruded through the capillary wall resulted in a localized saccular outpouching. By injecting a variety of lipids into the veins of cats, Cook[193] demonstrated collections of lipid in retinal capillaries associated with multiple vascular outpouching. Chester and Banker,[104] in a study of diabetic retinopathy, demonstrated that the microaneurysm generally arose from acellular capillaries or arterioles. The vessels from which the microaneurysms arose were either occluded by lipid or were acellular branches of the occluded vessel. Based upon these findings, they suggested that vascular occlusion led to ischemia of the distal capillaries with subsequent loss of endothelial and mural cells. They[104] postulated that the occlusive phenomena led to localized dilatation at the site of thrombosis with subsequent sacculation and aneurysm formation in the acellular vessels. The demonstration of capillary occlusion in patients with diabetic retinopathy by the use of fluorescein angiography offers clinical support for that concept.[194]

The fact that microaneurysms occur in diseases other than diabetes is well known and suggests the presence of a common denominator of the basic lesion. That vascular occlusion occurs in many of the diseases associated with retinal microaneurysm formation is well known. Such diseases include retinal vein occlusion in man and in the experimental animal,[152] sickle cell disease,[195] and malignant hypertension [103, 196] Microscopic study of the trypsin–digested retina of patients with accelerated hypertension demonstrates that the microaneurysm, as in the diabetic, arises from acellular or occluded capillaries. In malignant hypertension the occlusive material has the staining characteristics of fibrin.[103, 104]

No evidence to support the concept relating vascular occlusion to microaneurysm formation can be found in the few recent histologic studies of the retina in Waldenström's macroglobulinemia and multiple myeloma by Ashton and coworkers.[171, 172] They demonstrated the presence of lipid–filled microaneurysms in those diseases without evidence of occlusive disease.

In animals, microaneurysms have been demonstrated in experimentally induced diabetes mellitus[197-201] as well as in spontaneously occurring disease.[202] Injection of egg albumin into the vitreous of cats[203] and the production of the Schwartzman reaction in rabbits[204] have been associated with the presence of retinal microaneurysms. Despite the successful production of such lesions in the laboratory animal, little has been added to the understanding of the mechanism of their production.

THE MICROANEURYSM AND CLINICAL STATES

The microaneurysm occurs most commonly in patients with diabetes mellitus. Less frequently retinal aneurysms are found in central retinal vein occlusion,[150, 152] malignant hypertension,[103, 196, 205] pernicious anemia,[197] thrombotic glaucoma, retinoblastoma, choroidal melanoma, uveitis,[205] multiple myeloma,[172] Waldenström's macroglobulinemia,[171] sickle cell disease,[195] the vasculitis of Eale's disease,[96] angiomatosis retinae,[206] and pulseless disease.[70, 75]

While microaneurysms are described in many diseases, their dominant cause is diabetes mellitus. Therefore, that diagnosis should be considered first whenever retinal aneurysms are observed. Although overt diabetes was not detected in the majority of the case reports of microaneurysms in the above diseases, glucose tolerance tests were infrequently performed. This oversight may be significant since retinal aneurysms may be observed in the diabetic before the disease becomes obvious through its usual clinical manifestations. Characteristically, venous abnormalities accompany the microaneurysm in diabetes mellitus. Eventually hard exudates, cotton wool patches, hemorrhage, and neovascularization are noted as well. Massive vitreous hemorrhage and proliferative retinopathy may obscure the underlying retina.

ANNOTATED BIBLIOGRAPHY

The Microaneurysm

Ashton, N.: *Studies of the Retinal Capillaries in Relation to Diabetic and Other Retinopathies,* Br. J. Ophthalmol., **47:** 521, 1963. A provocative discussion of retinal capillary disease and some views of microaneurysm formation.

Ashton, N.: *Diabetic Micro-Angiopathy,* Bibl. Ophthalmol., **52:** 1, 1958; also Adv. Ophthalmol., **8:** 1, 1958. An excellent review of what was known of the microvascular diseases in diabetes mellitus at that date. The discussion of the microaneurysm presents some of the author's views of its pathogenesis.

Ballantyne, A. J. and Loewenstein, A.: *The Pathology of Diabetic Retinopathy,* Trans. Ophthalmol. Soc. U. K., **63:** 95, 1943. One of the excellent early clinical pathological correlations of the microaneurysm.

Bloodworth, J. M. B., Jr.: *Diabetic Microangiopathy,* Diabetes, **12:** 99, 1963. Presentation of the electron-microscopic changes of the retinal and glomerular capillaries in diabetes mellitus.

Chester, E. M. and Banker, B. Q.: *The Role of Lipid Thrombi in the Pathogenesis of Diabetic Retinopathy,* Arch. Intern. Med., **120:** 397, 1967. An attempt to relate arteriolar and capillary occlusion as the cause of microaneurysm formation.

Cogan, D. G., Toussaint, D., and Kuwabara, T.: *Retinal Vascular Patterns. Part IV, Diabetic Retinopathy,* Arch. Ophthalmol., **66:** 366, 1961. The authors, utilizing the technique of trypsin digestion of the retina, present evidence to support their concept of damage to the mural cell of capillaries as the prime cause of microaneurysm formation in diabetes mellitus.

Cogan, D. G.: *Diabetic Retinopathy,* N. Engl. J. Med., **270:** 787, 1964. A further expression of the importance of mural cell damage and the development of arteriolar–venular shunts in the formation of microaneurysms.

Kohner, E. M. and Henkind, P.: *Correlation of Fluorescein Angiogram and Retinal Digest in Diabetic Retinopathy,* Am. J. Ophthalmol., **69:** 403, 1970. An attempt to correlate the fluorescein angiographic changes of the retina with those observed in retinal digests in diabetic retinopathy.

Stary, H. C.: *Disease of Small Blood Vessels in Diabetes Mellitus,* Am. J. Med. Sci., **252:** 357, 1966. A detailed discussion of the abnormalities of the small blood vessels in diabetes mellitus.

Chapter VI
NEOVASCULARIZATION AND PROLIFERATIVE RETINOPATHY

NEOVASCULARIZATION (NEW VESSEL FORMATION)

Neovascularization of the retina and optic nerve can be defined as the abnormal development of new blood vessels in those structures in response to certain disease states. By definition neovascularization excludes congenital vascular anomalies and persistent fetal hyaloid vessels which normally disappear at or before birth.

It will be apparent in our subsequent discussion of neovascularization of the retina and optic nerve that this pathological process mimics the normal development of the human retinal circulation. A review of the current concepts of normal fetal retinal angiogenesis is presented next as a basis for understanding its pathological counterpart.

Fetal Retinal Angiogenesis in Man

In man, the intrinsic circulatory system of the retina begins to develop at approximately the fifteenth week of intrauterine life. At that time, according to Ashton,[207] mesenchymal cells, which he calls spindle cells, appear in the vicinity of the hyaloid artery. These cells are believed to arise from the adventitia of the hyaloid artery and from venous channels on either side of that vessel. The mesenchymal cells proliferate into the optic nerve and nerve fiber layer of the retina. These primitive cells then differentiate into endothelial cells and form solid cords which canalize and become primitive capillaries. As blood flows through these primitive vessels some of them enlarge to form arteries and veins.[207, 208] By the eighth month the process of retinal vascularization in the fetus is complete.

The above concept of fetal retinal angiogenesis differs from the previously held views offered by Michaelson[209] which stated that:

1. The process originates as vascular buds which arise from a bulbous swelling of the hyaloid artery.
2. The vascular buds, originally solid, become canalized and differentiate directly into arteries and veins.
3. Capillaries develop only from veins.

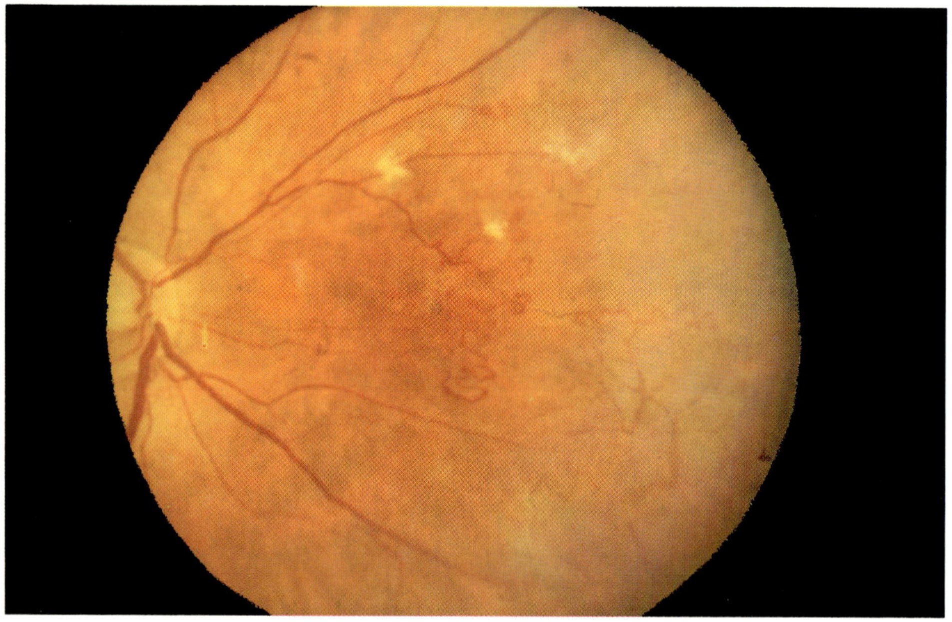

Plate 154. O.D. Nasal. Network of loosely arranged, tortuous vessels on nasal side of the disc. Note irregular white patches overlying blood vessels superior and nasal to disc (spontaneously obliterated new vessels, see p. 139). Cotton wool patches are present at 5 o'clock, 4 disc diameters from the disc.

Plate 155. An enlarged view of a cluster of abnormal new vessels noted in Plate 154.

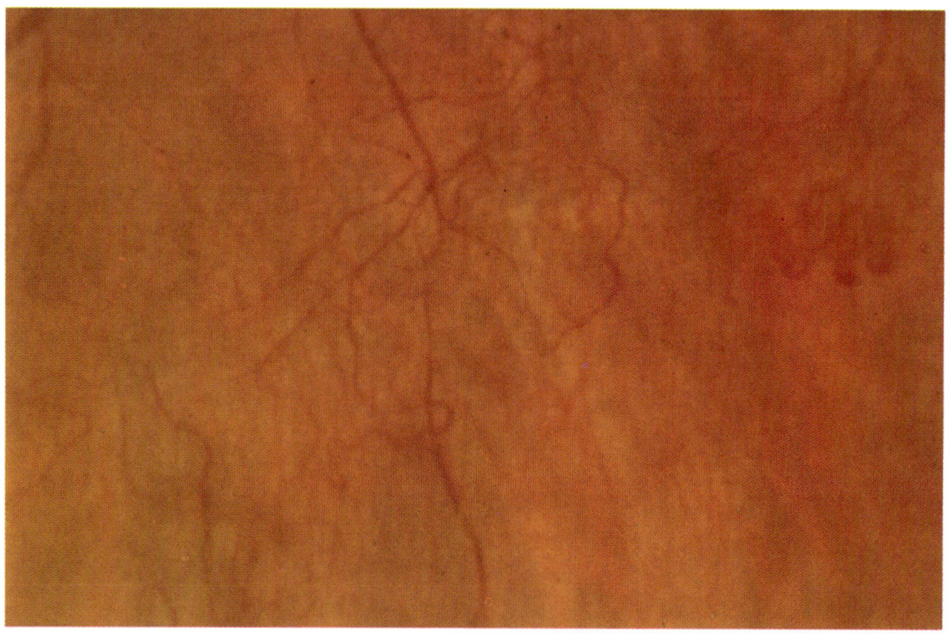

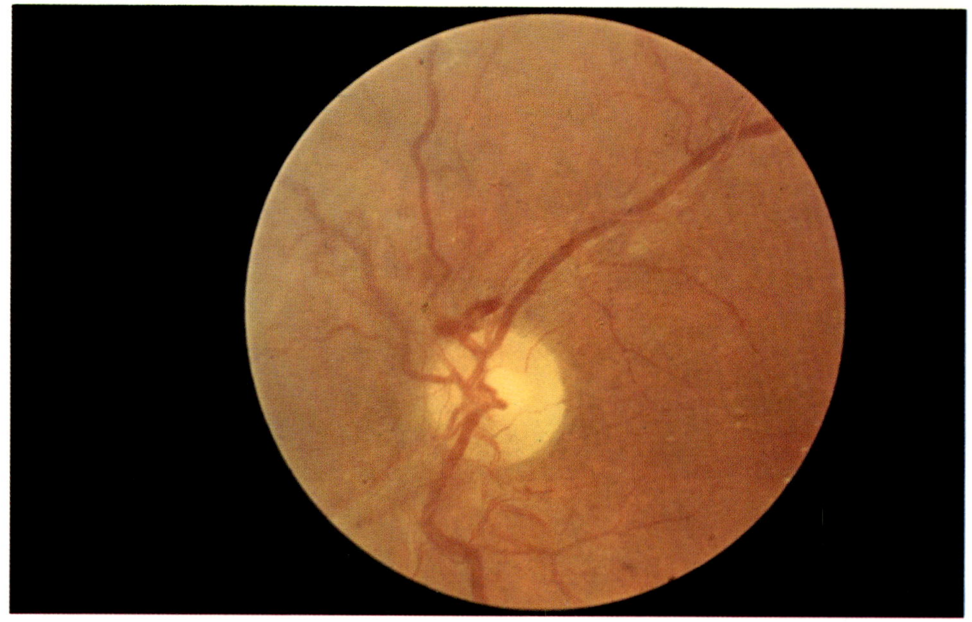

Plate 156. O.S. Central and slightly temporal. New vessel formation inferior and temporal to disc. Did you notice? (1) The venous tortuosity and arteriovenous compression; (2) Two flame–shaped hemorrhages above the disc, one of which is a Roth spot; (3) Several linear hard exudates close to and within the visible portion of the macula.

Plate 157. Enlarged view. Convoluted mass of new vessels (rete mirabile) behind retinal venule.

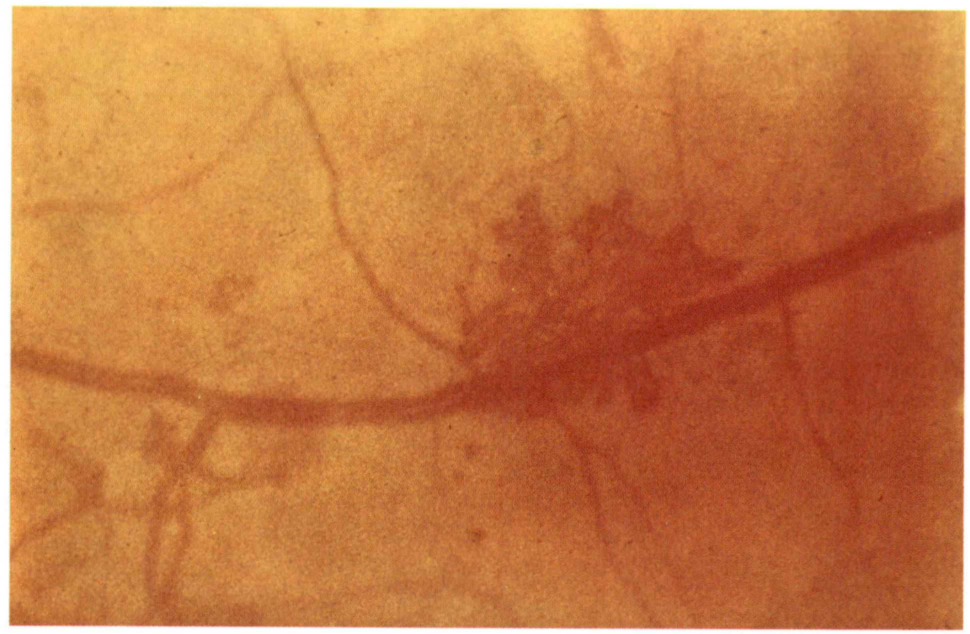

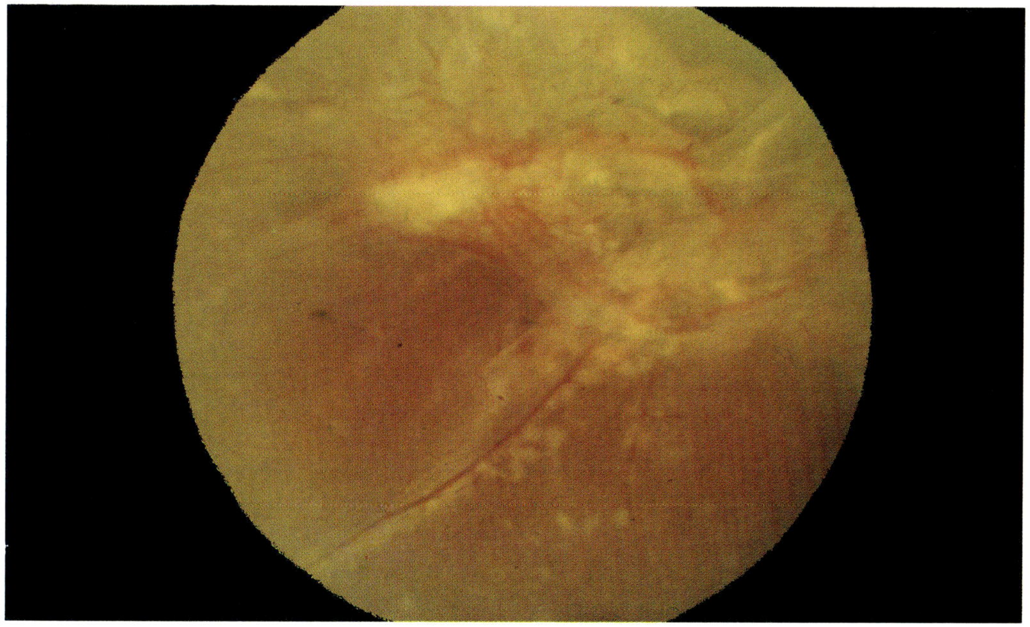

Plate 158. A fine network of new vessels overlie sheets of glistening scar tissue (a good example of proliferative retinopathy). The neovascularization appears to be preretinal. Many hard exudates are also present.

Neovascularization of the Retina

CLINICAL APPEARANCE

Intraretinal new blood vessels appear as a disorderly cluster of fine vascular twigs. They arise from veins and generally cross over the parent vessels, often connecting two or more veins (Plates 154 and 155). Their apparently purposeless course does not appear to lead to surrounding arterioles. The abnormal vessels may be brushlike, rosette–shaped, or just a series of fine vessels curved like a hairpin (Plate 156). The term *rete mirabile* is applied to a mass of interconnected and convoluted vessels (Plate 157).

Preretinal new vessels are anterior to the internal limiting membrane and appear as tufts, fan–shaped masses, or coils of tortuous vessels which extend anteriorly into the vitreous cavity (Plate 158). The vessels which enter the vitreous cavity are generally accompanied by sheets or fan–shaped bands of fibrous tissue, the classic clinical finding of proliferative retinopathy (Plate 158). Although neovascularization is not found in the macular area, it may occur in any other part of the retina which normally contains blood vessels. Newly developed intraretinal vessels may disappear and leave no visible clinical residua. According to Davis,[210] the regression may be incomplete, leaving a tuft of white tissue overlying a retinal vein (Plates 154 and 159). Venous sheathing which progresses to complete vascular obliteration, appearing as white lines without a visible blood column, may also be observed as an end result (Plate 159 and Drawing 159).

Plate 159. A band of scar tissue extends through the central and inferior part of the photograph. The network of white lines represents obliteration of new vessels. Parallel sheathing of the "y" shaped blood vessel is observed. The normal landmarks of the retina are distorted as a result of the neovascularization and proliferation of fibrous tissue (proliferative retinopathy).

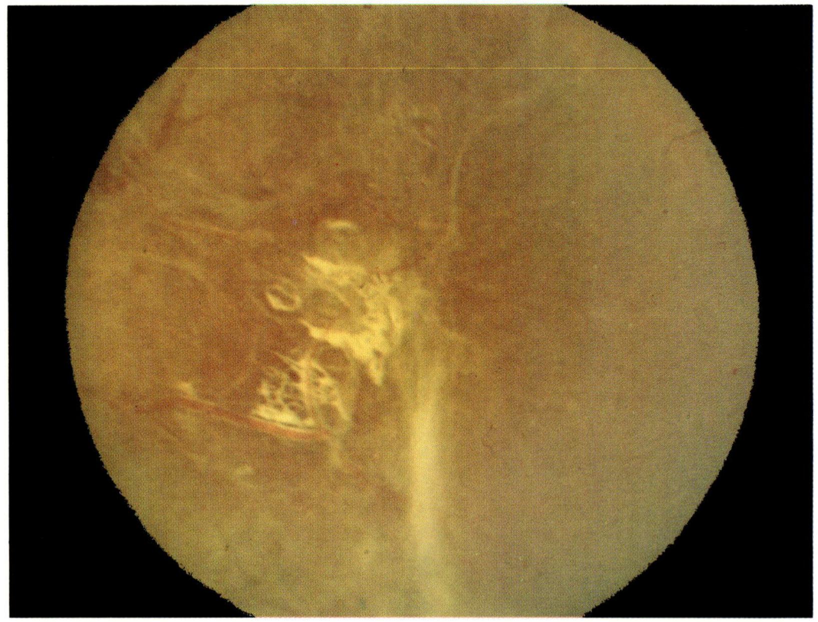

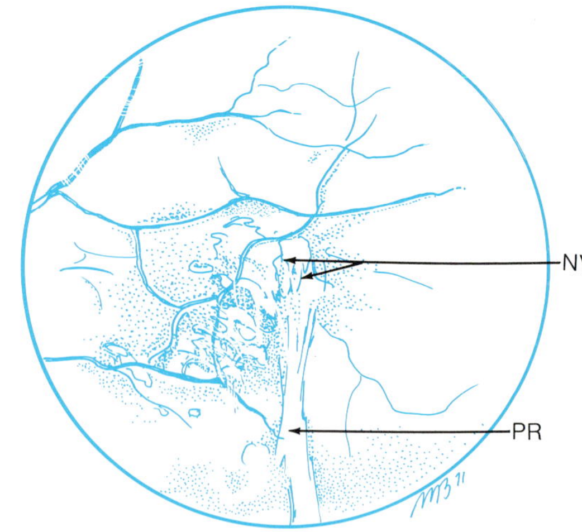

Drawing 159. Plate 159 (PR, proliferative retinopathy; NV, neovascularization).

Plate 160. O.D. Diabetic retinopathy. A network of tortuous new vessels extends from the disc into all four quadrants of the retina. Did you notice? (1) Multiple hemorrhages and microaneurysms visible in the area which extends from 8 to 3 o'clock; (2) Cotton wool patches present at 12 o'clock; (3) Hard exudates at 9 and 1 o'clock in the peripheral part of the retina; (4) Venular tortuosity.

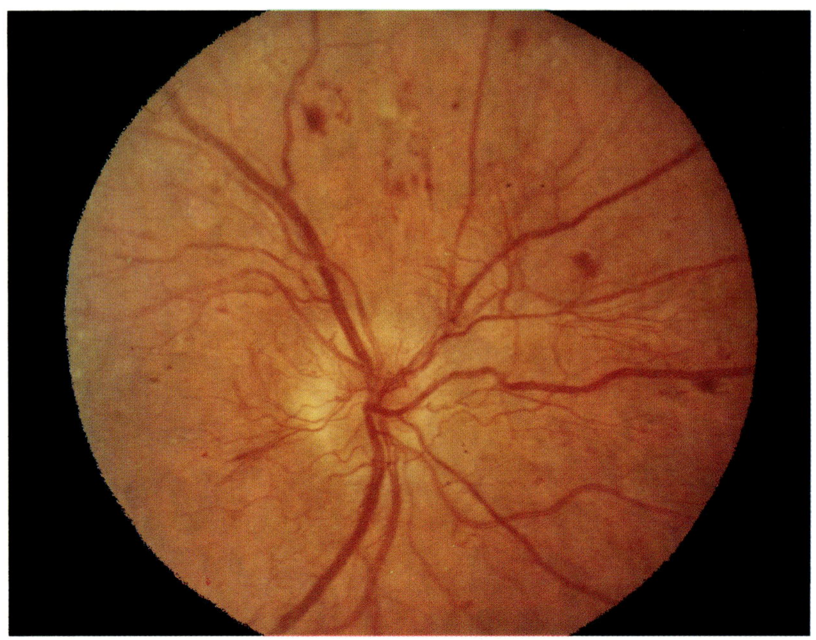

Drawing 160. Plate 160 (NV, neovascularization; HEM, hemorrhage; MA, microaneurysm; V, venular tortuosity; CWP, cotton wool patch; HE, hard exudate).

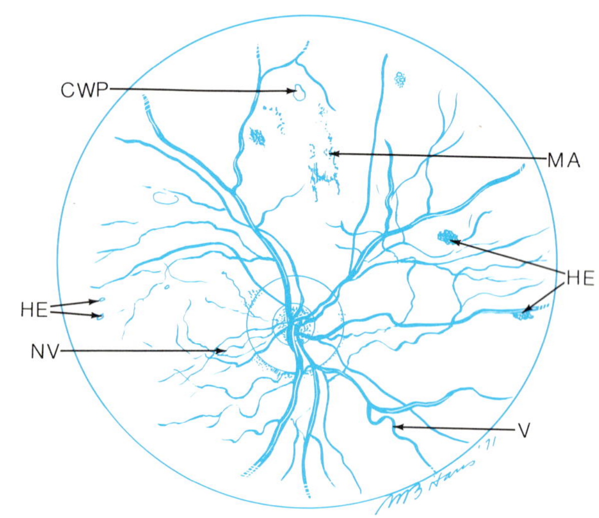

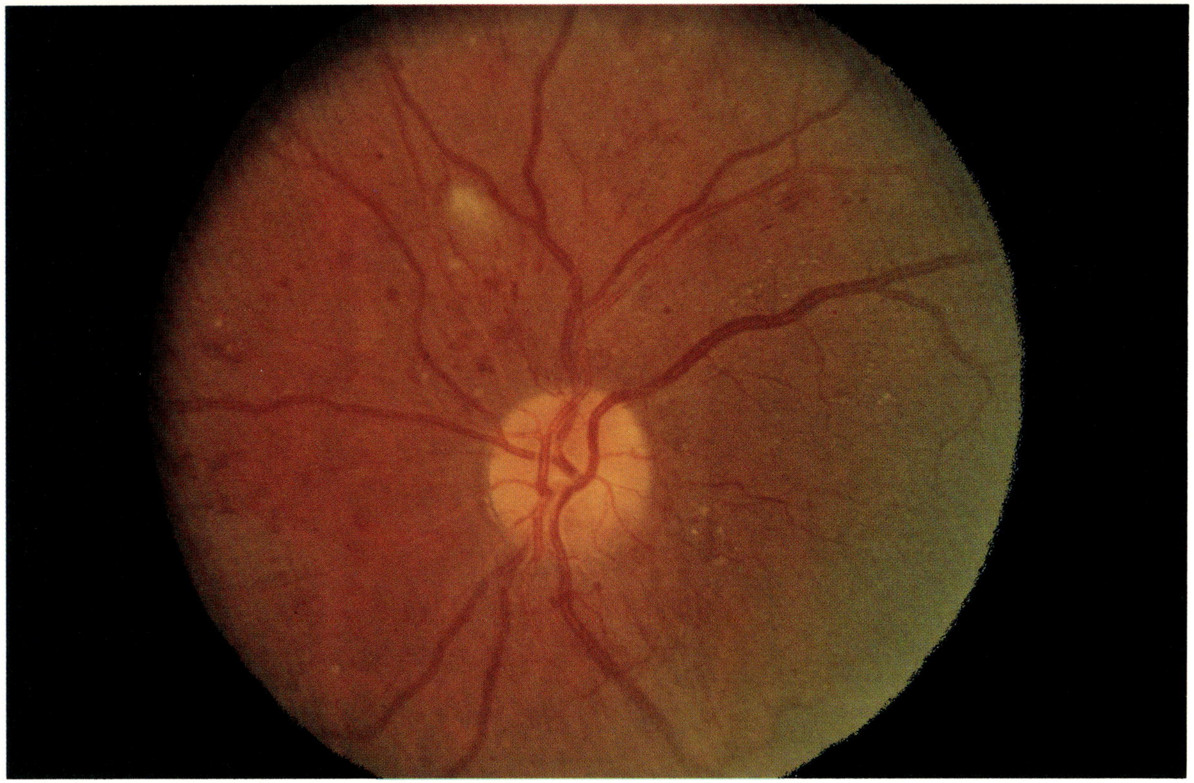

Plate 161. O. S. Diabetic retinopathy. Neovascularization is present at 6 o'clock immediately below the disc. Microaneurysms arise from the new vessels at that site. Another network of new vessels is noted at the superior margin of the disc. Venous tortuousity, multiple hemorrhages, hard exudates, and microaneurysms are also observed. A cotton wool patch is present at 11 o'clock, two disc diameters above the disc.

Neovascularization of the Optic Disc

CLINICAL APPEARANCE

Neovascularization of the disc may manifest itself as no more than an increased number of visible small vessels in the nerve head (Plate 160 and Drawing 160). The newly developed vessels on the disc may be tortuous, coiled, or folded with hairpin–like curves, and often contain bulbous ends which resemble microaneurysms[211, 212] (Plate 161 and Drawing 161). The abnormal vessels often appear as varicosities and resemble hemorrhage. Serial funduscopic examination demonstrates that the neovascularization persists indefinitely, whereas hemorrhage generally disappears within a period of several weeks. Because the internal limiting membrane does not extend over the optic disc, no barrier is offered to its proliferating new vessels and vitreous penetration results.[213]

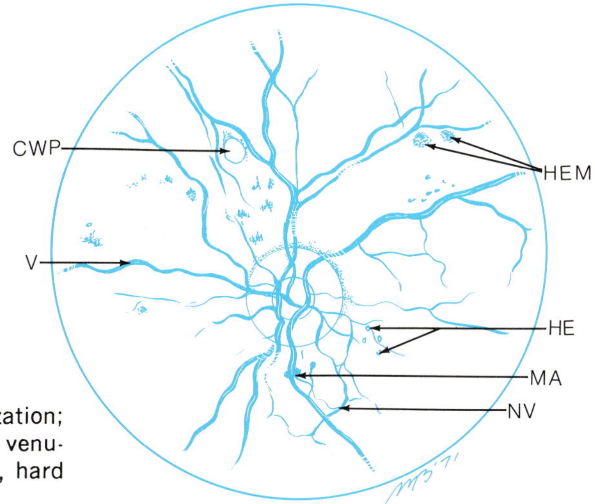

Drawing 161. Plate 161 (NV, neovascularization; MA, microaneurysm; HEM, hemorrhage; V, venular tortuosity; CWP, cotton wool patch; HE, hard exudate).

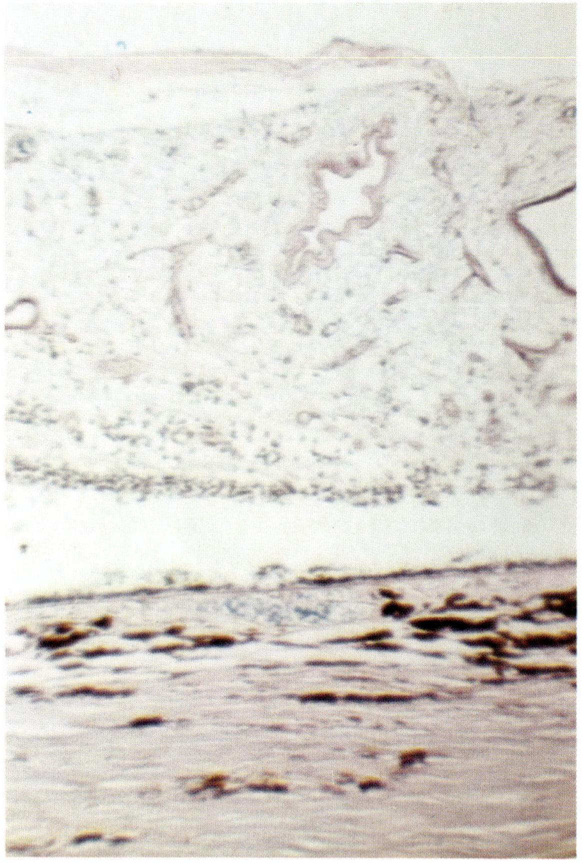

Plate 162. Increase in number of blood vessels throughout anterior 2/3 of retina. Note band of fibrous tissue extending anteriorly from nerve fiber layer (LFB, approx. × 80).

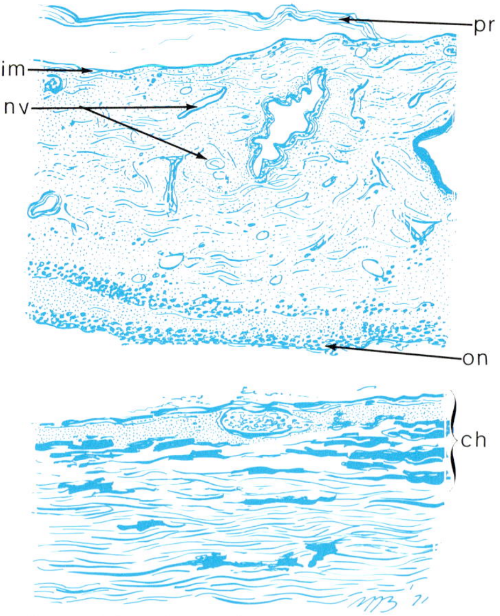

Drawing 162. Plate 162 (pr, proliferative retinopathy; im, internal limiting membrane; nv, neovascularization; on, outer nuclear layer; ch, choroid).

Drawing 163. Plate 163 (nv, neovascularization; im, internal limiting membrane; a, thick-walled arteriole; nf, nerve fiber layer).

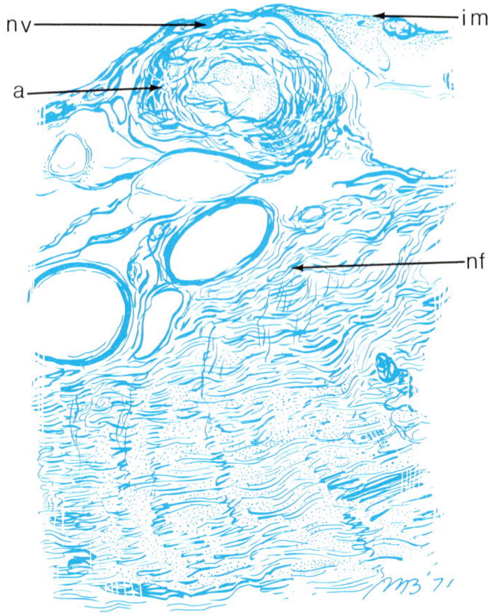

Plate 163. Multiple capillaries beneath internal limiting membrane (LFB, approx. × 80).

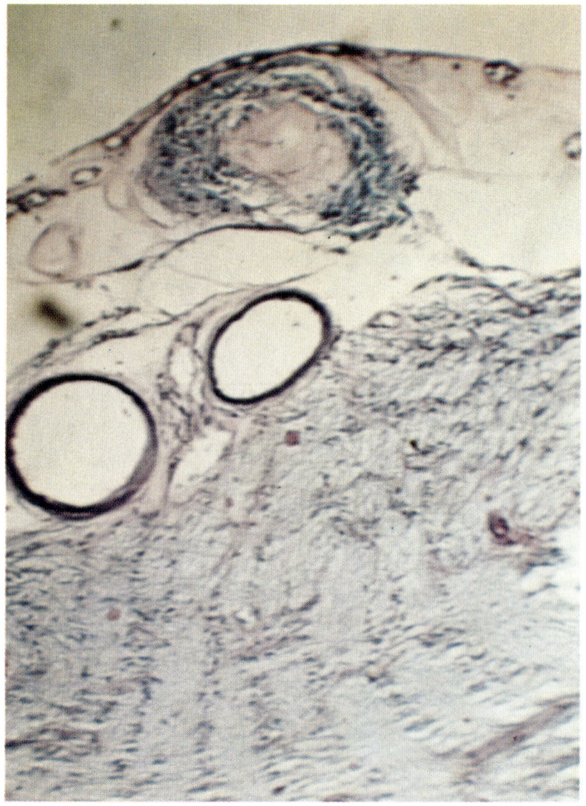

Pathology

The histologic changes of neovascularization are well illustrated by the abnormalities found in retrolental fibroplasia. As described by Ashton,[214] the initial findings consist of a diffuse thickening resulting from the development of small nests of endothelial cells within the nerve fiber layer of the retina. The proliferating endothelial cells canalize, penetrate the internal limiting membrane, extend along the surface of the retina beneath the hyaloid membrane, and penetrate the vitreous. In diabetes mellitus, the most common condition associated with neovascularization, the histologic changes are found to be an increased number of blood vessels of the anterior two-thirds of the retina (Plate 162 and Drawing 162). The new vessels may be confined to the nerve fiber layer and remain behind the internal limiting membrane (Plate 163 and Drawing 163). If penetration of the internal limiting membrane occurs the new vessels are found anterior to that structure (Plate 164 and Drawing 164). Hemorrhage frequently develops from these fragile new vessels with subsequent organization (Plate 165 and Drawing 165). Contracture and retinal detachment follow.[215] According to Ashton,[214] fibroblasts proliferate and accompany the angioblastic tissue which invades the vitreous. As a result fibrous strands develop in the vitreous. In essence, this is the pathologic change of proliferative retinopathy which will be discussed in detail (see pp. 146–52).

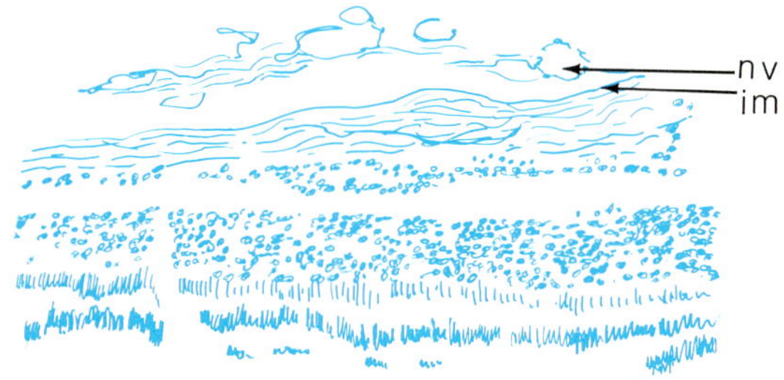

Drawing 164. Plate 164 (im, internal limiting membrane; nv, neovascularization).

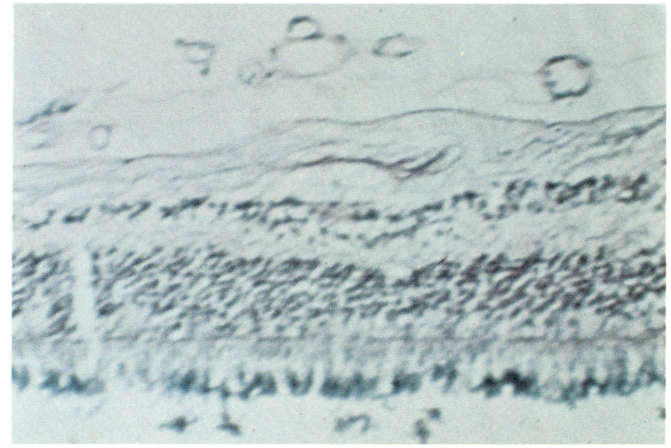

Plate 164. Many small blood vessels and fibrous tissue, anterior to the internal limiting membrane (LFB, approx. × 20).

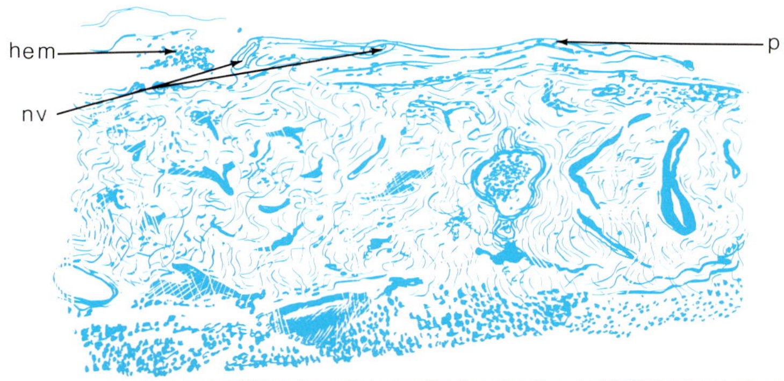

Drawing 165. Plate 165 (pr, proliferative retinopathy (fibrosis); hem, hemorrhage; nv, neovascularization).

Plate 165. Fibrous tissue, new vessel formation, and hemorrhage anterior to the internal limiting membrane (LFB, × 80).

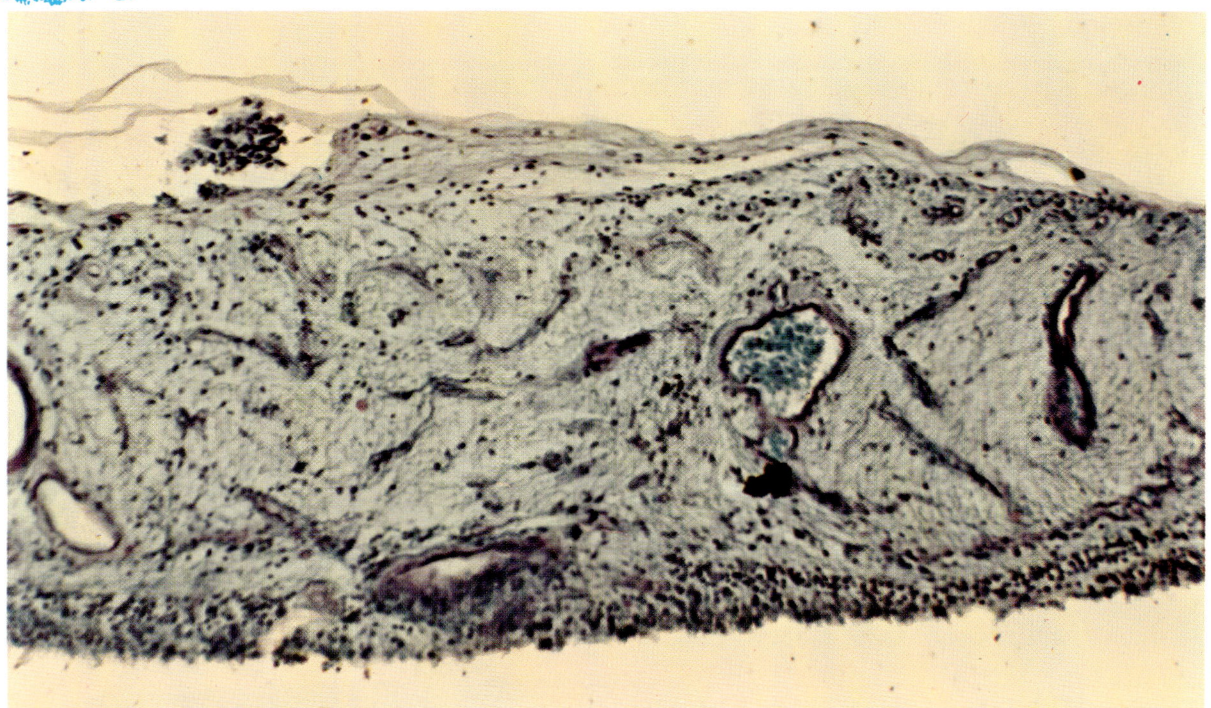

Pathogenesis

Ashton *et al.*[216] produced retinal vaso-obliteration in newborn kittens by exposing them to high oxygen concentrations. When the animals were then allowed to breathe room air, retinal neovascularization, which extended into the vitreous, was observed. Histologically the new vessel growth in the retinae of the kittens duplicated the findings of retrolental fibroplasia in the infant. Studies of chick embryo tissue culture[217] and rabbit ear chamber preparation[218] demonstrated the importance of endothelial outgrowth and migration from pre–existing vessels in neovascularization. Such observations coupled with the experimental evidence relating variation of oxygen concentration to vasoproliferation led Ashton[219] to ask whether endothelial cells are directly sensitive to oxygen. He suggests that endothelial cells may multiply at low oxygen concentration, rest at normal levels, and die at high concentration. Most investigators, however, agree that some extracellular substance may be responsible for neovascularization.[212] Ashton[219] suggests that the presence of living tissue, low oxygen tension, and poor venous drainage are necessary prerequisites. Under these conditions one could postulate that certain retinal diseases lead to local hypoxia and altered tissue metabolism. As a result a metabolite capable of stimulating new vessel formation develops. If venous drainage is impaired, as in central retinal vein occlusion, the abnormal metabolite could accumulate and promote neovascularization. Imre[220] believes that lactic acid is the specific metabolite that stimulates new vessel formation. His concept can be summarized as follows. Retinal disease which leads to local hypoxia promotes anaerobic glycolysis and increased lactic acid formation. If venous drainage is impaired, excess lactate accumulates.*

Successful experimental production of neovascularization has been limited to the young animal with an immature retinal vascular system. Ashton[219] has noted the inability to produce capillary obliteration or endothelial injury in the mature animal with exposure to high oxygen concentrations under pressure. He adds that separation of the retina from the choroid, leading to diminution of retinal oxygen supply, produces profuse neovascularization in the immature retina with extension into the vitreous. Identical trauma in the adult animal is not followed by any new vessel formation. Yet, vasoproliferation occurs in the human adult in certain pathologic states as well as in the premature infant.

Neovascularization and Clinical States

In the adult, retinal neovascularization is observed most frequently in patients with diabetes mellitus.[210, 212, 213] Most frequently it is associated with a combination of lesions which include hemorrhage, cotton wool patches, hard exudates, and microaneurysms. Occasionally the new vessel formation will be accompanied by only the venous changes of engorgement, segmentation, and tortuosity. In some instances, the fan–shaped intravitreal bands of fibrous tissue, characteristic of proliferative retinopathy, may be observed. Massive retinal or preretinal hemorrhage may obscure the underlying neovascularization.

Less frequent causes of new vessel formation in the adult include venous branch occlusion,[212] the vasculitis of Eale's disease,[212] sickle cell disease,[195, 221] pulseless disease,[71] and macroglobulinemia.[222] Retrolental fibroplasia[223] is the most common cause of new vessel formation in the infant.

Neovascularization of the optic disc is commonly associated with central retinal vein occlusion[152] and diabetes mellitus.[210, 213]

As previously noted, the abnormal new vessels may, on rare occasions, disappear spontaneously. Generally, the fragile new vessels persist and are believed to be a source of retinal and preretinal hemorrhage, particularly in diabetic retinopathy. In an attempt to prevent that complication pituitary ablation and retinal photocoagulation have been employed. The abnormal vessels may disappear after pituitary ablation.[224-226] Vascular obliteration can be accomplished by photocoagulation.[227-229]

In the latter form of therapy, a beam of light is focused on the retina through a dilated pupil. The light which is absorbed by the pigment cells of the retina and choroid generates sufficient heat to produce tissue coagulation and a chorioretinal scar is formed.[230, 231] The early funduscopic changes after photocoagulation (within one week) consist of marked pallor and a clear view of the neovascularization (Plate 166 and Drawing 166). Several weeks later the clinical appearance is similar to that of chorioretinitis (Plate 167 and Drawing 167). The scar obliterates capillaries in the treated area and reduces

*His concept is based upon the results of intravitreal injection of one eye of kittens with different concentrations of lactic, acetic, and pyruvic acid. The other eye, injected only with diluent, served as a control and showed no evidence of neovascularization. Of the 16 eyes injected with 0.1% lactic acid, 8 demonstrated new vessel formation extending from the region of the optic disc into the vitreous. If the effect was specific for lactic acid, one wonders why no such response was elicited with 0.05% injection, or why 0.5% solution produced only an "avascular fibroplastic" reaction in the vitreous. That response was also elicited with 0.5% acetic acid, as well. Moreover 0.1% intravitreal pyruvic acid produced neovascularization in 1 of 3 eyes. The conclusion that lactic acid is the offending agent can certainly be questioned.

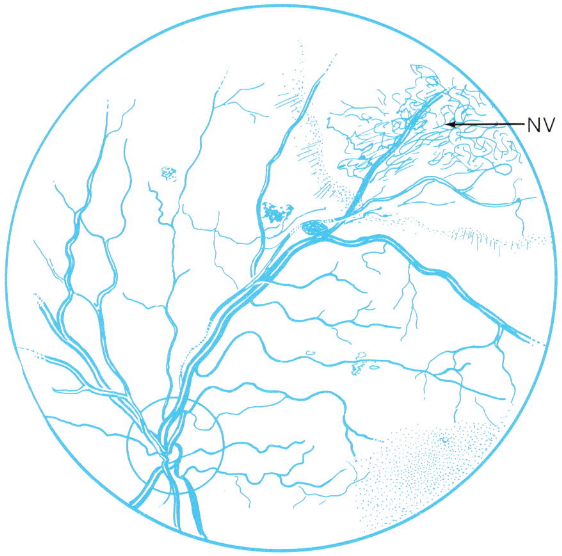

Drawing 166. Plate 166 (NV, neovascularization).

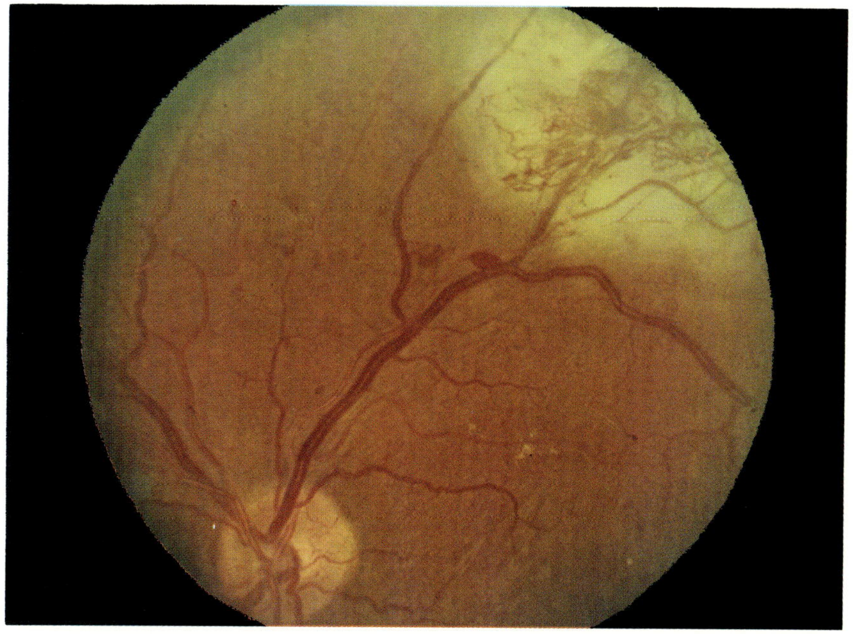

Plate 166. O.S. Superior temporal. One week after photocoagulation. Note the large irregular white area which contains a large collection of tortuous and intertwined new blood vessels. Several hemorrhages are present above the disc. Did you notice the venular tortuosity and hard exudates?

Drawing 167. Plate 167 (CHR, chorioretinal scar; CHV, choroidal blood vessels).

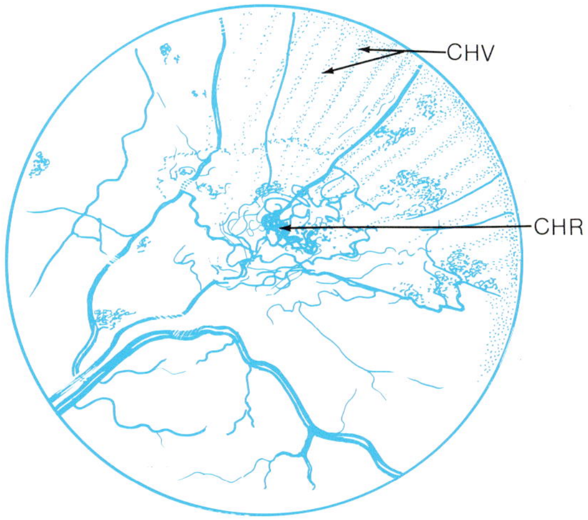

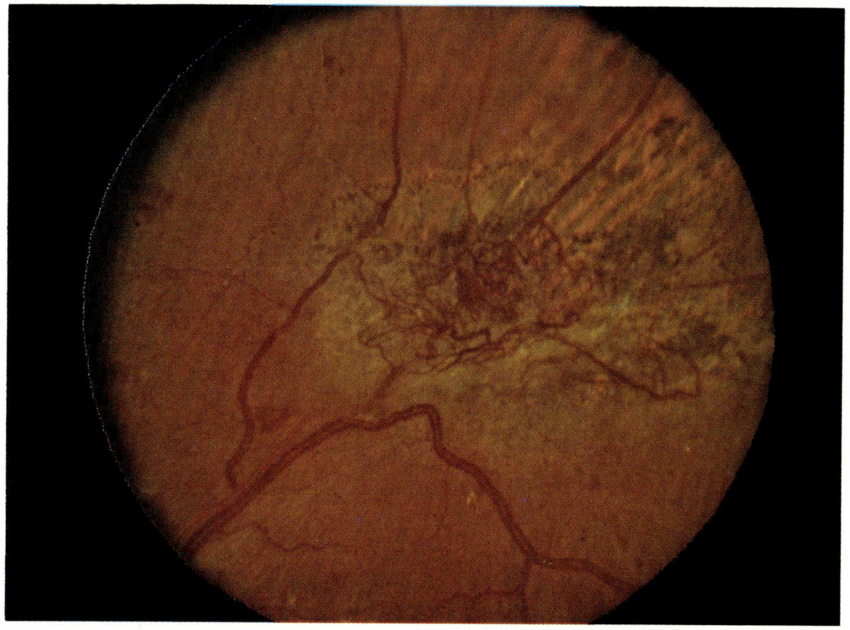

Plate 167. O.S. Superior temporal. The same patient as Plate 166, 1 month later. Note that the previously described white area has regained an orange–red reflex and contains large amounts of brown–black pigment. Choroidal blood vessels radiate upward from the involved area. The changes represent the chorioretinal scar which follows photocoagulation of the retina. The lesion simulates the findings of chorioretinitis.

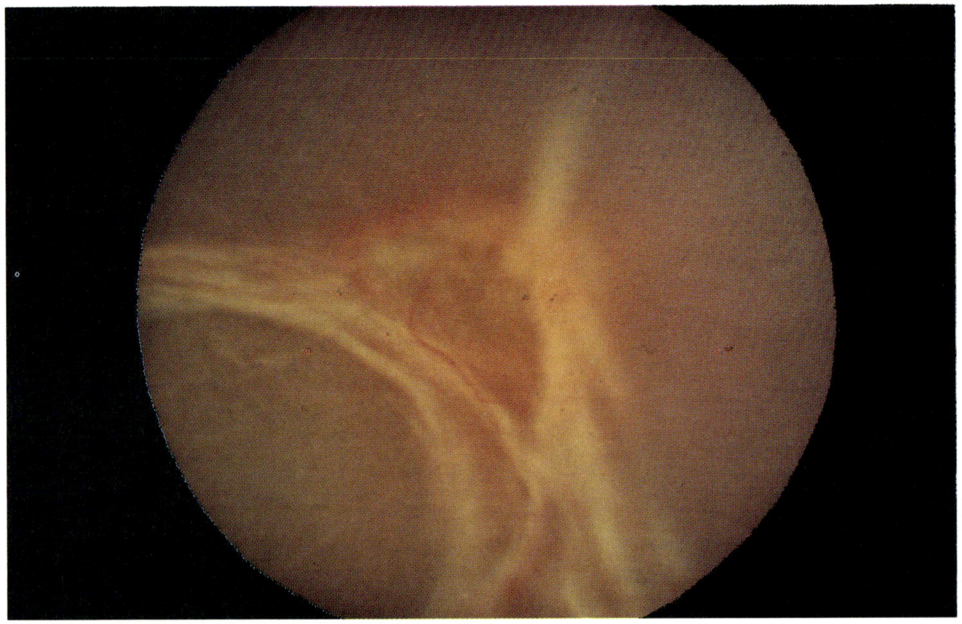

Plate 168. Photograph taken at depth of the vitreous demonstrating interlacing bands of fibrous tissue and neovascularization.

Plate 169. Note how the bands of fibrous tissue, newly formed vessels, and unidentified oval yellow areas obscure the normal retinal landmarks.

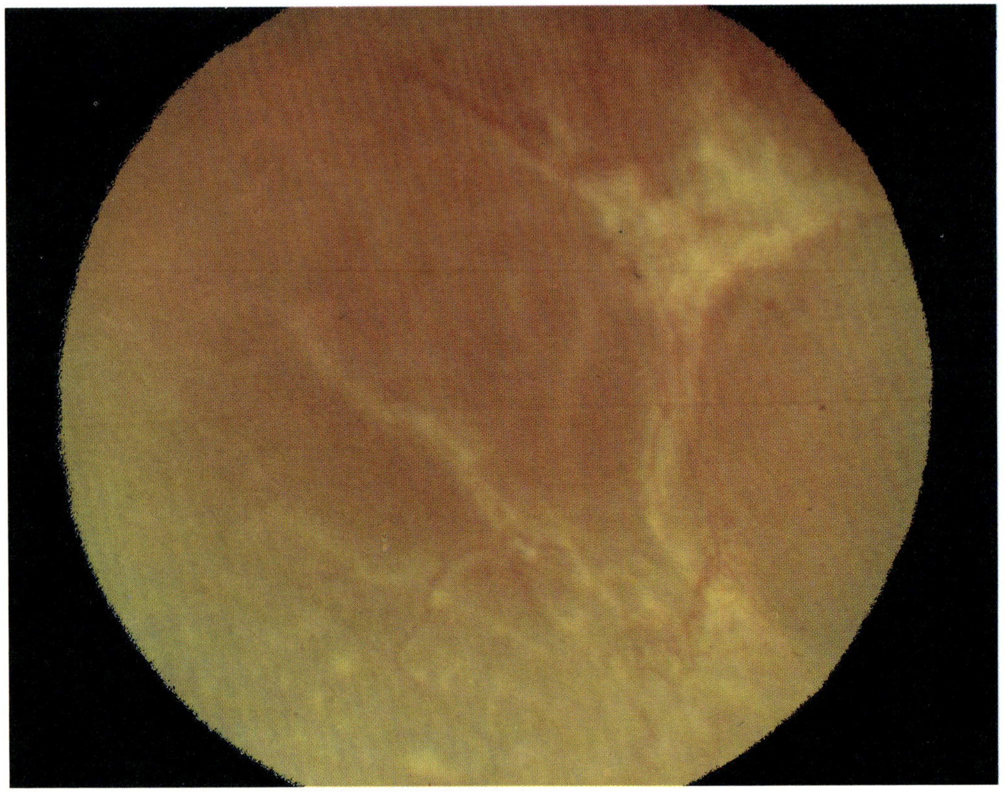

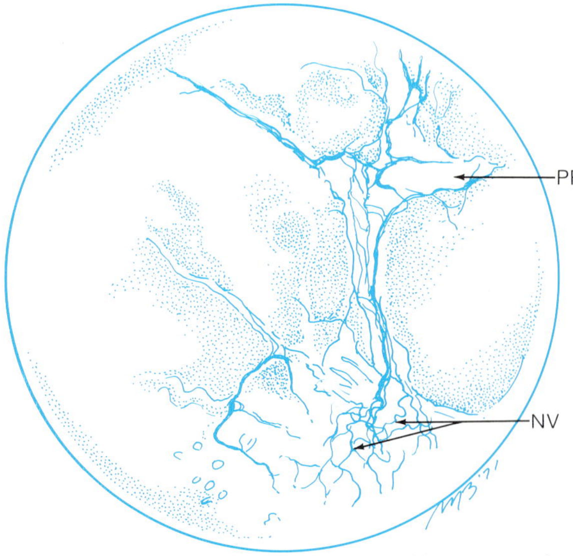

Drawing 169. Plate 169 (PR, proliferative retinopathy; NV, neovascularization).

the likelihood of retinal and vitreous hemorrhage.[227, 230, 231] Despite the reported successes with both photocoagulation and pituitary ablation, the long range effects are difficult to evaluate in the absence of well–controlled studies.

PROLIFERATIVE RETINOPATHY (RETINITIS PROLIFERANS)

Clinical Appearance

Proliferative retinopathy is characterized by the presence of retinal and preretinal fibrous tissue, and neovascularization. Using a positive lens of the ophthalmoscope, generally in the range between +8 and +2, white bands of scar tissue and blood vessels are observed in the vitreous cavity (Plate 168). Under such circumstances the underlying retina is often partly obscured (Plate 169 and Drawing 169). The veil–like bands of white tissue seem to arise from the optic nerve, spread peripherally in the form of a fan (Plate 170 and Drawing 170), and often envelop segments of normal retina (Plate 171). By careful serial funduscopic observations, Dobree[232] demonstrated that the development of these changes took several years and could be divided into the following three stages:

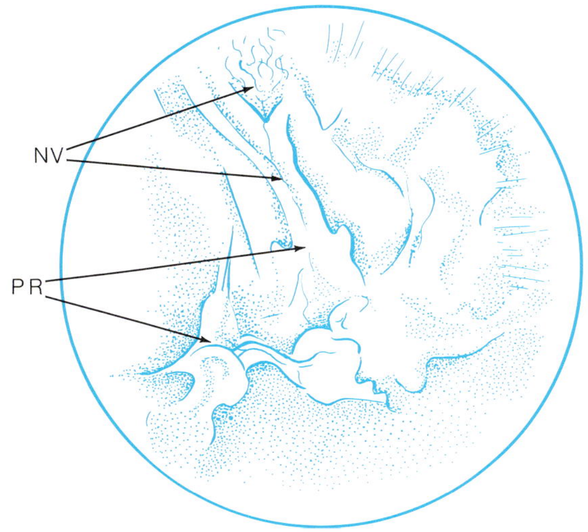

Drawing 170. Plate 170 (PR, proliferative retinopathy; NV, neovascularization).

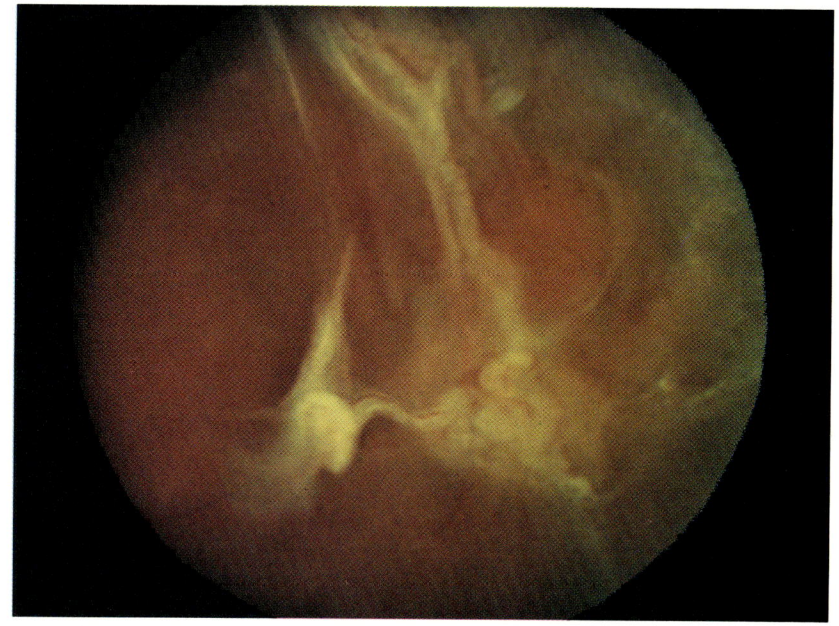

Plate 170. O.D. Central. Note the bands of white tissue which extend from the barely visible optic disc.

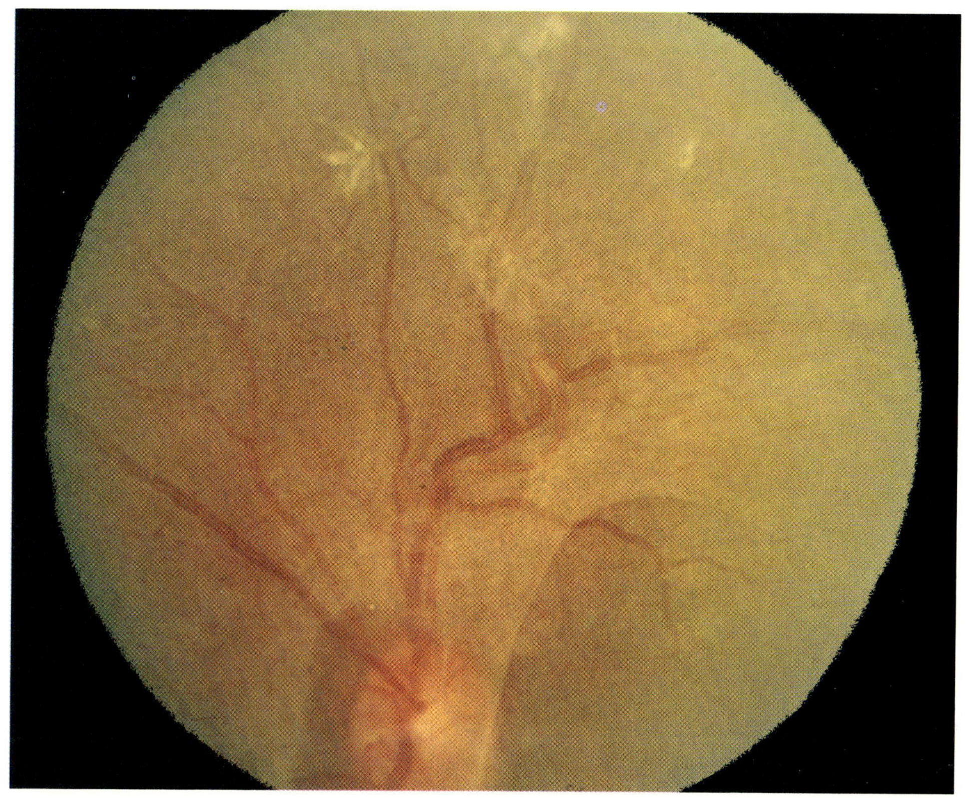

Plate 171. Veil-like band of white tissue arising from disc. Fibrous tissue sharply outlines segment of normal retina. White scars result from obliteration of newly formed vessels.

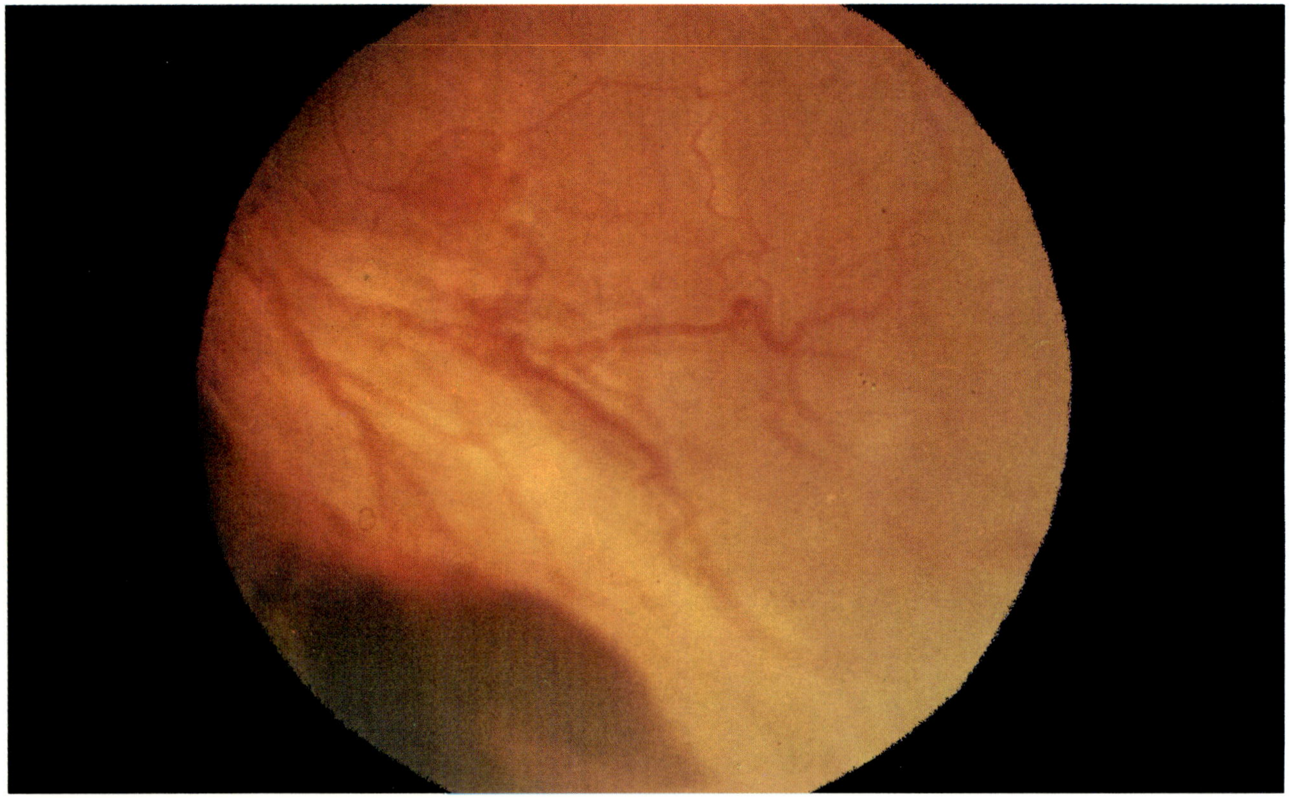

Plate 172. Large network of new vessels and preretinal hemorrhage (the sharply outlined brown–black mass of blood). (Circular white area is an artefact.)

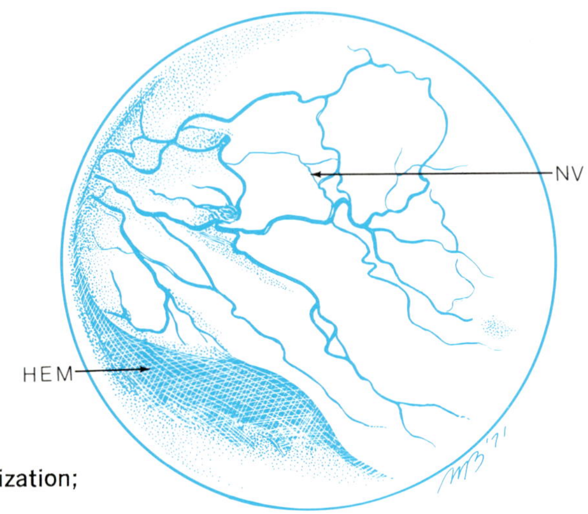

Drawing 172. Plate 172 (NV, neovascularization; HEM, hemorrhage).

STAGE 1

The formation of naked vessels

Initially a brushlike arrangement of the new vessels formed on the optic disc. Shortly thereafter, this network established connections with larger veins on the disc and extended into the subhyaloid space. Hemorrhage was observed as the networks became larger (Plate 172 and Drawing 172). During this stage, which lasted 6 to 18 months, no connective tissue formation was observed. Although Davis[210] agreed that new vessels generally arose from the disc, he noted that they could also arise anywhere in the retina except at the macula.

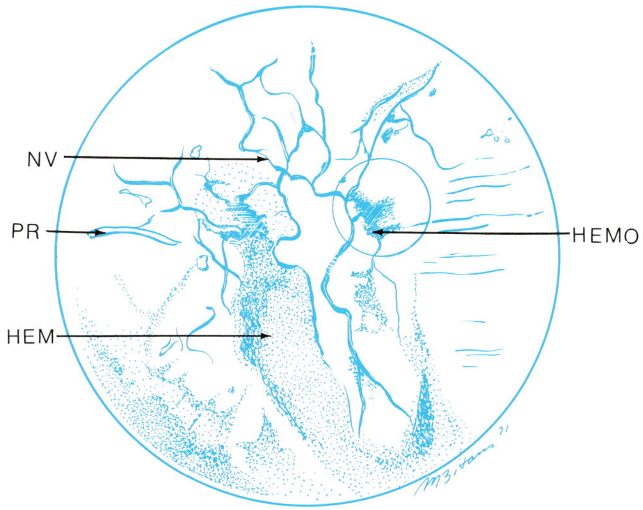

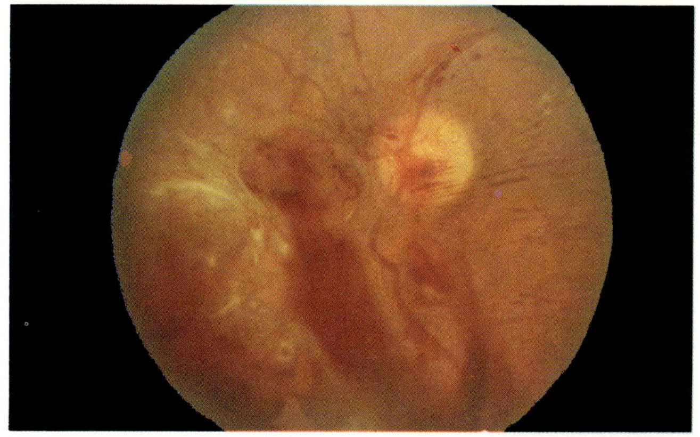

Plate 173. O.S. Preretinal and retinal hemorrhage. Neovascularization and fibrous tissue formation.

Drawing 173. Plate 173 (HEMO, hemorrhage in optic nerve; HEM, preretinal hemorrhage; NV, neovascularization; PR, proliferative retinopathy).

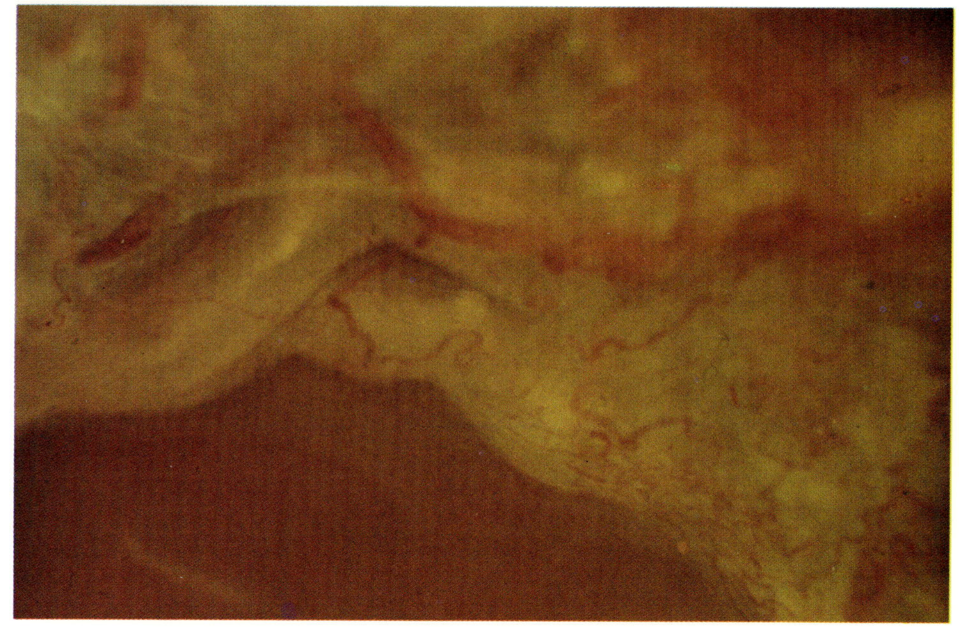

Plate 174. Enlarged view. Massive preretinal hemorrhage, fibrosis, and neovascularization.

STAGE 2

Vascular proliferation and connective tissue formation

Extension of the neovascularization into the retina along the vessels and vitreous was observed. Throughout this stage bands of connective tissue developed in the retina and vitreous among the newly formed vessels (Plate 171). Retinal, subhyaloid, and vitreous hemcrrhage occurred frequently (Plates 173 and 174 and Drawings 173 and 174). This phase lasted 1 to 2 years and gradually merged into the third stage.

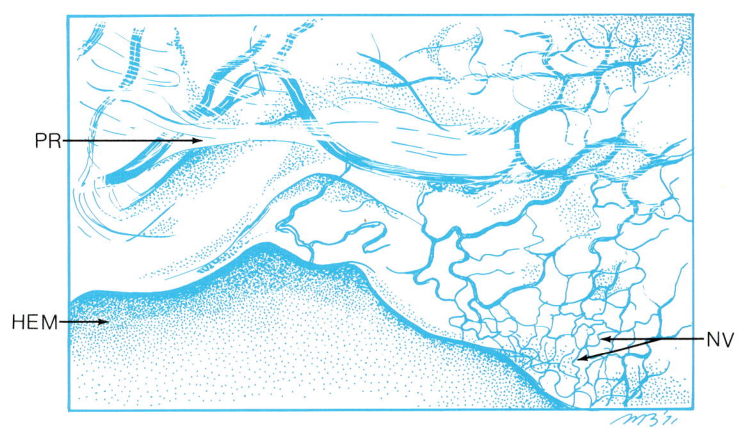

Drawing 174. Plate 174 (HEM, preretinal hemorrhage; PR, proliferative retinopathy; NV, neovascularization).

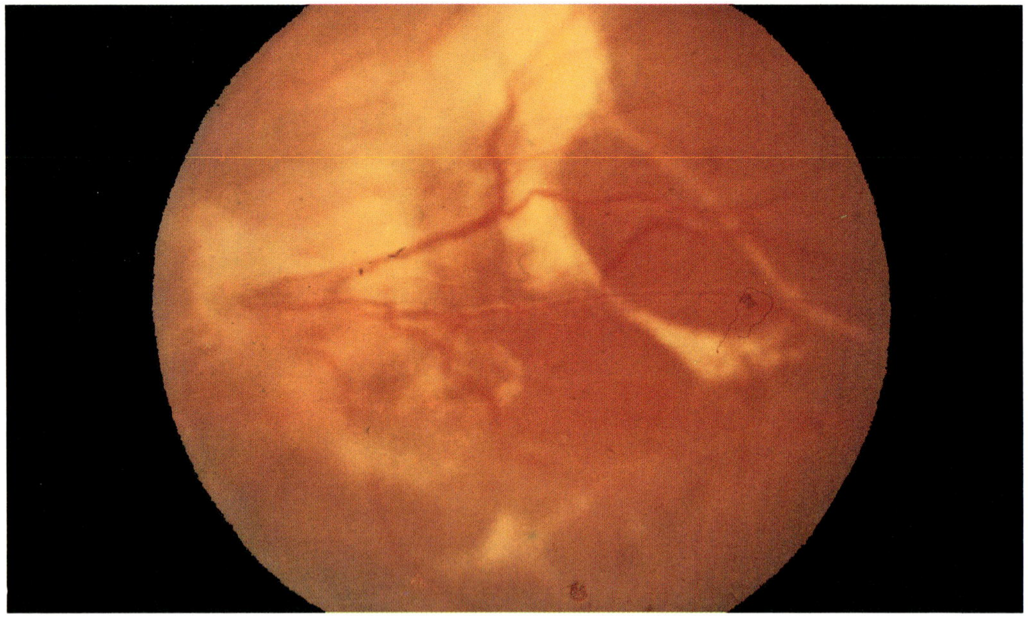

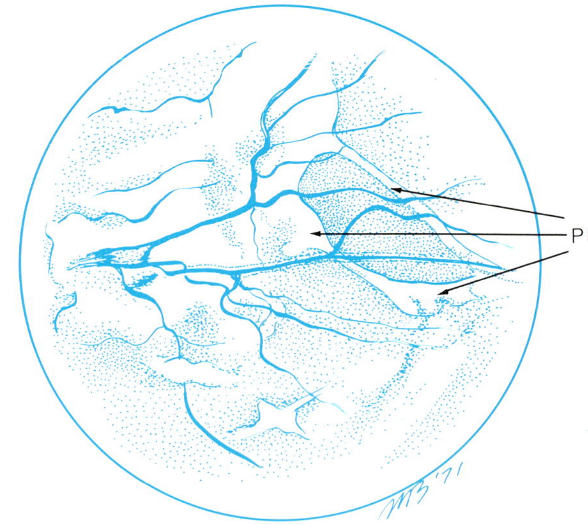

Plate 175. Massive scar tissue formation and neovascularization.

Drawing 175. Plate 175 (PR, proliferative retinopathy).

Plate 176. Massive scar tissue formation and neovascularization. Note distortion of architecture of the underlying retina.

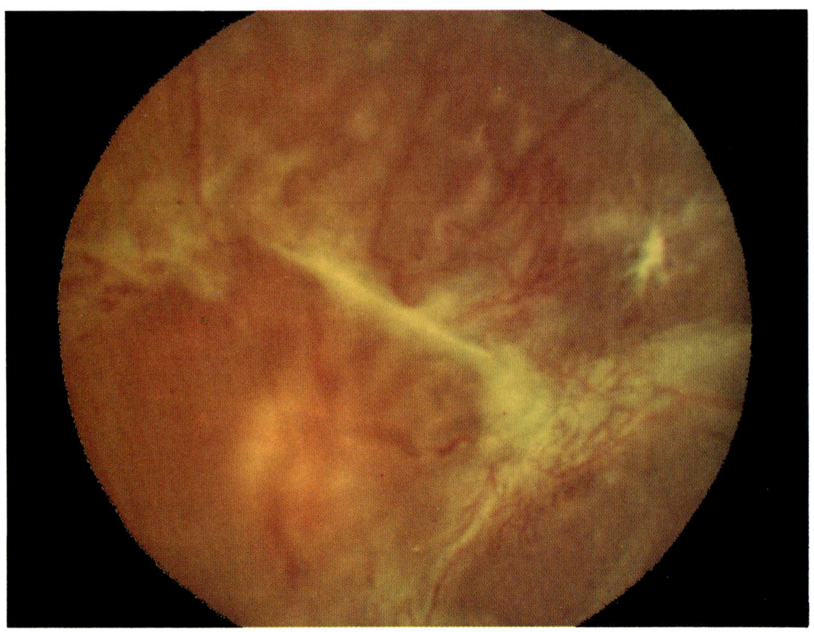

Drawing 176. Plate 176 (PR, proliferative retinopathy; NV, neovascularization).

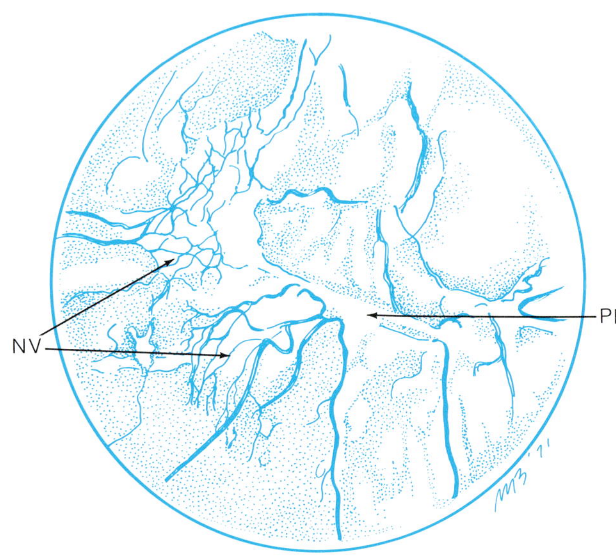

STAGE 3

Regression of the vascular systems and connective tissue contracture

The abnormal vessels slowly atrophied while the connective tissue became more prominent, providing a view dominated by white sheets of tissue containing relatively few vessels (Plate 170). As the connective tissue contracted, alterations of the course of retinal vessels were observed. Further observations disclosed renewed evidence of neovascularization (Plates 175 and 176 and Drawings 175 and 176). Although hemorrhage was less common, defects in vision developed due to mechanical obstruction by connective tissue and the effects of traction leading to retinal detachment (see pp. 152–55).

Pathology

The early histologic changes consist of proliferation of hyperplastic foci of endothelial and spindle cells. Clusters of the former differentiate into vascular channels, as previously described (see p. 143). The origin and characteristics of the spindle cells have been viewed differently by various investigators. They have been called glial cells.[215, 233] More recently, Ashton[214] presented the view that the spindle cells were mesenchymal cells destined to become precursors of such vascular components as connective and smooth muscle tissue. He noted that as the proliferating angioblastic retinal tissue extended through the internal limiting membrane it was accompanied by protein transudate. Fibroblasts, originating from the mesenchymal cells, proliferated in the transudate which had entered the vitreous, and formed strands of fibrous tissue. The process continued with increased fibrosis. Ultimately, the fibrous tissue contracted and retinal detachment followed (Plates 177 and 178 and Drawings 177 and 178).

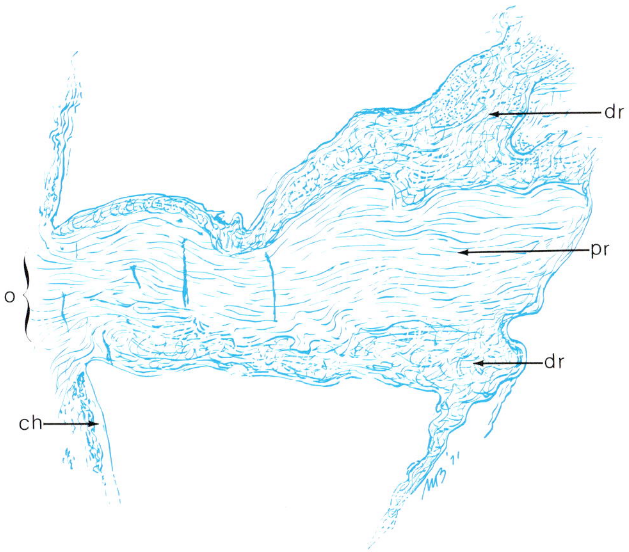

Drawing 177. Plate 177 (o, optic nerve; ch, choroid; pr, proliferative retinopathy; dr, detached retina).

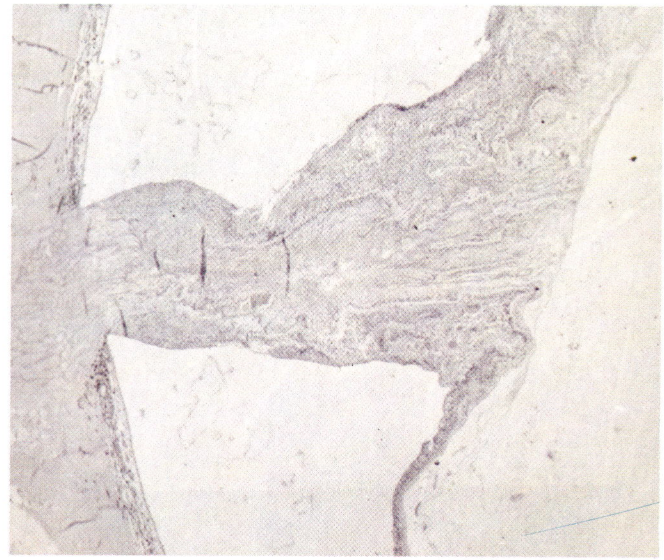

Plate 177. Microscopic section of lesion of patient represented in retinal photograph 178. Note mass of tissue extending anteriorly from the disc. The proliferative tissue contains blood vessels and fibrous tissue. As it extended anteriorly it pulled the retinal tissue away from the choroid (retinal detachment) (PAS, × 12).

Plate 178. Proliferating morning glory–like mass of fibrous tissue extending from the disc.

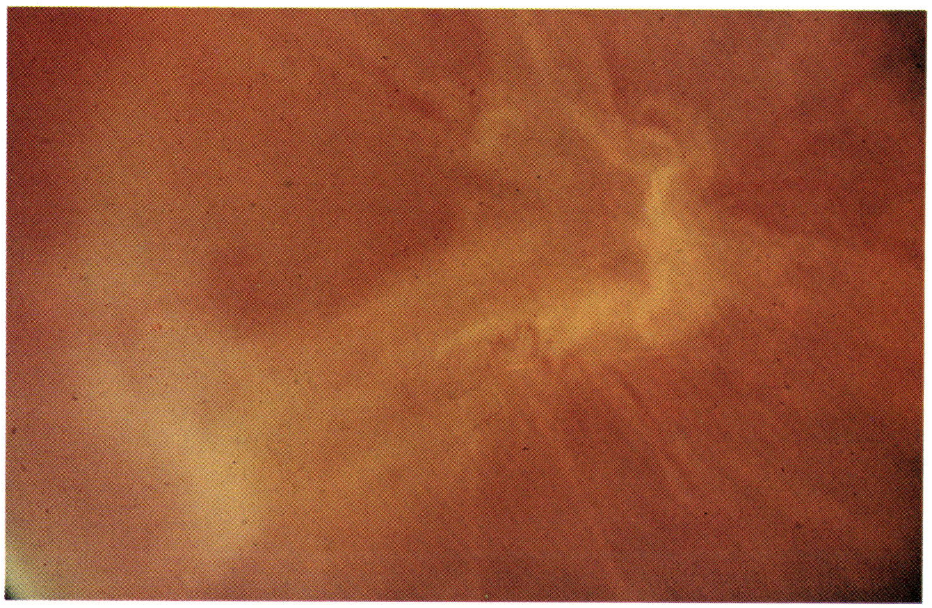

Drawing 178. Plate 178 (O, optic disc; PR, proliferative retinopathy).

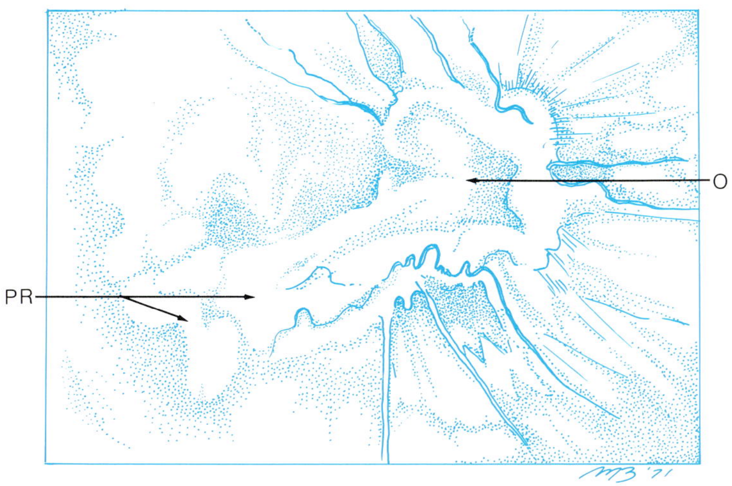

Pathogenesis

The proliferating blood vessels and fibrous tissue were originally considered to be the residua of organized granulation tissue in response to injury. It was assumed that hemorrhage originating in the retina perforated the internal limiting and hyaloid membranes and entered the vitreous.[234, 235] In response to such trauma, according to this concept, granulation tissue developed in the nerve fiber layer of the retina and extended into the vitreous.

It was suggested by Klien[235] that neovascularization, in the absence of hemorrhage, could also lead to proliferative retinopathy. Prolonged clinical studies of the natural history of diabetic retinopathy confirmed that concept[210, 232] and established that the newly formed vessels developed before retinal and preretinal hemorrhage became apparent. Davis[210] noted that vitreoretinal adhesions and neovascularization occurred together. He[210] and other workers[236] observed that posterior vitreous detachment followed. The resulting traction upon the vitreoretinal adhesions led to preretinal and vitreous hemorrhage and retinal detachment.

There is little doubt, at least in diabetic retinopathy, that neovascularization is generally the initial and basic lesion in proliferative retinopathy. Nevertheless, it is conceivable that hemorrhage may either serve to further stimulate fibrosis or it may even initiate the entire cycle of events.

Proliferative retinopathy is most frequently observed in patients with diabetes mellitus. Its incidence ranges between 6%[167] and approximately 20%[237] in patients with diabetic retinopathy. Generally detected in patients less than 60 years of age,[169] it rarely becomes apparent less than 10 years after the onset of overt diabetes. Although spontaneous arrest may occur with proliferative retinopathy, it usually is progressive. Any combination of associated changes such as venous alterations, cotton wool patches, hard exudates, microaneurysms, and retinal hemorrhage may be observed. However, as the proliferative changes progress, they often obscure the changes in the underlying retina. Because of its complications, which include vitreous hemorrhage, fibrosis, retinal detachment, and hemorrhagic glaucoma, proliferative retinopathy is a major cause of permanent visual loss.[227, 238]

Less common causes of proliferative retinopathy include sickle cell abnormalities (S–S and S–C)[76, 221, 239] and Eale's disease[212] (see p. 85). Proliferative retinopathy develops in approximately 25% of premature infants afflicted with retrolental fibroplasia.[85 (p. 189)]

Although it is difficult to evaluate the effects of pituitary ablation and photocoagulation in diabetic retinopathy, it is clear that no favorable changes are observed in the fibrosis of proliferative retinopathy.[170, 240, 241]

Complications

Retinal detachment and hemorrhagic glaucoma have been mentioned as complications of proliferative retinopathy. It would, therefore, now be appropriate to present brief discussions of those serious abnormalities.

RETINAL DETACHMENT

The term retinal detachment is applied when the rods and cones are separated from the pigment cells of the retina.[2 (pp. 549-568), 4 (pp. 379-409), 242 (pp. 2890-3926)] This seperation occurs at the line of cleavage of the two layers of the embryonic optic cup (Fig. IV) (see pp. 3–5). This form of retinal detachment is generally associated with the accumulation of fluid between the retina and choroid (subretinal fluid). The fluid may be a transudate, exudate, or blood which develops as a result of disease of the retina and/or choroid (Plate 179 and Drawing 179). Vitreous detachment may also lead to the accumulation of the subretinal fluid in the following manner. In vitreous detachment, the posterior part of the vitreous separates from the retina. The subvitreal space, the area between the vitreous body and the retina, then becomes filled with fluid. This fluid flows through an associated retinal tear or hole and accumulates in the subretinal space, between the rods and cones and the pigment cells of the retina.

In proliferative retinopathy, the contraction of the fibrous tissue pulls the retina away from the choroid. When that occurs, the entire retina, including the pigment cell layer, is detached (Drawing 177).

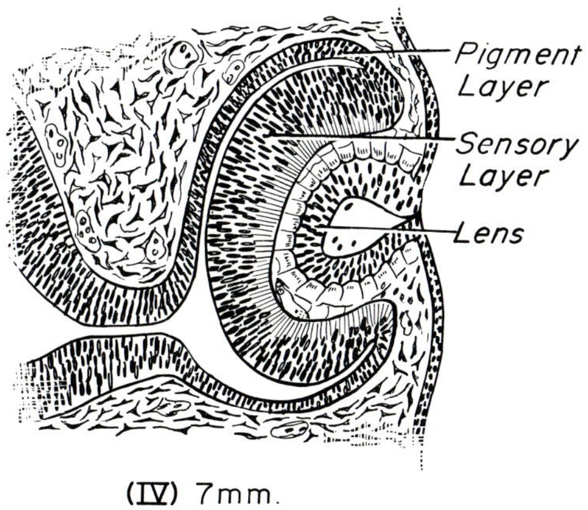

Figure IV. Drawing. Differentiation of optic cup (from Patten).

Plate 179. Note the accumulation of eosinophilic material between the rods and cones and the pigment cell layer of the retina. Thickened retinal arterioles, gliosis of the nerve fiber layer, and outer plexiform deposits of fibrin and red blood cells are also present (PTAH, approx. × 80).

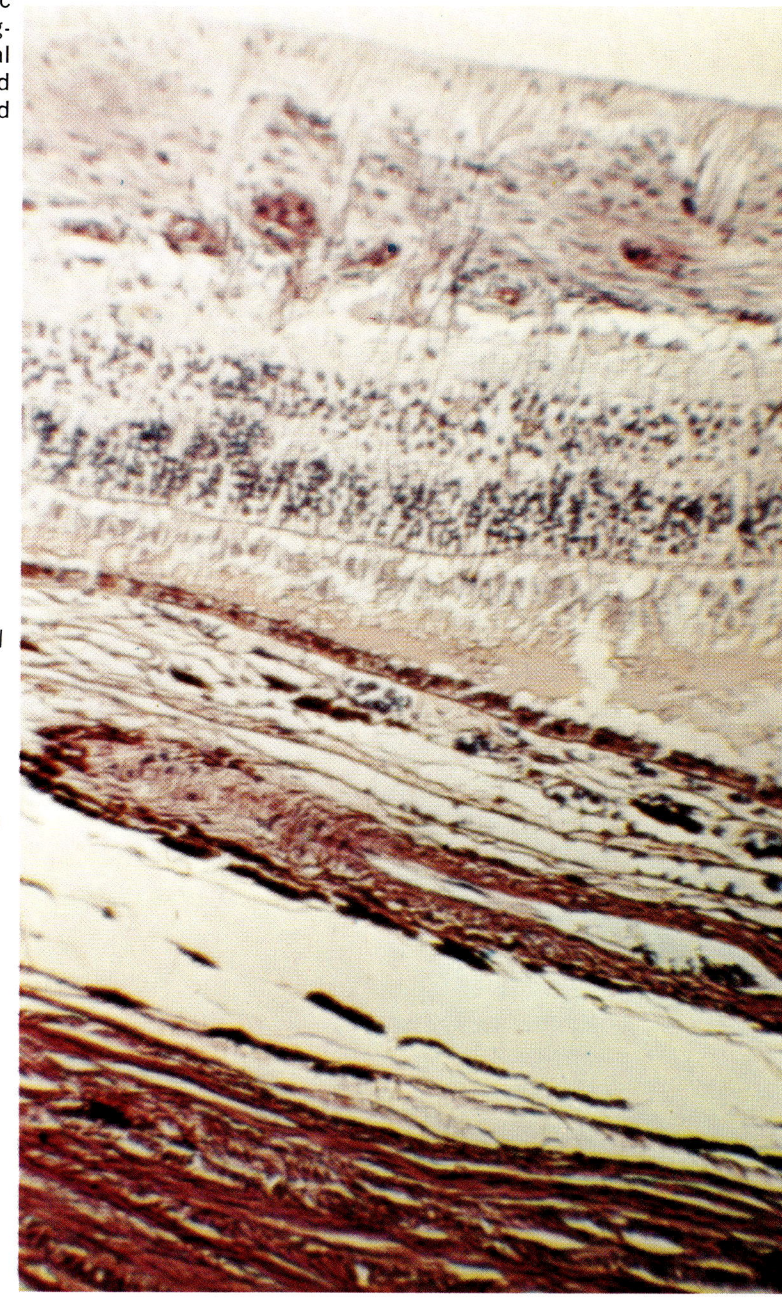

Drawing 179. Plate 179 (im, internal limiting membrane; em, external limiting membrane; pl, pigment cell layer; ch, choroid; nfgl, nerve fiber layer gliosis; t, subretinal transudate; a, arteriole; hem, hemorrhage in outer plexiform layer).

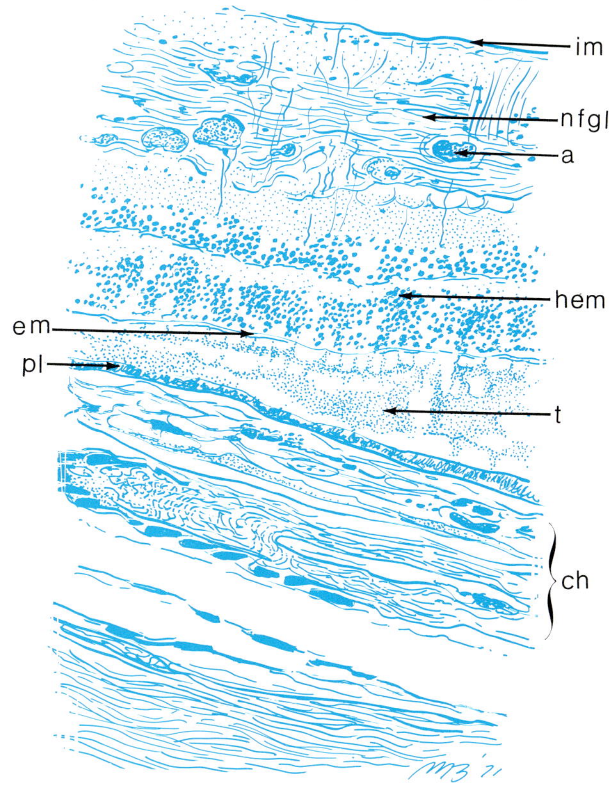

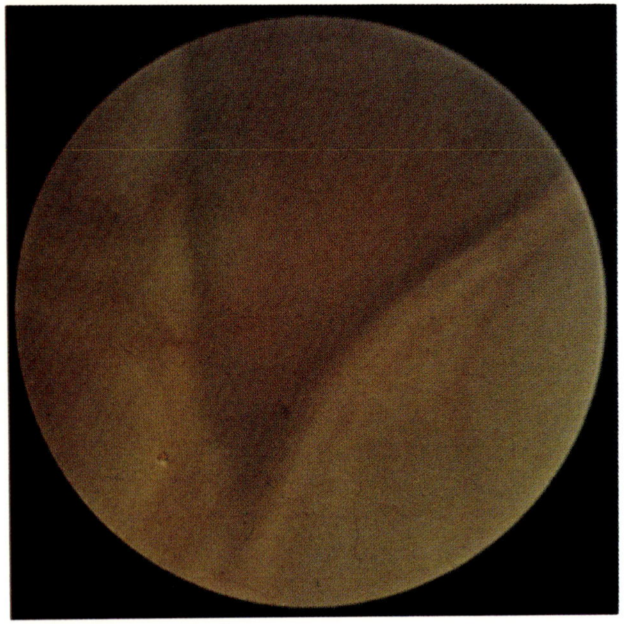

Plate 181. A portion of normal retina (again out of focus) is observed between two white "clouds" of tissue. Blood vessels overlie the veils of white.

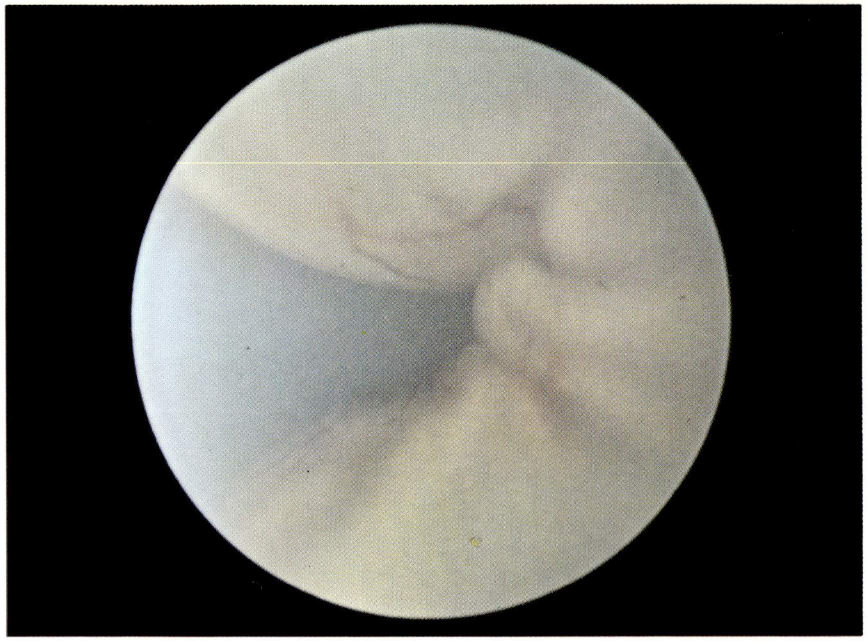

Plate 180. Detached retina. A white, cloudlike tissue which contains several overlying blood vessels occupies 3/4 of the field. The blue color of the remaining part of the photograph is an artefact. It represents normal retina, which is out of focus.

Plate 182. A white, domelike mass apepars to float towards the viewer and occupy the lower 1/2 of the field. Blood vessels are visible on the top of the lesion. The remainder of the retina is out of focus.

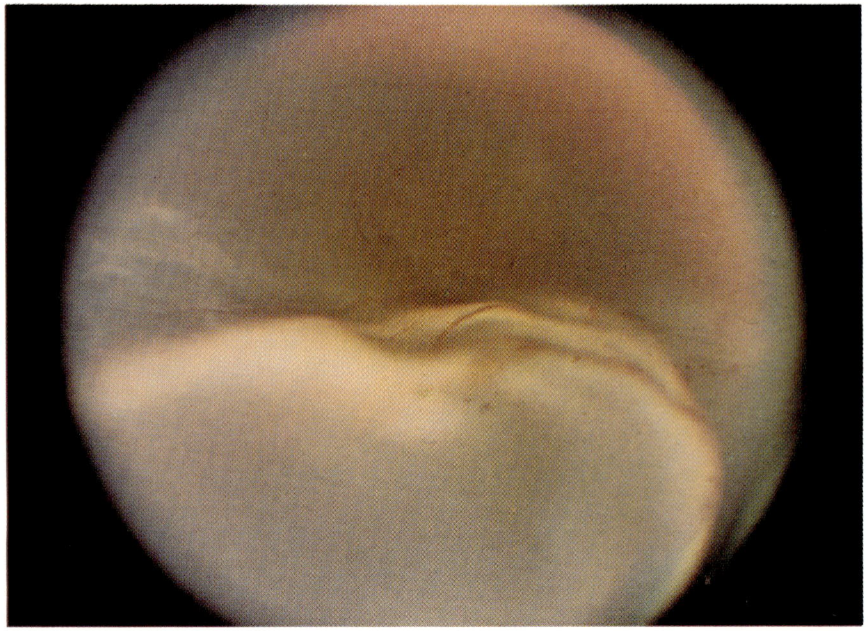

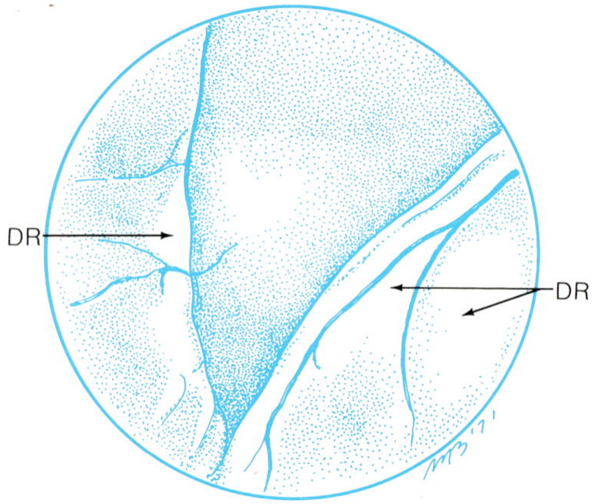

Drawing 181. Plate 181 (DR, detached retina).

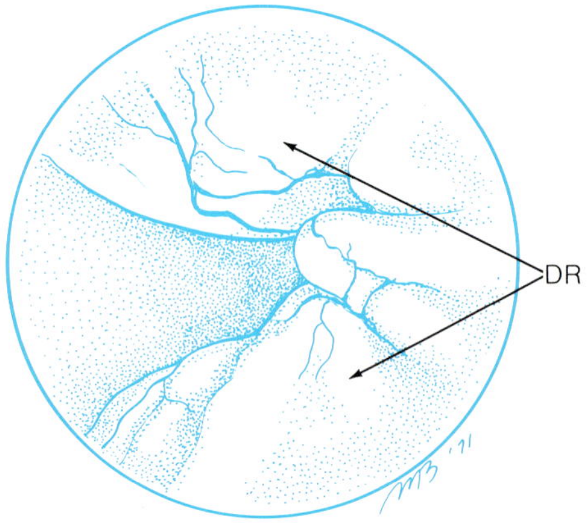

Drawing 180. Plate 180 (DR, detached retina).

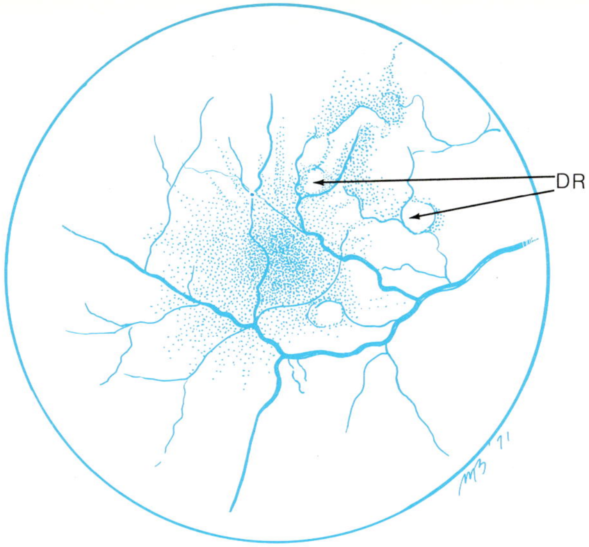

Drawing 183. Plate 183 (DR, detached retina).

Plate 183. Reattachment of detachment noted on Plate 182. The retina appears to have reattached itself. Three white, irregular areas are visible. These may represent small areas of detachment. Note the absence of a scar after reattachment, in contrast to Plate 184.

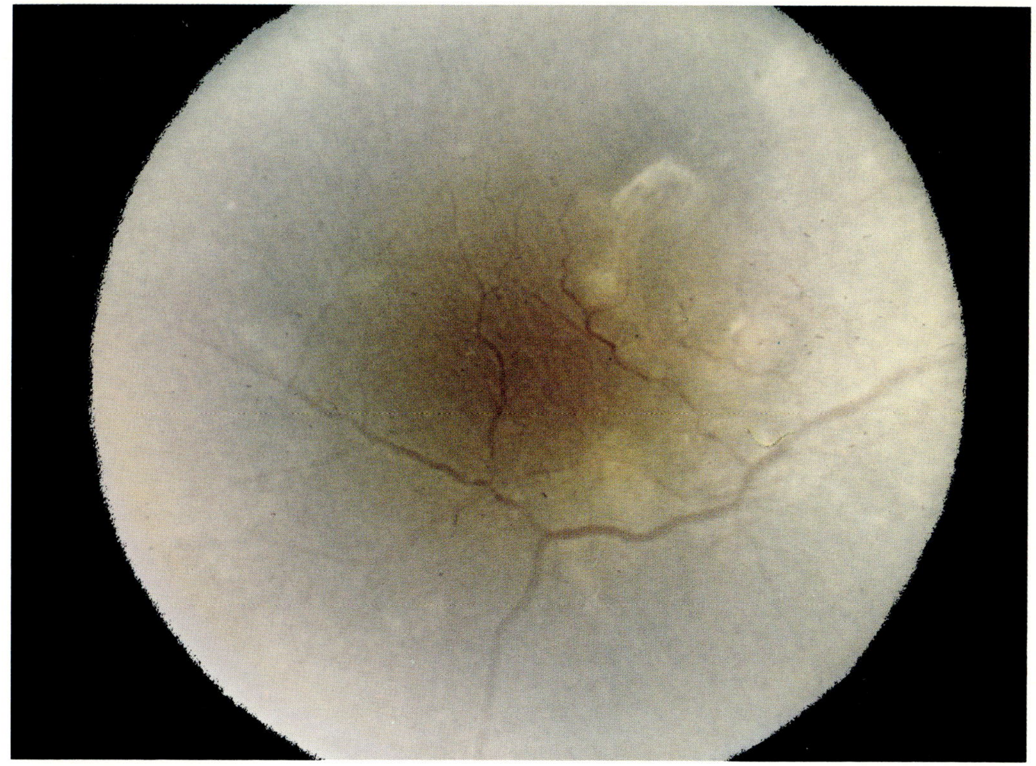

Clinical Findings

The major symptom of retinal detachment is painless visual loss, often preceded by flashes of light, dark spots, or cloudy vision.

Funduscopy discloses partial replacement of the red reflex by a gray membrane. The detached retina is gray or white. It is folded, often dome–shaped, and it may oscillate with movement of the eye (Plates 180–182 and Drawings 180 and 181). Blood vessels over it lose their light reflex and may appear to be black. Hemorrhage may be present. A hole or tear of the retina may be visible. Patches of chorioretinitis or vascular and extravascular lesions may be seen when retinal detachment results from inflammatory or vascular disease of the choroid and/or the retina.

The retina may become reattached spontaneously (Plates 183 and 184 and Drawings 183 and 184).

Although spontaneous reattachment may occur, surgical correction, in some form, is the treatment of choice.

Plate 184. O.D. Spontaneous reattachment of detachment of retina noted in Plate 180. An elliptical lesion extends from the temporal part of the optic disc. The walls of the abnormality are pigmented; closer to the disc, the borders are formed, in part, by a white streak. Blood vessels appear to be elevated as they cross the borders and enter the normal retina which is enclosed within the elliptical scar. It represents the scar which may be visible at the site of the retinal reattachment. This abnormality frequently results when reattachment occurs after long standing retinal detachment. Histologically, the lesion represents the adhesions between retina and choroid.

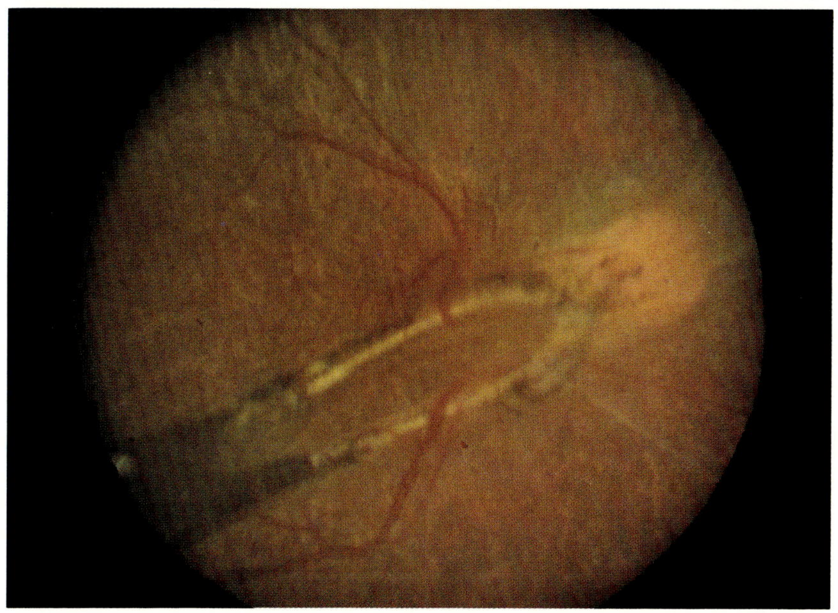

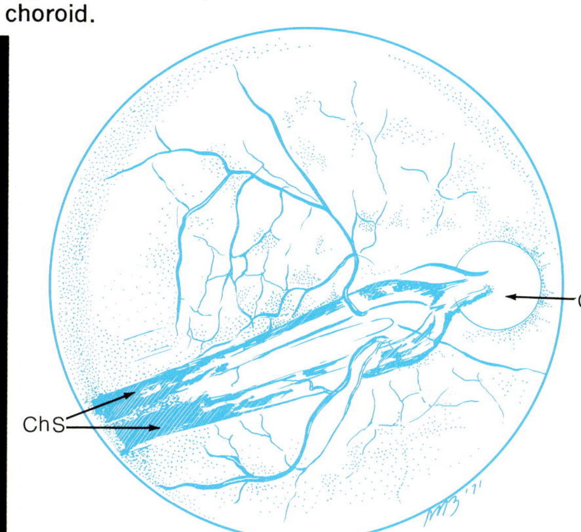

Drawing 184. Plate 184 (CHS, chorioretinal scar; O, optic disc).

HEMORRHAGIC GLAUCOMA

A brief review of the anatomy of the anterior chamber of the eye may help clarify the pathogenesis of the glaucoma associated with proliferative retinopathy. The anterior chamber lies between the anterior surface of the iris and lens and the posterior surface of the cornea (Drawing of Fig. VI). The recess formed by the insertion of the iris into the base of the ciliary body is known as the filtration angle of the eye. It is partially filled with a loose meshwork of trabeculae through which the aqueous humor flows. Proliferative diabetic retinopathy is often accompanied by neovascularization and fibrosis of the iris, known as rubeosis iridis. The distorted iris is pulled against the trabecular meshwork of the anterior chamber and closes the filtration angle. As a result, the flow of aqueous humor is impeded and intraocular pressure rises to abnormal levels. Often hemorrhage also occurs in the anterior chamber. The end result is a hemorrhagic glaucoma.[243 (pp. 175, 208), 244]

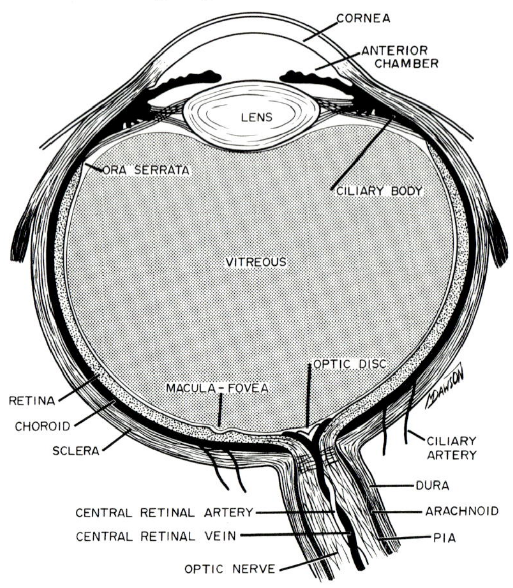

Figure VI

ANNOTATED BIBLIOGRAPHY

Neovascularization and Proliferative Retinopathy

Ashton, N., Ward, B., and Serpell, G.: *Effect of Oxygen on Developing Retinal Vessels with Particular Reference to the Problems of Retrolental Fibroplasia,* Br. J. Ophthalmol., **38:** 397, 1954. The authors present experimental evidence to support the concept that retinal vasoproliferation follows the vaso–obliteration induced by hyperoxia.

Ballantyne, A. J.: *New–Formed Vessels in the Fundus Oculi,* Ophthalmologica, **118:** 611, 1949. An excellent presentation of the clinical findings in retinal neovascularization.

Davis, M. D.: *Vitreous Contraction in Proliferative Diabetic Retinopathy,* Arch. Ophthalmol., **74:** 741, 1965. The development of the concept that neovascularization, vitreoretinal adhesions, and detachment of the vitreous were sequential changes in the development of proliferative retinopathy.

Dobree, J. H.: *Proliferative Diabetic Retinopathy. Evaluation of the Retinal Lesions,* Br. J. Ophthalmol., **48:** 637, 1964. An excellent clinical observation of the sequential changes in the development of abnormal new vessels and proliferative retinopathy.

Imre, G.: *Studies on the Mechanism of Retinal Neovascularization. Role of Lactic Acid,* Br. J. Ophthalmol., **48:** 75, 1964. An experimental effort to discover the metabolic product responsible for neovascularization.

Klien, B. A.: *Retinitis Proliferans. Clinical and Histologic Studies,* Arch. Ophthalmol., **20:** 427, 1938. The pathology of proliferative retinopathy is presented.

Michaelson, I. C.: *The Mode of Development of the Vascular System of the Retina, with Some Observations on Its Significance for Certain Retinal Diseases,* Trans. Ophthalmol. Soc. U.K., **68:** 137, 1948. A superb discussion of the normal development of the retinal circulation and its similarity to new vessel formation in disease.

Tolentino, F. I., Lee, P. F., and Schepens, C. L.: *Biomicroscopic Study of Vitreous Cavity in Diabetic Retinopathy,* Arch. Ophthalmol., **75:** 238, 1966. An excellent clinical study which supports the findings of Dobree and Davis.

Test Plates (unlabeled retinal photographs)

Questions and Answers C1–C14

Plate C1

Clinical findings: A 28–year–old male who has had insulin–dependent diabetes mellitus for 16 years. Bl. P. 170/120 mmHg. Plate C1 — O.D. — temporal and superior.

PLATE C1

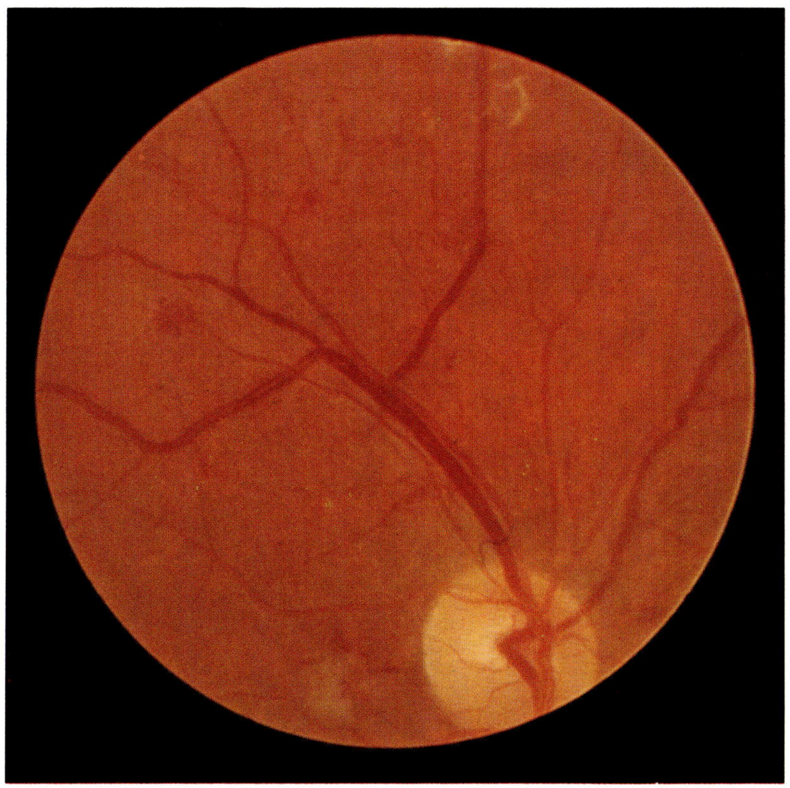

QUESTIONS — C1

Question 1. List abnormalities (see answer, this page).

Question 2. What are the common sites of neovascularization, as noted by funduscopy?

Question 3. Is neovascularization a static process?

Question 4. Is there any evidence of regression of neovascularization in this photograph?

Question 5. What are some of the complications of retinal neovascularization?

ANSWERS — C1

Answer 1. The disc is normal. The superior temporal venule is dilated and segmented. The arterioles are narrow. A cotton wool patch is present at 9 o'clock. A flame–shaped hemorrhage is noted above it. Neovascularization is observed between 10 and 11 o'clock, 3–4 disc diameters above the disc. Clusters of white, irregular areas are noted above the disc, approximately 4 disc diameters away.

Answer 2. The optic disc, the retina, and the vitreous cavity.

Answer 3. No. It appears to be progressive. However, regression may occur in parts of it, as other new vessels form.

Answer 4. Yes. The white, scarred areas noted above the disc probably represent obliterated new vessels.

Answer 5. Hemorrhage into the retina and vitreous is a serious complication. In addition, the fibrous tissue formation which appears to accompany neovascularization is one of the mechanisms by which proliferative retinopathy develops.

Reference

Davis, M. D.: *Vitreous Contraction in Proliferative Diabetic Retinopathy,* Arch. Ophthalmol., **74:** 741, 1965.

Plate C2

Clinical findings: A 57–year–old female who has had diabetes mellitus for 13 years. Treatment consisted of a calculated diet and oral hypoglycemic agents for 9 years. Four years ago, insulin was administered because the oral hypoglycemic agents were no longer effective. During the last 6 months, the patient noted marked fatigue. Physical examination disclosed pallor and splenomegaly. Bl. P. 180/110 mmHg. Hct. 26%; Hb, 8 gms/100 ml; WBC – 98,000/ $mm.^3$ Differential: polymorphonuclear leukocytes — 30; bands — 26; eosinophils — 20; basophils — 4; lymphocytes — 3; blast cells — 4; myelocytes — 13. Platelets — 186,000. Plate C2 — O.D. — temporal.

QUESTIONS — C2

Question 1. List abnormalities (see answer, p. 159).

Question 2. Would you expect the patient's vision to be altered by the lesions noted in the retina?

Queston 3. How can one differentiate retinal hemorrhage from the microaneurysm?

Question 4. What new diagnostic procedure may help answer Question 3?

Question 5. What produces the white dot at the site of a microaneurysm?

Question 6. What funduscopic abnormalities occur in patients with leukemia?

PLATE C2

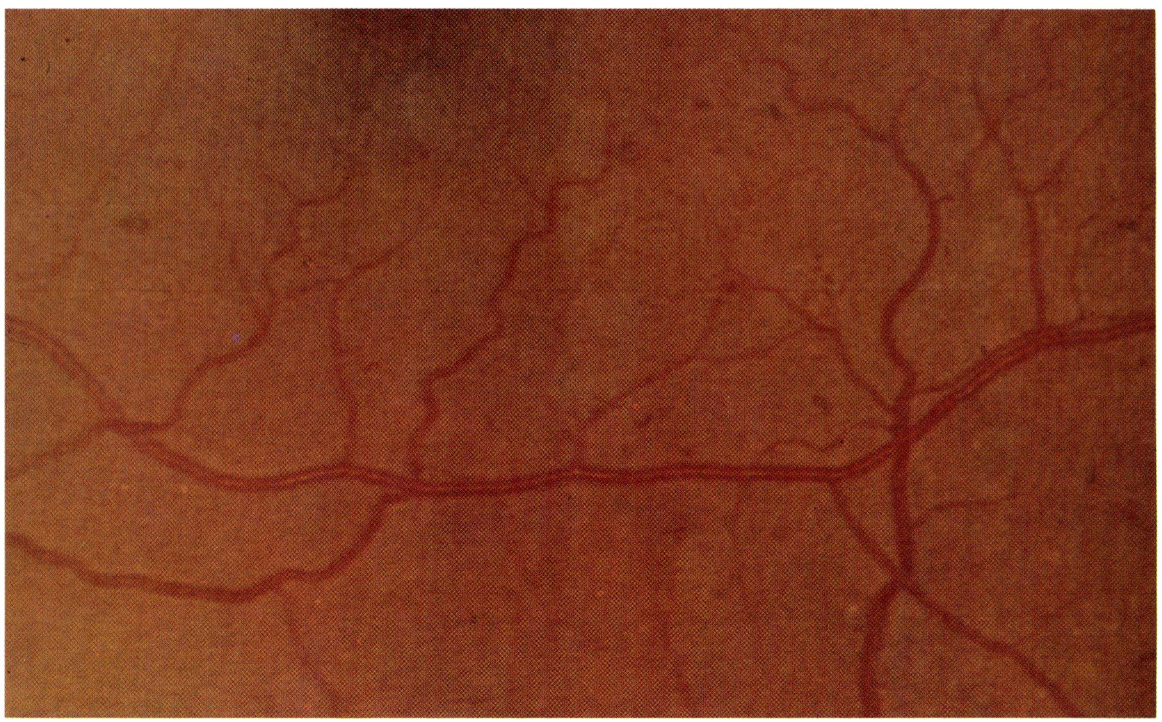

ANSWERS — C2

Answer 1. The macula can be identified in the inferior part of the field. There are several flame–shaped hemorrhages and microaneurysms. There are three discrete white dots above the arteriole. Venular tortuosity and "copper wire" arteriolar change are noted. A hard exudate is present in the upper portion of the macula.

Answer 2. Visual acuity was not decreased in this patient. The lesions are small and the fovea was spared.

Answer 3. The linear or flame–shaped hemorrhage differs in its shape from the round microaneurysm. The small, round hemorrhage in the deep layers of the retina resembles the microaneurysm. Hemorrhage is likely to disappear within several weeks. In contrast, the microaneurysm persists for months. When it disappears it may leave a small, white dot, as noted in this retinal photograph. In addition, the microaneurysm usually has a sharp outline, whereas the hemorrhage's borders may be slightly irregular.

Answer 4. Fluorescein angiography. The aneurysm, if not obliterated, will fill with the dye and its attachment to a vessel will be obvious. The hemorrhage is not likely to fluoresce.

Answer 5. Hyalinization and obliteration of its lumen.

Reference

Wagener, H. P.: *Retinal Microaneurysms,* Am. J. Med. Sci., **225:** 205, 1953.

Answer 6. Retinal hemorrhage is the most common finding in leukemia. Dominantly in the nerve fiber layer, it may penetrate the internal limiting membrane and become apparent as a subhyaloid or vitreous hemorrhage. If it dissects posteriorly it appears as the round hemorrhage of the outer plexiform layer. Even deeper penetration leads to the accumulation of blood between the pigment cell layer and the rods and cones (subretinal) and results in retinal detachment. The white–centered hemorrhage (Roth spot) may develop in either the round or flame–shaped variety. Venous tortuosity, engorgement, and sheathing also occur commonly. Less frequently one may find cotton wool patches, hard exudates, and papilledema. Retinal abnormalities are more common in the acute or blast cell stage of leukemia.

References

Allen, R. A. and Straatsma, B. R.: *Ocular Involvement in Leukemia and Allied Disorders,* Arch. Ophthalmol., **66:** 490, 1961.

Holt, J. M. and Gordon–Smith, E. C.: *Retinal Abnormalities in Diseases of the Blood,* Br. J. Ophthalmol., **53:** 145, 1969.

Plate C3

Clinical findings: A 35–year–old, healthy, white male noted the inability to see a tennis ball above the level of his head while serving. Plate C3 — O.D.

PLATE C3

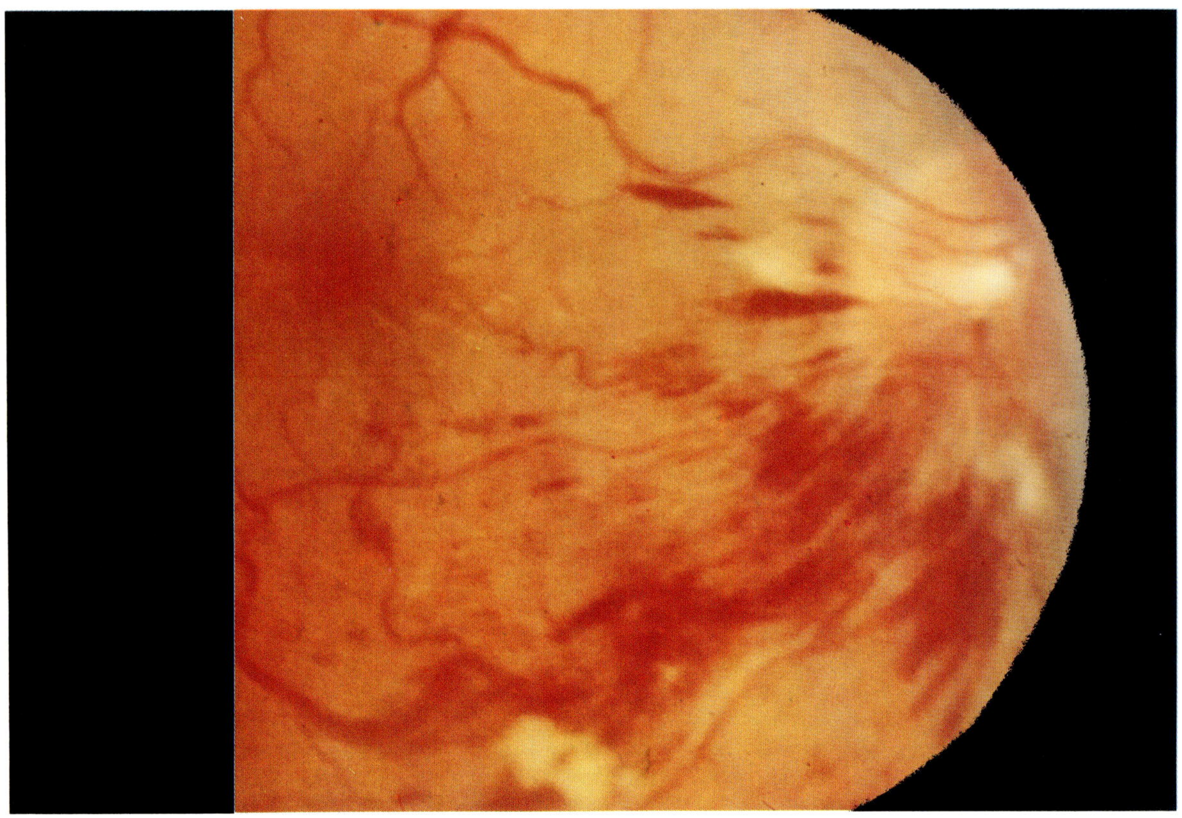

QUESTIONS — C3

Question 1. List abnormalities (see answer, p. 161).

Question 2. What is your diagnosis?

Question 3. What is believed to be the most common cause of venous branch occlusion?

Question 4. Based upon the findings in the retinal photograph, does that mechanism apply in this patient?

Question 5. What clinical data would help you determine the cause of central retinal vein or branch occlusion?

Question 6. What other clinical entities may produce a unilateral retinopathy characterized by hemorrhage and venous dilatation?

Question 7. What other diagnostic procedures may help establish the cause of venous occlusion or venous stasis retinopathy?

ANSWERS — C3

Answer 1. Slight hyperemia of the disc. Several hemorrhages inferior and temporal to the disc. Cotton wool patches are present at 9 and 7 o'clock along with engorgement and tortuosity of the inferior temporal venule. The arterioles are normal.

Answer 2. Occlusion of the inferior temporal vein.

Answer 3. Arteriovenous compression.

Answer 4. No. There is no evidence of A–V compression in this instance.

Answer 5. Hypertension, coronary artery disease, peripheral vascular disease, and diabetes mellitus are often associated abnormalities.

Answer 6. Carotid artery insufficiency due to atherosclerosis and pulseless disease may produce ipsilateral venous stasis retinopathy (hemorrhage and venous dilatation).

Answer 7.

a. Sickle cell preparation.
b. Serum proteins (multiple myeloma and macroglobulinemia).
c. Hematocrit, hemoglobin, erythrocyte and leukocyte count (polycythemia, leukemia).
d. Evidence of CO_2 retention (obstructive lung disease or respiratory depression).
e. Glucose tolerance test (diabetes mellitus).
f. This patient's clinical and laboratory studies disclosed no abnormalities.

The absence of any other detectable abnormality has been observed in a given number of patients with occlusive retinal venous disease.

References

Duke–Elder, W. S. and Dobree, J. H.: *Diseases of the Retina,* in: Duke–Elder, W. S. (ed.), *System of Ophthalmology,* Vol. X, pp. 98–120, Mosby, St. Louis, 1967.

Kearns, T. P. and Hollenhorst, R. W.: *Venous–Stasis Retinopathy of Occlusive Disease of the Carotid Artery,* Proc. Mayo Clin., **38:** 304, 1963.

Paton, A., Rubinstein, K., and Smith, V. H.: *Arterial Insufficiency in Retinal Venous Occlusion,* Trans. Ophthalmol. Soc. U. K., **84:** 559, 1964.

Plate C4

Clinical findings: A 35–year–old black male was known to have insulin dependent diabetes mellitus for 6 years. He was admitted to the hospital because of nausea, vomiting, polyuria, and drowsiness. He had retained no food for 12 hours. Examination disclosed that he was drowsy, confused, and dehydrated. He was breathing deeply at a rate of 30/minute. Bl. P. 140/80 mmHg. The remainder of the physical examination was normal except for the funduscopic examination. Laboratory findings: urine — 5% sugar; urine acetone — strongly positive; blood sugar—580 mgs/100 ml; serum acetone — positive in 1/80 dilution; CO_2 — 10 meq/100 ml; pH — 7.3. When the blood was drawn it was observed to be milky. Plate C4 — O.S. — taken 24 hours later.

PLATE C4

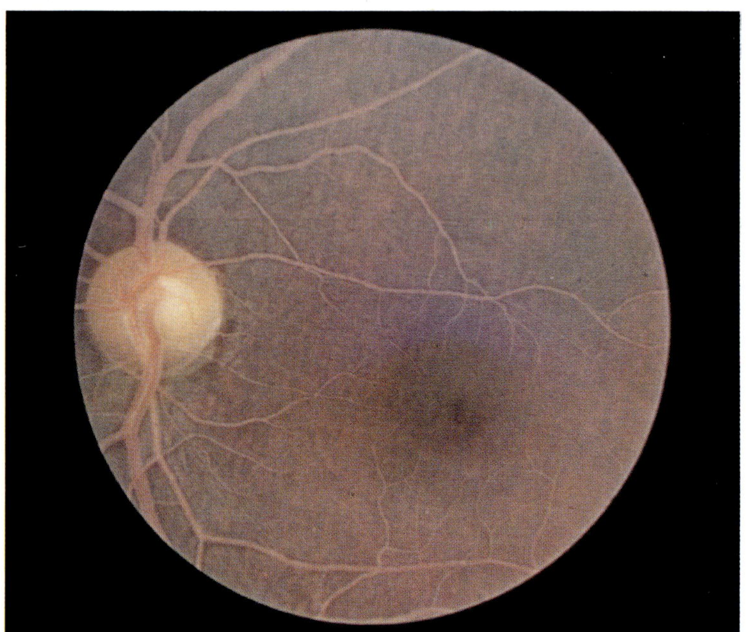

Plate C5

Retinal photograph C5 (O.S. — central superior) taken one week after admission.

PLATE C5

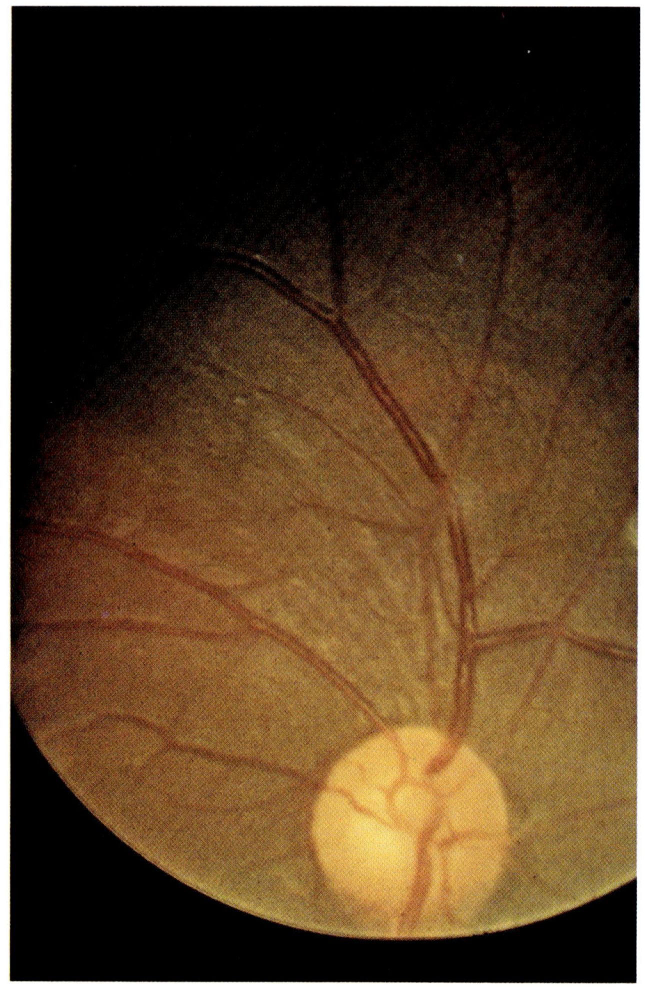

QUESTIONS — C4 AND C5

Question 1. Describe findings of Plate C4 (see answer, p. 163).

Question 2. What are the changes described above called?

Question 3. What lipid fraction of the blood is responsible? The patient responded readily to the administration of insulin, intravenous fluids, and electrolytes. Within 12 hours the ketoacidosis was controlled. The evidence of lipemia retinalis gradually diminished and disappeared after 5 days.

Question 4. Describe Plate 5 (see answer, p. 163).

Question 5. Does lipemia retinalis occur in diseases other than diabetes mellitus?

ANSWERS — C4 AND C5

Answer 1. The disc appears to be white and its margins are distinct. The arterioles and venules are pink and have a white central axial streak. The macula is normal. There are no extravascular lesions.

Answer 2. Lipemia retinalis.

Answer 3. Triglycerides. This patient had marked triglyceridemia which may be associated with uncontrolled diabetes mellitus.

Answer 4. The disc no longer appears to be white. The fundus reflex is the normal mixture of red and black. Minimal venular tortuosity is present. Arteriovenous compression is observed above the disc. It occurs at the first crossing. However, it may be significant since it is beyond 1 disc diameter away from the disc. The author has observed arteriovenous compression in patients with diabetes mellitus who did not have hypertension. To date, a specific arteriolar lesion which can be identified with diabetes mellitus has not been recognized.

Answer 5. Yes. Types I, III, IV, and V lipoproteinemia.

Reference

Fredrickson, D. S., Levy, R. I., and Lees, R. S.: *Fat Transport in Lipoproteins — An Integrated Approach to Mechanisms and Disorders,* N. Engl. J. Med., **276:** 148, 1967.

Plate C6

Clinical findings: A 39–year–old white male with insulin dependent diabetes mellitus for 23 years. Plate C6 — O. D. — central, nasal, and superior.

PLATE C6

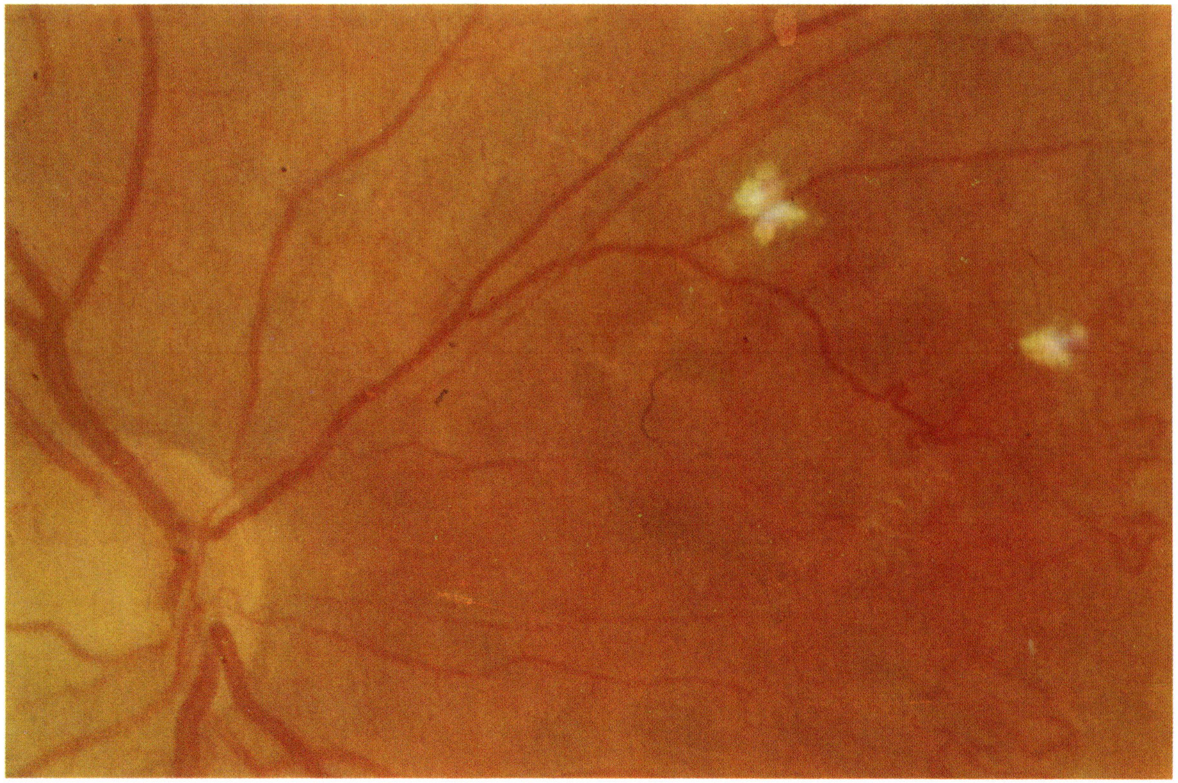

QUESTIONS — C6

Question 1. List abnormalities (see answer, this page).

Question 2. What are the white, scar–like areas?

Question 3. How else might one interpret the white areas?

ANSWERS — C6

Answer 1. The disc is normal. There are two white, irregular areas. One overlies a branch of the superior temporal venule. The other obscures and is interwoven with a mass of tortuous vessels which have an abnormal distribution, undoubtedly the product of new vessel formation.

Answer 2. These are probably the result of obliteration of masses of new vessels. According to Davis, this process of vascular obliteration is part of the sequence of events in neovascularization.

Answer 3. They resemble the cotton wool patch. Clinically it would be difficult to separate the two processes. The fact that the white lesions appear to be associated with neovascularization makes vascular obliteration more likely.

Reference

Davis, M. D.: *Vitreous Contraction in Proliferative Diabetic Retinopathy,* Arch. Ophthalmol., **74,** 741, 1965.

Plate C7

Clinical findings: A 28–year–old male who has had insulin dependent diabetes mellitus for 16 years. Bl. P. 170/120 mmHg. Plate C7 — O.S. — nasal.

QUESTIONS — C7

Question 1. List abnormalities (see answer, this page).

Question 2. What is your diagnosis?

Question 3. What complications may result from this abnormality?

Question 4. What are the mechanisms offered to explain the development of these abnormalities?

ANSWERS — C7

Answer 1. The nasal margin of disc appears to be normal. There is a small flame–shaped hemorrhage above it. Venular tortuosity is marked. A segment of normal retina, immediately adjacent to the disc, is outlined by a fanlike mass of white tissue and new vessel formation. A white mass (probably fibrous tissue) is visible at 8 o'clock on the nasal side, 3 disc diameters from the disc.

Answer 2. Proliferative retinopathy.

Answer 3.

a. Vitreous, preretinal, and retinal hemorrhage.

b. Retinal detachment (see pp. 152–155).

c. Glaucoma (see p. 156).

Answer 4.

a. and b. Hemorrhage is believed to originate from the newly formed, fragile vessels. Presumably, the retraction of the fibrous scar and the vitreous detachment put tension on these vessels and both hemorrhage and retinal detachment follow.

c. The glaucoma associated with proliferative retinopathy is the result of neovascularization and fibrosis of the iris and its trabeculae which lead to closure of the filtration angle of the anterior chamber.

PLATE C7

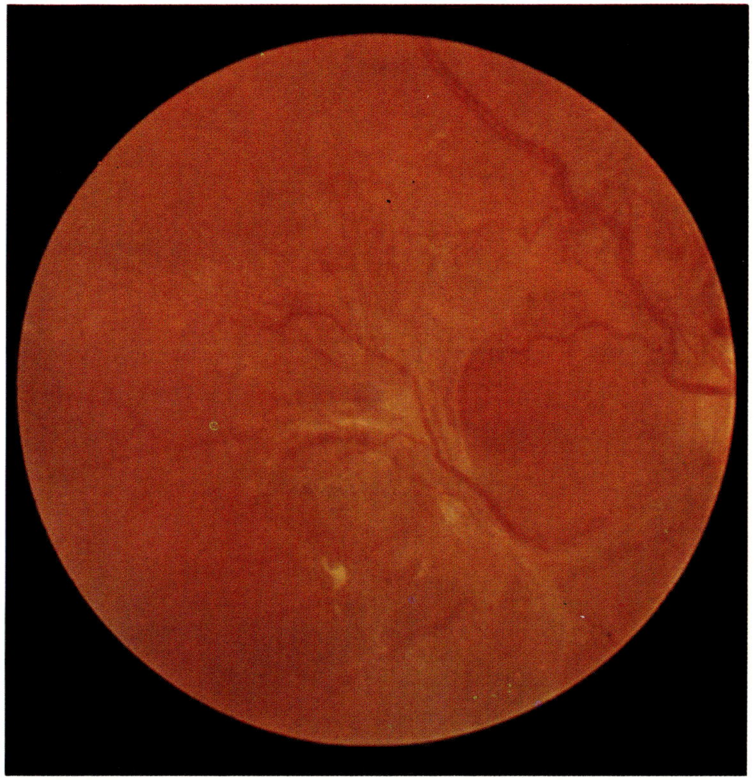

References

Becker, B. and Shaffer, R. N.: *Diagnosis and Therapy of the Glaucomas,* pp. 175, 208–209, Mosby, St. Louis, 1965.

Davis, M. D.: *Vitreous Contraction in Proliferative Diabetic Retinopathy,* Arch. Ophthalmol., **74:** 741, 1965.

Dobree, J. H.: *Proliferative Diabetic Retinopathy. Evolution of the Retinal Lesions,* Br. J. Ophthalmol., **48:** 637, 1964.

Hogan, M. J. and Zimmerman, L. E. (eds.): *Ophthalmic Pathology. An Atlas and Textbook,* 2nd ed., pp. 697–700, 710–711, Saunders, Philadelphia, 1962.

Tolentino, F. I., Lee, P. F., and Schepens, C. L.: *Biomicroscopic Study of Vitreous Cavity in Diabetic Retinopathy,* Arch. Ophthalmol., **75:** 288, 1966.

Plate C8

Clinical findings: A 45–year–old slender male known to have diabetes for 15 years. Dietary restriction and oral hypoglycemic agents provided good control. There were no episodes of diabetic ketoacidosis. Plate C8 — O.S. — magnified view of the macular area.

Plate C9

Clinical findings: An obese female known to have diabetes for 12 years. Dietary restriction and oral hypoglycemic agents effectively controlled levels of blood and urine sugar until 6 years ago. At that time the patient developed insulin resistant disease following a hysterectomy for fibromyomata. She has had repeated episodes of ketoacidosis since then. Her insulin requirements have ranged as high as 1,000 to 2,000 units per day. The insulin resistance has been treated successfully with steroids. Her current dose of insulin of approximately 100 units per day affords satisfactory control. Plate C9 — O.S. — inferior and central magnified view.

Plate C10

Clinical findings: A 35–year–old male with well–controlled insulin sensitive diabetes for 20 years. No episodes of ketoacidosis have occurred over that period of time. Plate C10 — O.S. — nasal.

Plate C11

Clinical findings: A 40–year–old male with poorly controlled insulin dependent diabetes for 15 years. Several episodes of ketoacidosis have been recorded. Plate C11 — O.D. — inferior central magnified view.

PLATES C8 THROUGH C11 (see Answers p. 167)

Question C8. List abnormalities.

Question C9. List abnormalities.

Question C10. List abnormalities.

Question C11. List abnormalities.

PLATE C8

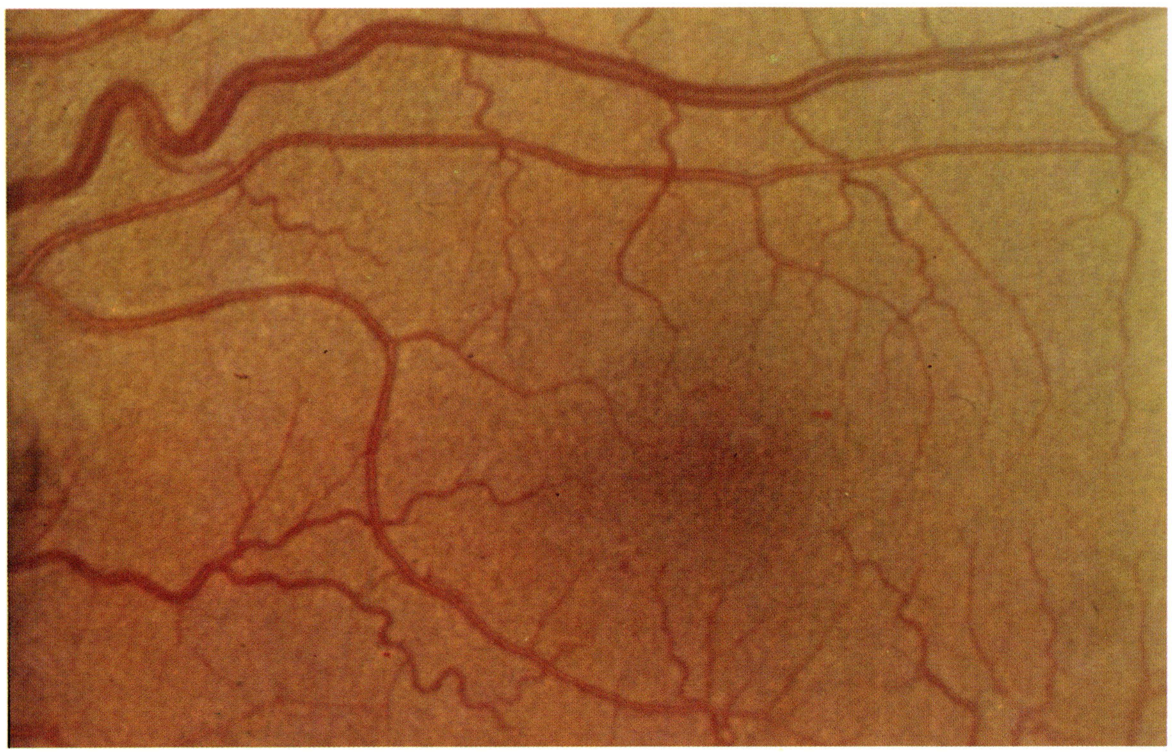

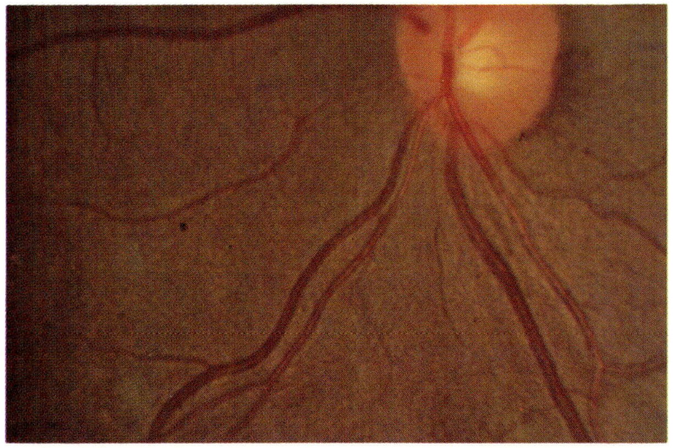

PLATE C9

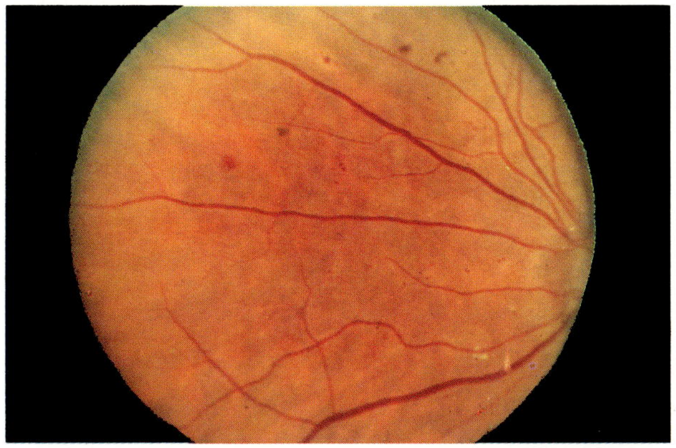

PLATE C10

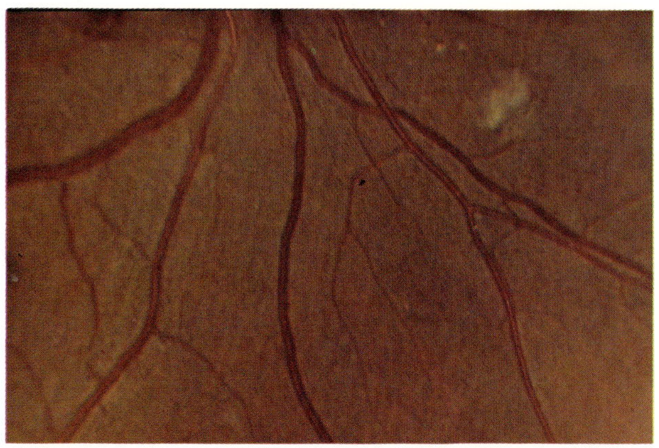

PLATE C11

ANSWERS TO QUESTIONS C8 THROUGH C11

Answer C8. There is marked venular tortuosity. The macula is well outlined and the foveal reflex is normal. There are several hard exudates within the macula and one microaneurysm below it.

Answer C9. The disc is normal. "Copper wire" arteriolar change and slight venular tortuosity are present. A solitary microaneurysm is visible below a venule, between 7 and 8 o'clock, 2 disc diameters from the nerve head.

Answer C10. The small visible portion of the nasal border of the disc is normal. Venular tortuosity is present. There are several microaneurysms and several oval hemorrhages in the peripheral portions of the nasal retina. Two hard exudates are visible near the disc, between 8 and 9 o'clock. Brown pigment envelops a small arteriole at 7 o'clock.

Answer C11. The arterioles and venules are normal. A cotton wool patch and several hard exudates are visible. A solitary microaneurysm can be identified beneath a small arteriole and close to the center of the Plate.

GENERAL QUESTIONS — C8 THROUGH C11

Question 1. If one accepts that the four case reports are fairly typical of the relationship of diabetic retinopathy to duration of overt disease and degree of control, what conclusions can be drawn?

Question 2. What other clinical abnormalities are frequently observed when retinopathy is present in the diabetic patient?

Question 3. Based upon clinical findings, what is the order of frequency of the retinopathy, peripheral neuropathy, and nephropathy?

ANSWERS TO GENERAL QUESTIONS — C8 THROUGH C11

Answer 1. a. Manifestations of diabetic retinopathy, which include venous abnormalities, microaneurysms, hemorrhage, cotton wool patches, and hard exudates, are generally observed 10 years or more after overt disease is discovered.
b. Although differences of opinion exist, it appears that control of diabetes, as measured by degree of hyperglycemia and glycosuria, is not the determining factor in the development of diabetic retinopathy.

Answer 2. Peripheral neuropathy and intracapilllary glomerulosclerosis.

Answer 3. Order of frequency. Retinopathy is most common; neuropathy is next; and nephropathy is least commonly observed clinically.

Reference

Adnitt, P. I. and Taylor, E.: *Progression of Diabetic Retinopathy. Relationship to Blood–Sugar,* Lancet, **1:** 652, 1970.

Plate C12

Clinical findings: A 66-year-old female was admitted to the hospital because of fracture of the femoral neck following a fall. X-ray of the skeletal system, in addition to the above fracture, showed osteoporosis of vertebrae, pelvic bones, and both femurs. Laboratory findings included: Hb — 9.8 gm/100 ml; RBC — 3,000,000; Hct. 32%; WBC — 7,000/mm^3. Differential was normal. Rouleaux formation noted on smear and in red blood cell counting chamber. Ca — 9 meq/100 ml; P — 3 meq/100 ml; alkaline phosphatase — 3.5 units/100 ml; total proteins — 9.7 gms/100 ml; albumin 3.5; -globulin — 6.2. Bone marrow — aspiration biopsy disclosed an increased number of plasma cells.

A diagnosis of multiple myeloma was made.

QUESTIONS — C12

Question 1. Describe findings in Plate C12 (see answer, p. 169).

Question 2. Are the abnormalities described specific for multiple myeloma?

PLATE C12

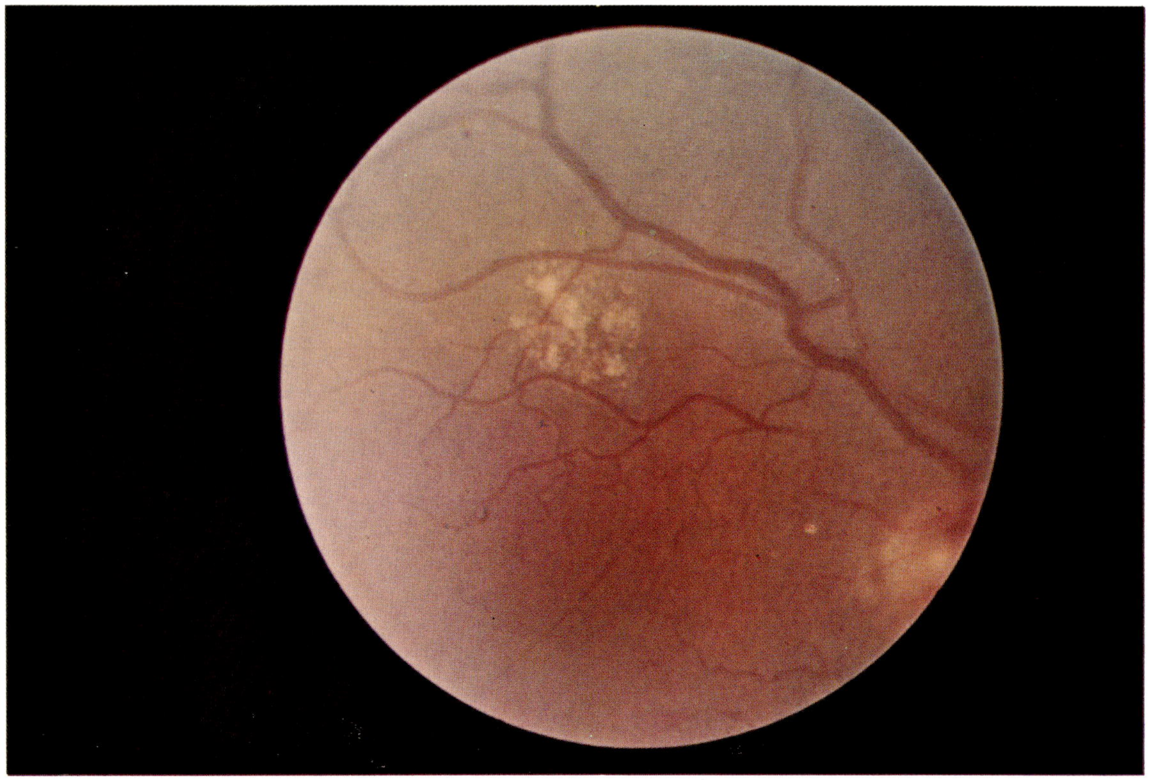

ANSWERS — C12

Answer 1. The visible nasal portion of the disc is normal. There is a moderate degree of tortuosity and engorgement of the superior nasal vein. A cluster of hard exudates is visible at 10 o'clock, 2–3 disc diameters from the nerve head. A solitary hard exudate is noted close to the disc.

Answer 2. No. The venous changes and extravascular lesions are present in a wide group of hematologic disorders, particularly when anemia is present (see pp. 64, 76, 92, 93, 126).

References

Allen, R. A. and Straatsma, B. R.: *Ocular Involvement in Leukemia and Allied Disorders,* Arch. Ophthalmol., **66:** 490, 1961.

Holt, J. M. and Gordon–Smith, E. C.: *Retinal Abnormalities in Diseases of the Blood,* Br. J. Ophthalmol., **53:** 145, 1969.

Plate C13

Clinical findings: A 39–year–old male with insulin dependent diabetes mellitus since age 16. In addition to the retinopathy, as noted in retinal photograph, Plate C13, there was evidence of peripheral neuropathy. The BUN was 22 mg/100 ml; Bl. P. 160/100 mmHg; vision was 20/40 O.D. and 20/200 O.S. Plate C13 — O.D. — macular area.

Plate C14

Clinical findings: A 45–year–old male with insulin dependent diabetes mellitus for 25 years. During his last admission to the hospital, he was totally blind. There was evidence of peripheral neuropathy. The BUN was 120 mgs/100 ml and the creatinine was 7.5 mgs/100 ml. Marked proteinuria was present. Bl. P. 180/110 mmHg. Plate C14 — O.D. — central and nasal.

PLATE C13

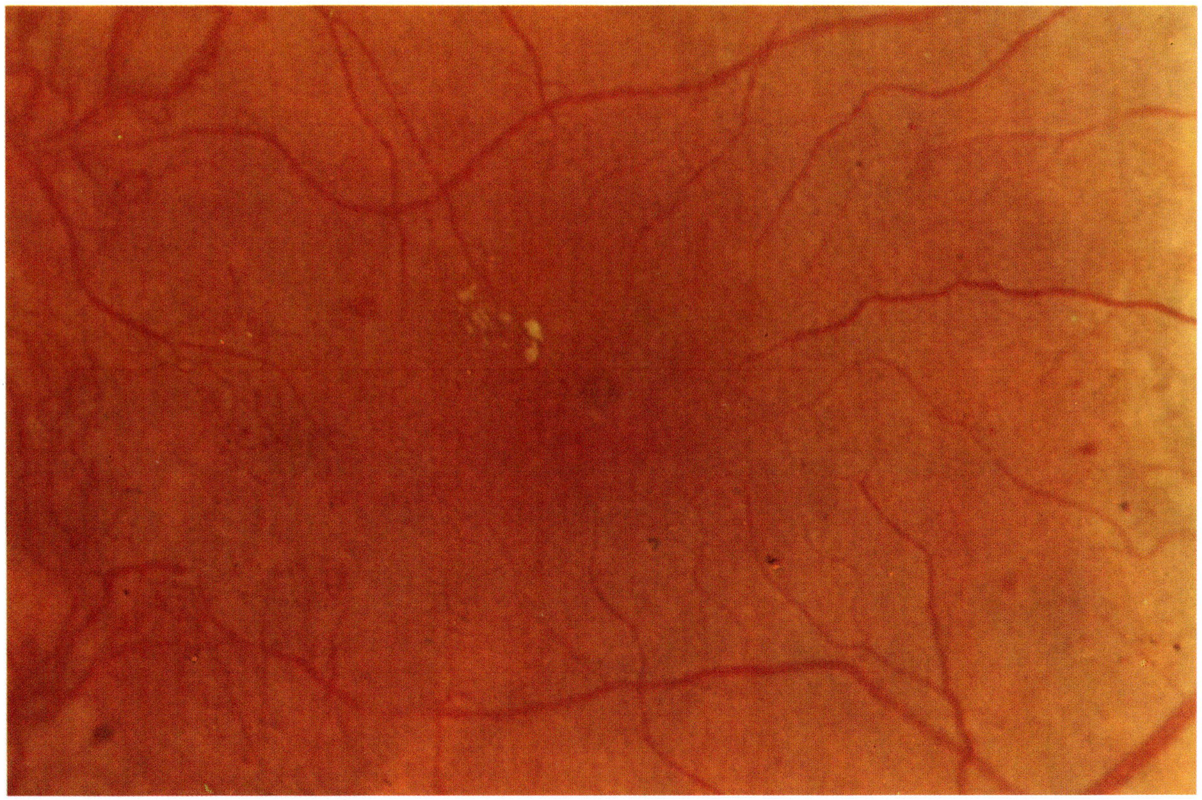

PLATE C14

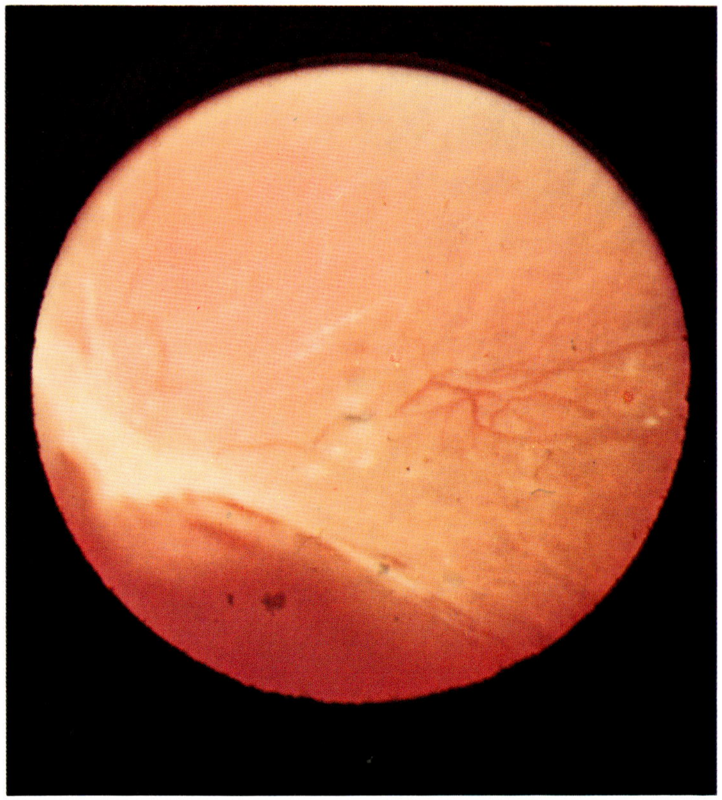

QUESTIONS — C13 AND C14

Question 1. List abnormalities in Plate C13 (see answer, this page).

Question 2. List abnormalities in Plate C14 (see answer, this page).

Question 3. Where would you place the large hemorrhage observed in Plate C14? Consider Plates C13 and C14 as examples of severe diabetic retinopathy. Each presents neovascularization. In Plate C14, there is marked proliferation of fibrous tissue and massive hemorrhage as well. In addition, patient C14 is blind. In each of the two patients the changes noted were approximately the same in both eyes.

Question 4. What effect upon the retinal changes in each of these patients could be expected if pituitary ablation were performed?

Question 5. What other operative approach can be used in an attempt to control diabetic retinopathy?

Question 6. Which of the changes observed in retinal photographs, Plates C13 and C14, are likely to be responsive to photocoagulation?

ANSWERS — C13 AND C14

Answer 1. The fovea appears to be encircled by either hemorrhage or pigment. Slightly above it, at 11 o'clock, there are several hard exudates. There are numerous, abnormally distributed, new vessels temporal to the macula. Numerous microaneurysms and a few flame–shaped hemorrhages are visible. Venular tortuosity is evident.

Answer 2. A large, sharply outlined hemorrhage obscures the lower portion of the field. A small, linear hemorrhage is also present. Bands of scar tissue radiate peripherally from a point above the large hemorrhage. Neovascularization appears to originate from the same region. The disease process has either obscured or destroyed the normal architecture of the retina.

Answer 3. Since it obscures the retinal structures under it, it is preretinal. In all likelihood, it is in the vitreous cavity.

Answer 4. Regresson of neovascularization and hemorrhage may occur. The fibrous tissue does not appear to be affected by this procedure.

Answer 5. Retinal photocoagulation (see pp. 144, 147).

Answer 6. Neovascularization.

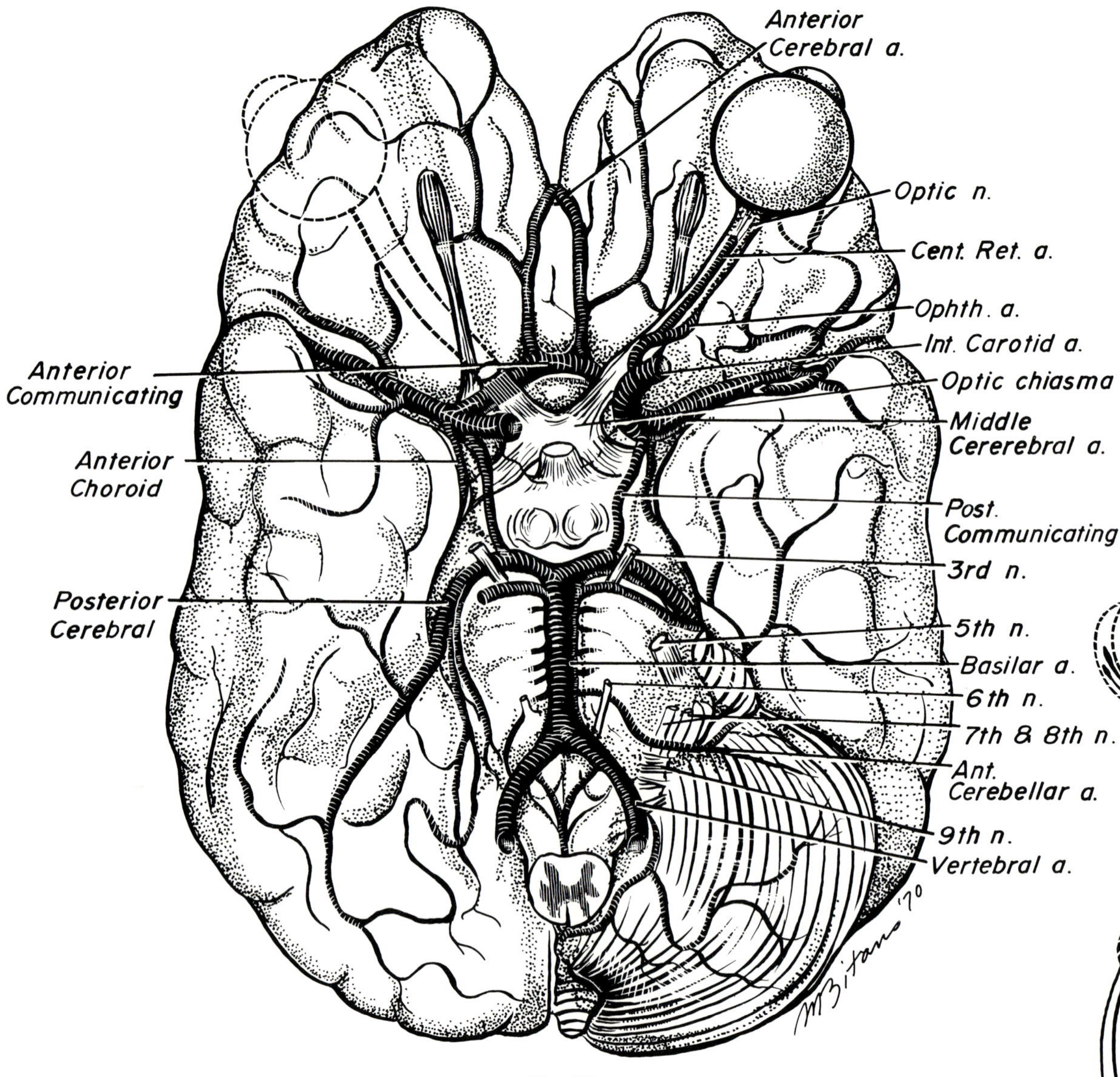
Anterior Cerebral a.
Optic n.
Cent. Ret. a.
Ophth. a.
Int. Carotid a.
Optic chiasma
Anterior Communicating
Middle Cererebral a.
Anterior Choroid
Post. Communicating
3rd n.
Posterior Cerebral
5th n.
Basilar a.
6th n.
7th & 8th n.
Ant. Cerebellar a.
9th n.
Vertebral a.

Fig. IX

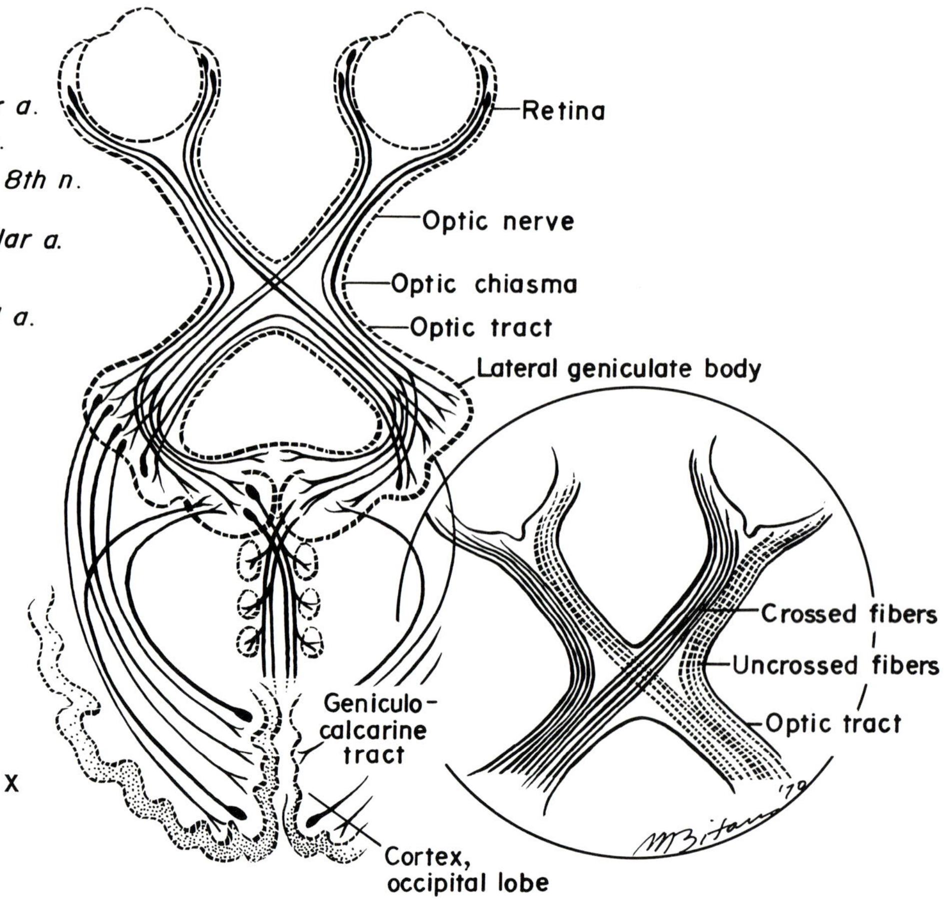
Retina
Optic nerve
Optic chiasma
Optic tract
Lateral geniculate body
Crossed fibers
Uncrossed fibers
Optic tract
Geniculo-calcarine tract
Cortex, occipital lobe

Fig. X

Chapter **VII**
DISEASE OF THE OPTIC NERVE

THE OPTIC NERVE

The optic nerve is formed by the axons of the ganglion cells of the retina (see pp. 9–10). These nonmyelinated fibers converge to form the optic papilla. The axons pierce the lamina cribrosa, acquire myelin sheaths, and emerge from the globe as a compact nerve. Anatomically, the optic nerve is divided into four segments: intraocular, intraorbital, intracanalicular, and intracranial.

The intraocular portion consists of the nonmyelinated fibers of the optic papilla. These axons are formed into bundles and extend through the lamina cribrosa (Drawing 4). The nerve fibers which leave the globe are myelinated and form the intraorbital segment. This portion extends to the optic foramen and is enveloped by the dural, arachnoid, and pial membranes of the brain. After the nerve leaves the orbit, it extends along the lesser wing of the sphenoid bone for a short distance, the intracanalicular portion. The next segment, the intracranial portion, courses backward to join the opposite optic nerve and forms the optic chiasm in the region of the sella turcica (Fig. IX). Beyond the chiasm the optic nerve fibers continue as the optic tracts (Fig. X). The majority of the nerve fibers of the optic tracts terminate in the lateral geniculate bodies. From that relay station, the visual impulse is transmitted, via the geniculocalcarine tract, to the visual cortex of the occipital lobe.

Throughout its course the optic nerve is closely related to many important structures (Fig. IX). Initially it is related to many structures within the orbit. Its intracranial portion extends under the posterior end of the olfactory nerve and above the ophthalmic and internal carotid arteries and the diaphragm of the sella. The chiasm is in the immediate vicinity of the sella turcica and its contents, the internal carotid arteries, the circle of Willis, and the third ventricle. The importance of these anatomic relationships will become evident in the discussion of abnormalities of the optic nerve since many of them result from the alterations of the adjacent structures.

Abnormalities of the optic nerve include papilledema, optic neuritis, optic atrophy, congenital anomalies, and tumor. Only the first three will be discussed in this book. The reader is referred to standard textbooks of ophthalmology for a presentation of congenital anomalies and tumors of the optic nerve.

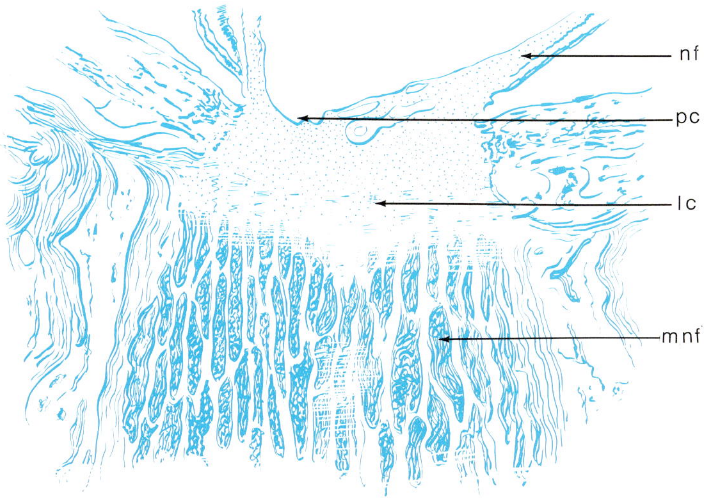

Drawing 4. Plate 4 (nf, nerve fiber layer; pc, physiologic cup; lc, lamina cribrosa; mnf, myelinated nerve fibers).

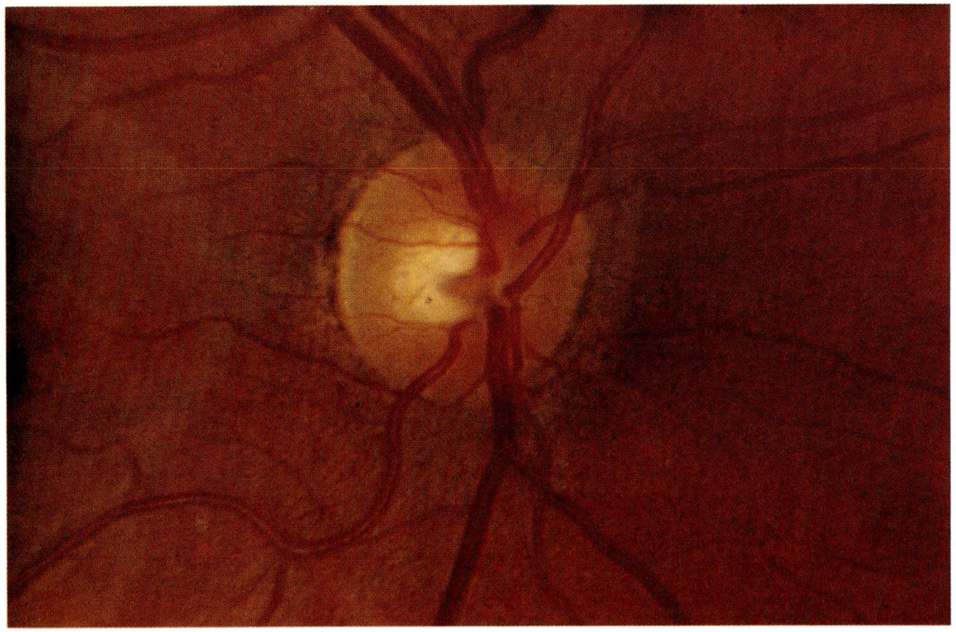

Plate 185. O.S. An enlarged view of the normal optic disc. The disc margins are distinct. The temporal margin is sharper than the nasal one. The disc is not elevated. The blood vessels above it are straight and in the same plane as the nerve head. The disc is pink except for the white physiologic cup. A sunburst effect is created by the retinal fibers as they enter the nerve head.

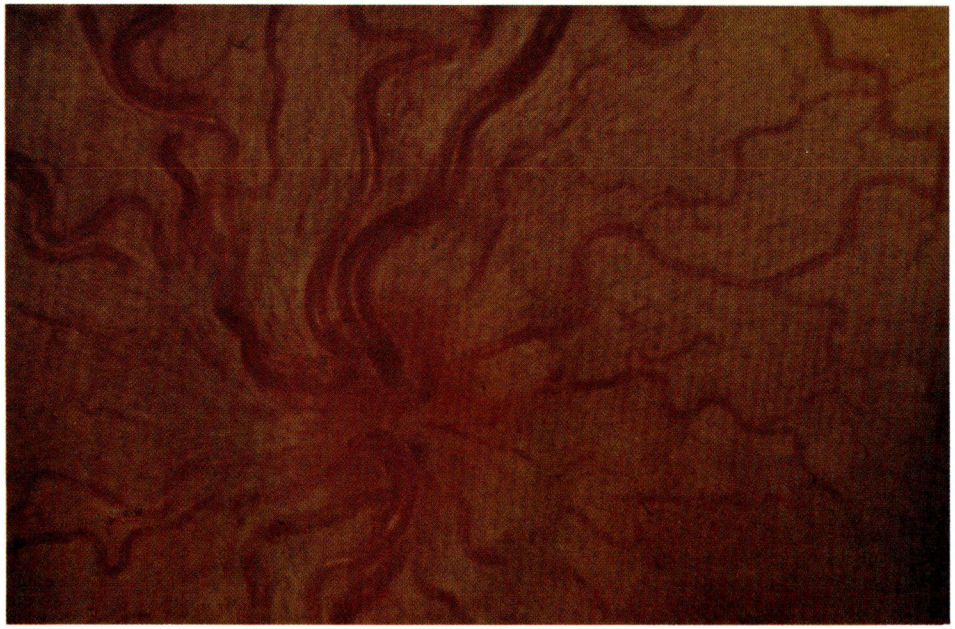

Plate 186. O.S. Hyperemia of disc. Elevation of vessels over the nerve head. Loss of disc margins and temporal halo. Venous engorgement and tortuosity.

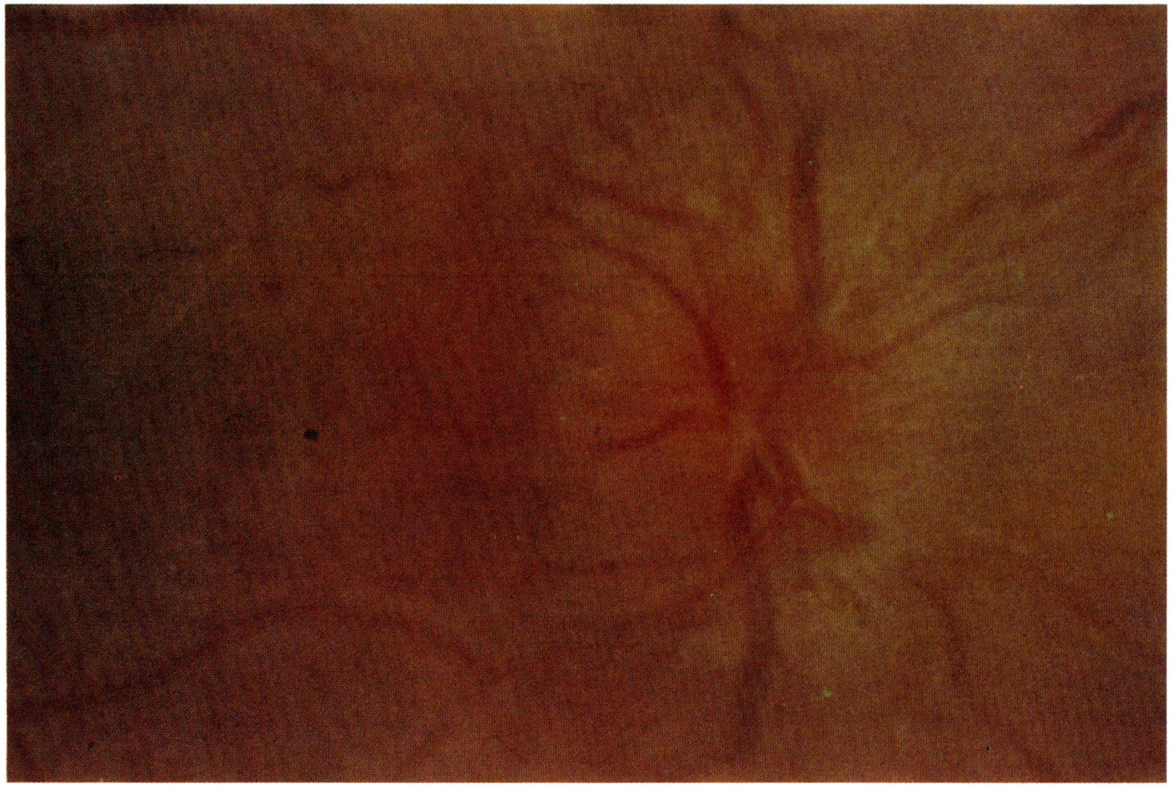

Plate 187. O.S. Loss of disc margins. Hyperemia of disc.

Papilledema

Papilledema is a noninflammatory edema of the optic disc. The synonym, choked disc, is used frequently in reference to patients who have evidence of increased intracranial pressure. When the process extends from the optic disc to the adjacent retina, the term neuroretinal edema is applied.[245]

CLINICAL APPEARANCE

Before the clinical findings of papilledema are considered, it would be profitable to review the ophthalmoscopic appearance of the normal optic disc (Plate 185). When papilledema is present the changes in the optic disc include hyperemia, elevation, indistinct margins, nerve fiber separation at its borders, and obliteration of the physiologic cup (Plates 186–192). As the hyperemia progresses the disc develops a diffuse pink blush (Plates 186–190). The margins are eventually lost and the nerve fibers which converge on the disc are widely separated (Plates 188–191). Progressive protrusion of the nerve head is observed, often as much as 6–8 diopters.* The elevated and engorged retinal veins appear to drop abruptly over the swollen nerve head (Plates 186, 187, and 192). Venous pulsation can no longer be elicited even after external pressure is applied to the eyeball. Concentric rings (halos) may develop around the disc (Plates 186–188). Striate or linear hemorrhage and cotton wool patches may develop in the disc or in the immediately adjacent retina (Plates 188–190, and 192). The spread of edema temporally may produce a macular fan or star (Plates 190 and 191).

*The elevation of the disc is measured in the following manner. Begin the examination with a high positive lens of the ophthalmoscope. Decrease the lens power until you focus on the most forward protrusion of the disc; then alter the lens until the retinal vessels close to the disc come into focus. The difference in lens power used to bring those two areas into focus measures the elevation in diopters.[3 (pp. 137-138)] Approximately 3 diopters equal 1 millimeter.

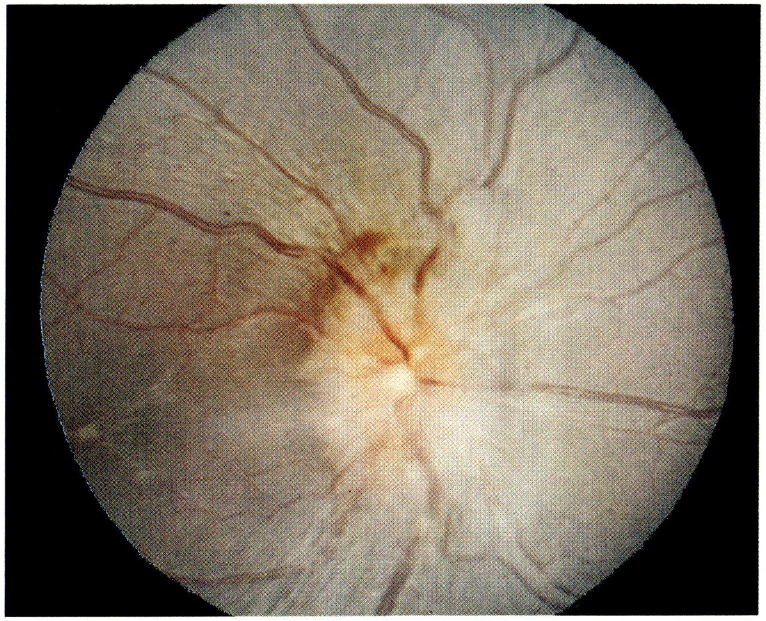

Plate 188. O.D. Hyperemia, loss of disc margins, halo, and nerve fiber separation. Venular tortuosity; narrowed arterioles with segmental "silver wire" change. Linear hemorrhage above disc. Did you notice a partial macular star?

Plate 189. O.S. Hyperemia of disc, halo, indistinct margins, nerve fiber separation, and cotton wool patches.

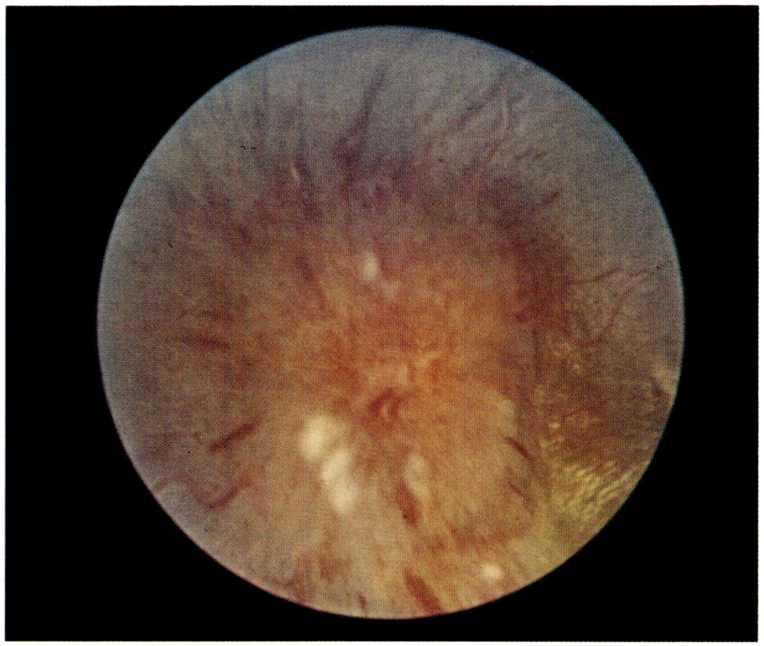

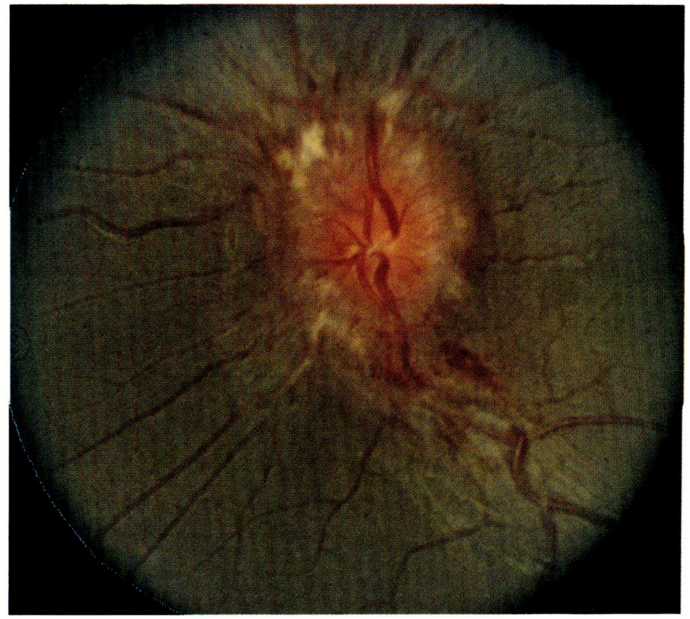

Plate 190. O.S. Hyperemia, elevation, and loss of disc margins. Hemorrhage and cotton wool patches in and close to nerve head. Macular fan.

Plate 191. O.S. Slight hyperemia, loss of margins, and nerve fiber separation over superior nasal part of disc. Note the hemorrhage, macular star, and cotton wool patch. "Copper and silver wire" arteriolar changes. Did you notice the cilioretinal vessel at 5 o'clock?

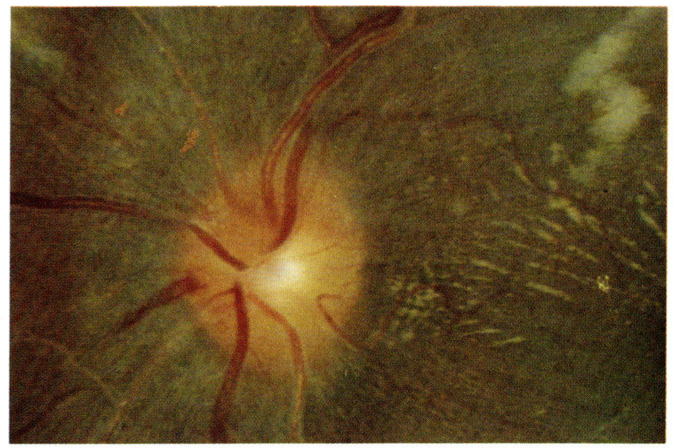

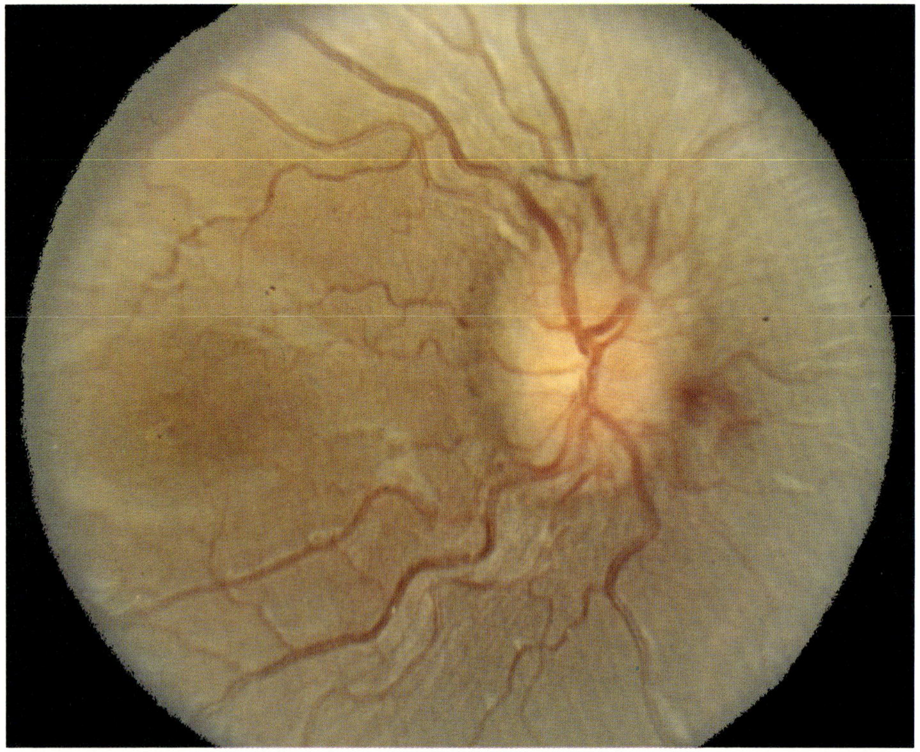

Plate 192. O.D. Papilledema in a patient with aqueductal stenosis and hydrocephalus. Did you notice the hemorrhage at 4 o'clock, the cotton wool patch at 11 o'clock and the retinal sheen?

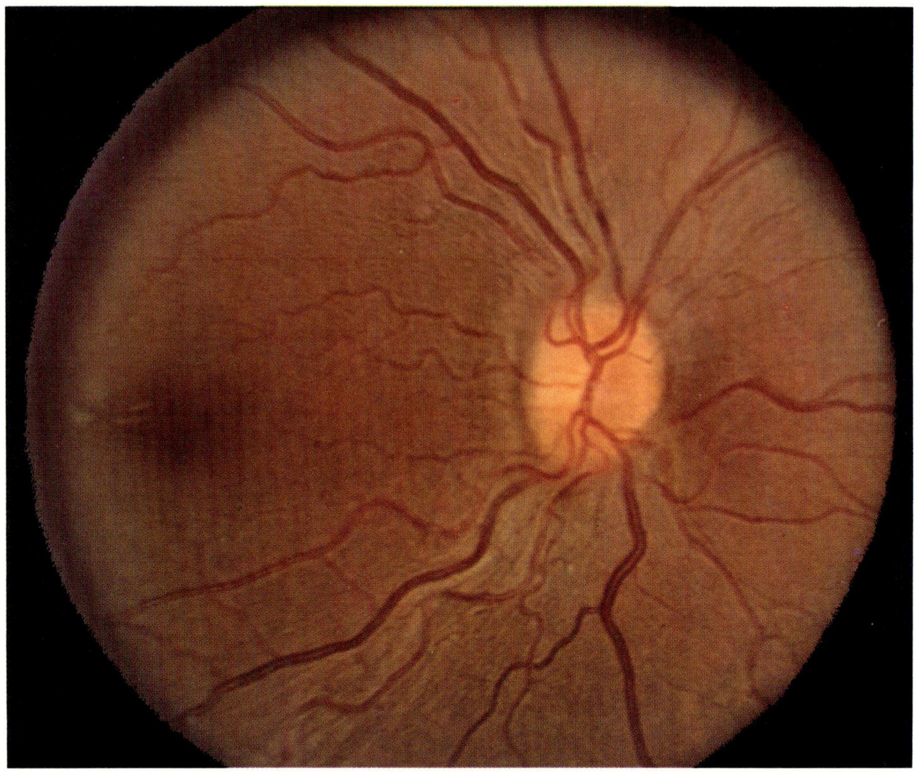

Plate 193. O.D. Same patient as Plate 192 2 months after decompression by means of a ventricular–atrial shunt. The disc margins are distinct. The hemorrhage and cotton wool patch are no longer present and the venous tortuosity is less marked.

The clinical recognition of overt papilledema, as described above, offers little challenge. In contrast, the early and subtle manifestations may be difficult to detect. The examiner must remember that newly developed and progressive changes of the optic disc, such as hyperemia, loss of distinct disc margins, and absence of central retinal vein pulsation, particularly in a patient with known or suspected intracranial disease, may be early indications of papilledema. As a rule the loss of disc margins begins first at the upper and lower borders. This change is followed by the loss of the nasal and temporal margins, in that order. Generally such a sequence of events occurs over a period of days or weeks. During that period the florid, classic changes may become evident. Characteristic changes can be demonstrated with fluorescein angiography in the presence of papilledema. The extensive and dilated capillary network on the disc becomes fluorescent during the arterial phase. The dye leaks from the capillaries and within 10 minutes the nerve head becomes fluorescent.[246, 247]

In patients with increased intracranial pressure, regression of papilledema may occur spontaneously or after decompression in seven to ten days (Plates 192 and 193). The return to normal, over a period of 6 to 8 weeks, includes a gradual decrease in the elevation of the disc; the margins regain their sharp outline; nerve fiber separation and the peripapillary halo disappear. The venous engorgement disappears and the optic disc regains its normal appearance. Unfortunately papilledema, if prolonged, may be followed by secondary optic atrophy. The disc becomes pale and its margins distinct but irregular. The lamina cribrosa may be obliterated. Such changes may be associated with sheathing of arterioles and venules (see pp. 184–89).

The visual symptoms of papilledema are usually not prominent and are generally overshadowed by those of increased intracranial pressure such as headache, nausea, vomiting, alterations of state of consciousness, or loss of motor function. Examination of visual fields may show an enlarged blind spot. Severe deterioration of vision is the result of optic atrophy.

The ophthalmoscopic findings in optic neuritis (papillitis) simulate those of papilledema. Optic neuritis is generally unilateral and, in contrast to papilledema, there is marked visual loss. The central scotoma, found in papillitis, affects color more than white. The course is shorter and recovery is usually spontaneous in papillitis. As a rule, the elevation of the disc is slight in optic neuritis, generally measuring no more than three diopters. Hemorrhage and venous engorgement may be more prominent in papillitis than in papilledema.[4 (p. 648)]

The terms pseudo–neuritis and pseudo–papilledema are applied to the ophthalmoscopic findings in patients with hypermetropia. Although the disc margins are indistinct and the nerve head elevation may reach six diopters, venous engorgement, hemorrhage, and cotton wool patches are not observed in pseudo–papilledema. Even more important is the static nature of the appearance of the disc in the latter. The character of the refractive error and the absence of clinical and laboratory evidence of intracranial disease help distinguish the optic nerve alteration of hypermetropia from papilledema.

Drusen or hyaline bodies of the disc may be mistaken for papilledema since they cause elevation of the nerve head and blurring of its margins (Plate 194). These rare abnormalities appear as multiple, ovoid, translucent, white masses, chiefly at the edges of the disc. Hyperemia, hemorrhage, areas of degeneration, and venous engorgement are absent. Drusen of the disc are generally bilateral and static. Although the blind spot may be increased, vision is not seriously impaired unless the process spreads into the adjacent retina or ruptures into the vitreous. Histologic examination discloses the presence of deposits anterior to the lamina cribrosa (Plate 195 and Drawing 195). They are generally located on the nasal side of the disc, although the central and temporal areas may also be involved. The lesions consist of masses of calcium and an amorphous material which resembles hyaline.[248] Their genesis is not known and they do not appear to be related to the drusen bodies found on Bruch's membrane.

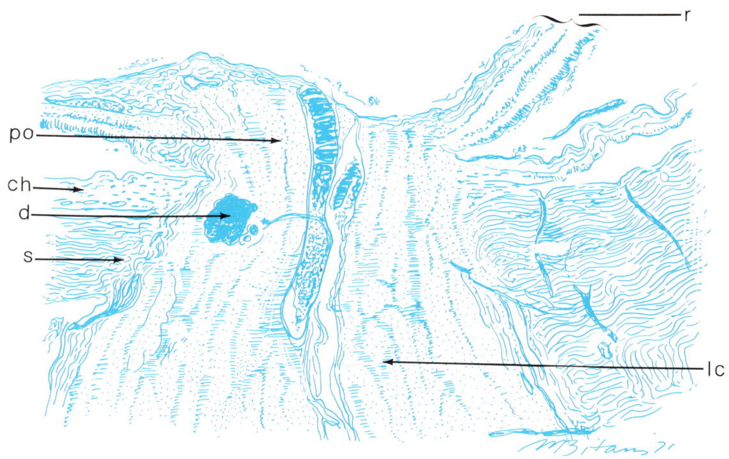

Drawing 195. Plate 195 (po, optic papilla; r, retina; lc, lamina cribrosa; ch, choroid; d, drusen; s, sclera).

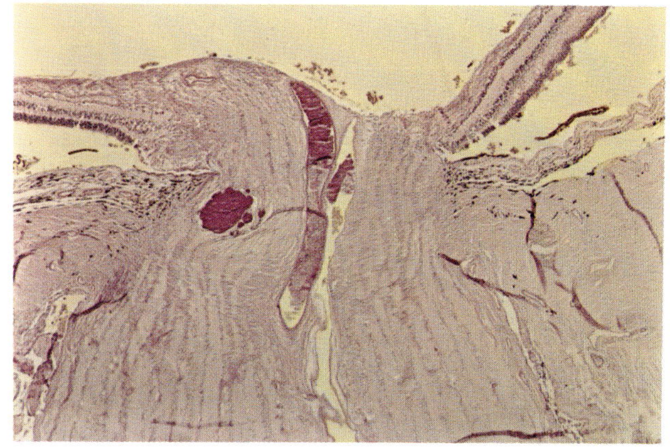

Plate 195. Drusen of the optic nerve. A PAS positive mass of amorphous material is present anterior to the lamina cribrosa (PAS, × 20).

Plate 194. Drusen of disc. Disc margins are indistinct. Several small oval bodies are visible on the disc extending to the margins. Note the absence of venous engorgement or tortuosity.

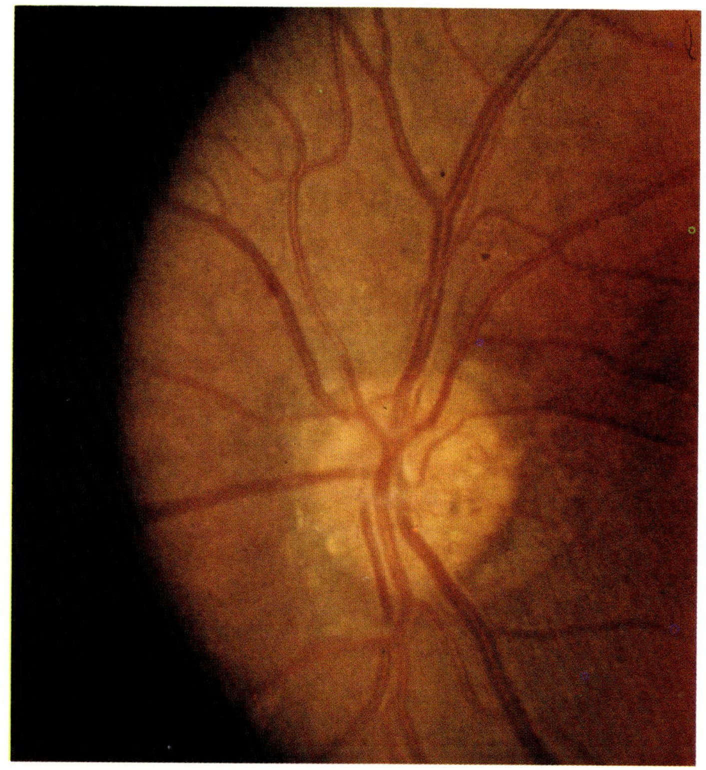

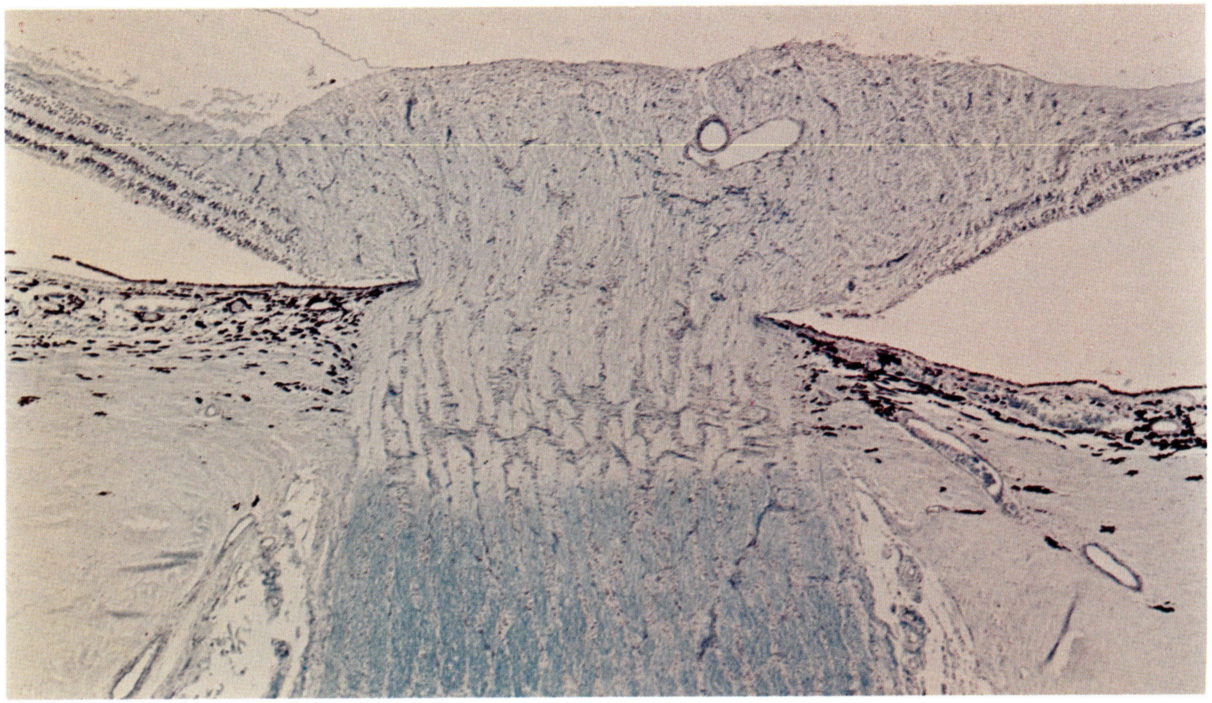

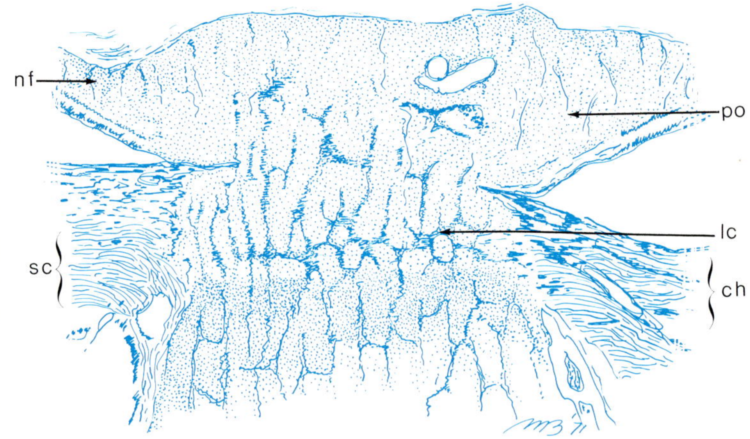

Drawing 196. Plate 196 (po, optic papilla; lc, lamina cribrosa; ch, choroid; sc, sclera; nf, nerve fibers).

Plate 196. Marked swelling of the papilla extending laterally. The nerve fibers anterior to the lamina cribrosa are separated and pale. Fibers of lamina are bowed proximally (LFB, × 12).

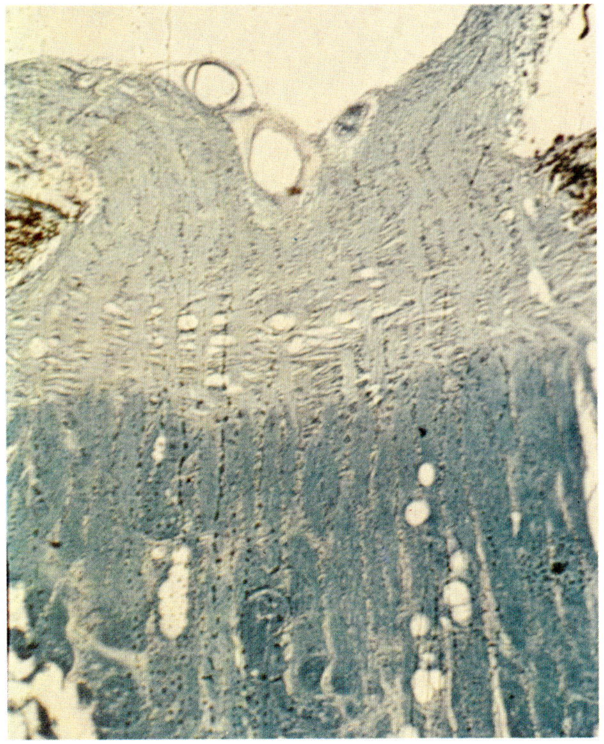

Plate 197. Compare with Plate 196. Normal nerve head. Note physiologic cup (Plate 197), the absence of swelling, and normal alignment of lamina cribrosa (LFB, × 20).

Drawing 197. Plate 197 (pc, physiologic cup; nf, nerve fiber layer; po, optic papilla; lc, lamina cribrosa; mnf, myelinated nerve fibers; fs, fibrous septa).

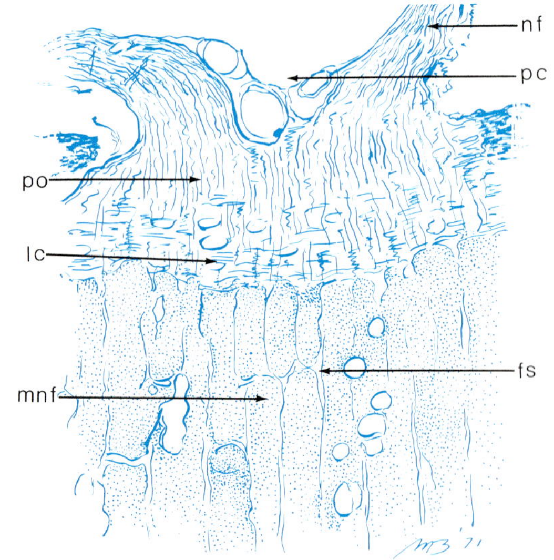

PATHOLOGY

The major histologic changes consist of vascular engorgement and swelling of the portion of the optic nerve which lies anterior to the lamina cribrosa and the adjacent retina. The edematous papilla increases in size in all directions (Plate 196 and Drawing 196). Compare 196 with the normal (Plate 197 and Drawing 197). It bulges forward, compresses, and often narrows or obliterates the physiologic cup. As the swelling spreads laterally it displaces the retina and either lifts it away from the pigment cell layer or by compression produces a series of concentric folds adjacent to the disc. The nerve fibers of the papilla and adjacent retina are separated, swollen, and pale–staining. The fibers of the lamina cribrosa are markedly separated and frequently develop a forward convexity. The edema may spread to the papillo–macular bundle or accumulate in the outer plexiform layer of the macula. Edema may be present under the pia in the portion of the optic nerve proximal to the lamina cribrosa.[249] When present, it is diminished at the entrance site of the central retinal vessels and generally disappears proximal to that point.

Venous and capillary congestion and hemorrhage of the papilla and adjacent retina are common findings (Plate 198 and Drawing 198). The red blood cells are frequently scattered in small clumps lying along and amongst the nérve fibers. Less commonly the hemorrhage may be more extensive and may accumulate under the internal limiting membrane of the adjacent retina or in the outer plexiform layer. Cellular infiltration is unusual and is more likely to be present in long standing papilledema.

In rare instances, these changes of papilledema may completely disappear with no resi-

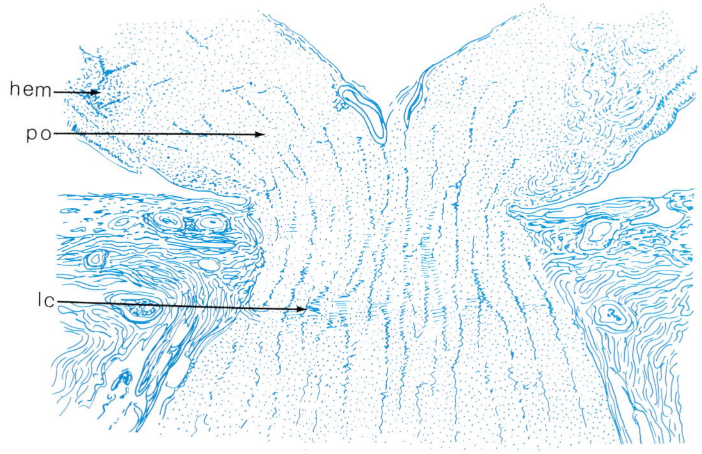

Drawing 198. Plate 198 (hem, hemorrhage; po, optic papilla; lc, lamina cribrosa).

Plate 198. Hemorrhage and papilledema. Note small hemorrhage among nerve fibers of a markedly edematous optic papilla (PTAH, × 25).

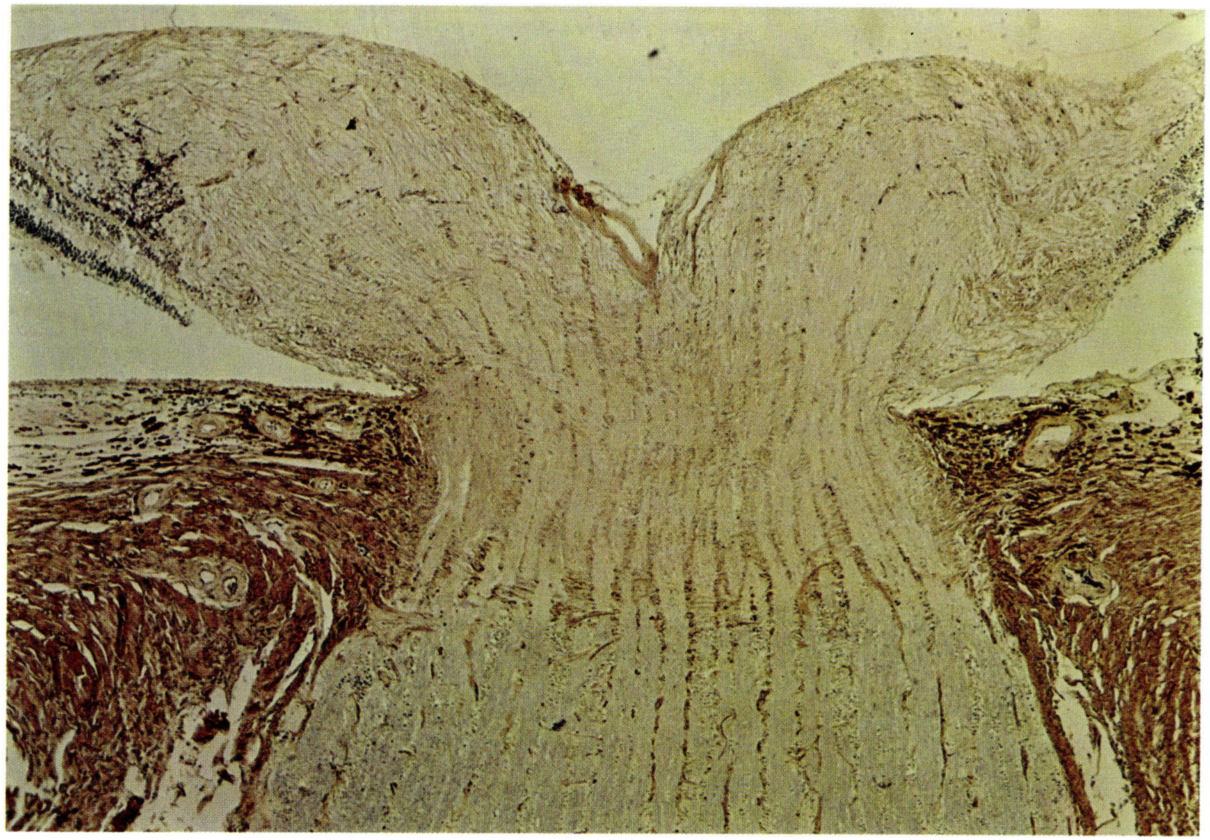

dua. When the changes persist, cytoid bodies may develop within either the papilla or wherever the nerve fiber swelling and displacement are marked. When papilledema is prolonged, optic atrophy may follow. This alteration may begin even while there is still considerable swelling of the papilla. It consists of a decrease in both size and number of nerve fibers along with proliferation of microglia and perivascular connective tissue.[249] The walls of the central vessels and their branches may become hyalinized and thickened or obliterated. Round cells and leukocytes may infiltrate around the vessel walls (see p. 190).

THE CLINICAL PATHOLOGICAL CORRELATION OF PAPILLEDEMA

The pathologic changes of papilledema correlate well with the clinical manifestations. The vascular congestion produces the hyperemia and venous tortuosity; the disc elevation and obliteration of the physiologic cup can be accounted for by anterior projection of the edematous papilla; the loss of margins and nerve fiber separation are the result of the lateral extension of the nerve head to the adjacent retina and the histologically observed swelling and separation of the nerve fibers. The halos or concentric rings are believed to be the result of the folds produced in the retina as the swelling spreads from the papilla. The spread of edema to the macular area accounts for the macular fan. Since the retinal nerve fibers of the papilla retain their parallel arrangement, papillary hemorrhage is linear. Cytoid bodies in the papilla are the basis for the cotton wool patches in the disc.

PATHOGENESIS

Papilledema is most often observed in patients with elevated intracranial pressure. Since the vaginal space which envelops the optic nerve communicates directly with the subarachnoid space, there is free communication of cerebrospinal fluid. When intracranial pressure is elevated, the pressure of the cerebrospinal fluid is increased in the sheath of the optic nerve as well as in the brain. It has been proposed that increased pressure in the vaginal sheath of the optic nerve could rise to or above the level of the pressure in the central retinal vein and impede its flow when intracranial pressure is elevated. Paton and Holmes,[249] who offered this concept, stated that the resulting venous stasis and increased pressure produced the edema of the optic nerve. Leinfelder[250] suggested that the elevated pressure in the central retinal vein impeded return flow from the capillaries of the nerve head which arose from the circle of Zinn–Haller. In his view, the congestion and stasis of the capillaries of that circle provide the mechanism for the development of the edema of the optic nerve and for its location in the fibers anterior to the lamina cribrosa.

Experimental evidence of the relationship of retarded blood flow in the central retinal vein, increased cerebrospinal fluid pressure, and distention of the optic nerve sheath with papilledema was provided by Cushing and Bordley,[251] who produced such changes in the dog by raising intracranial pressure. Further supportive data have been developed by Hayreh,[252] who placed inflated balloons in the subdural space of rhesus monkeys and noted that papilledema developed in 3 to 7 days in animals whose cerebrospinal fluid pressure was elevated. When a window was made in the optic nerve sheath on one side and increased intracranial pressure was induced, papilledema developed only in the eye with the intact optic nerve sheath. When the identical procedure was performed in the presence of bilateral papilledema and the elevated intracranial pressure maintained, regression of the optic nerve changes occurred only on the side where the nerve sheath window had been created.

Factual evidence is lacking to support either the concept that cerebrospinal fluid under pressure is forced into the substances of the optic nerve or that the edema of the papilla is a manifestation of edema of the brain. The absence of significant histologic evidence of cellular response in papilledema minimizes the role of inflammation as a causal factor.

Sudden drastic decrease in intraocular tension following trauma or ocular trephine, in the absence of increased cerebrospinal pressure, may produce papilledema.[2, (p. 587)] The mechanism responsible for swelling of the optic disc under those circumstances is not clear.

PAPILLEDEMA AND CLINICAL STATES

Lesions which produce increased intracranial pressure are the most common causes of papilledema. These include brain tumor, cerebral abscess and aneurysm, venous sinus thrombosis, subdural hematoma, subarachnoid hemorrhage, meningitis, malignant hypertension, lead poisoning, and pseudo–tumor cerebri.[245 (pp. 189-190)] Less common causes which may be accompanied by increased spinal fluid pressure include high cervical spinal cord tumor,[253, 254] chronic respiratory disorders with hypoventilation and hypercapnia,[255, 256] hypoparathyroidism,[257] leukemia,[258] hypochromic anemia,[259] poliomyelitis,[260] and the Guillain–Barré syndrome.[261]

Orbital tumors and unilateral alterations of intraocular pressure[2 (p. 587)] are associated with unilateral papilledema. A sudden fall of intraocular pressure, following ocular trephine or trauma, produces swelling of the optic disc in a very soft eye (papilledema ex vacuo[262]). Sudden rise in intraocular pressure in glaucoma is another rare cause, presumably on the basis of interference of venous return.[2 (p. 587)] Although not a constant finding, papilledema may follow central retinal vein occlusion.

Optic Neuritis

The alterations of the optic nerve which result from inflammation, demyelinization, or degeneration are called *optic neuritis.* When the disease processes affect the ophthalmoscopically visible portion of the optic nerve the term *papillitis* is used. If, in addition, the retina is involved, the alteration is called *optic neuroretinitis.* Disease of the portion of the optic nerve behind the lamina cribrosa is called *retrobulbar neuritis.* Although the term neuritis is entrenched in medical usage, optic or retrobulbar *neuropathy* would be more appropriate, for those forms of disease that are noninflammatory in nature. *Optic perineuritis* results from inflammation of the optic nerve sheaths.

CLINICAL FINDINGS

The initial symptom is a rapidly evolving painless loss of vision, usually monocular. In some patients pain may be elicited either by palpation or by movement of the eyeball. As a rule the pain subsides after several days. The pupil of the affected eye may be enlarged and fail to react to direct light stimulation. There is a varying degree of visual loss, especially for color. Visual field testing discloses central, paracentral, or centrocecal scotomas, i.e., an island of visual loss within the visual field. In perineuritis, a contraction of the field occurs rather than a scotoma. Although visual acuity generally returns to normal within a few weeks, recovery may not be complete and a scotoma may persist.

The visual loss precedes the characteristic funduscopic changes. In some cases the latter may never become evident. The disc is hyperemic and the elevation is slight or moderate; its margins are indistinct (Plate 199). (Compare appearance of the normal optic disc of Plate 200 with that of 199.) In inflammatory papillitis, the vitreous may be cloudy and/or contain clumps or strands of inflammatory cells. In neuroretinitis, peripapillary linear hemorrhages, cotton wool patches, and/or a macular star may be observed. In retrobulbar neuritis, the disc is usually normal initially. Later, when optic atrophy develops, pallor of the disc is observed.

Although the disc changes in optic neuritis may be similar to those of papilledema, the marked visual loss in the former is the major clinical difference between the two entities. The changes in the prepapillary structures (anterior chamber and vitreous) described in the inflammatory forms of papillitis are not observed in papilledema. The papilledema and neuroretinal edema of malignant hypertension, like some forms of optic neuroretinitis, commonly have accompanying extravascular lesions such as hemorrhage, cotton wool patches, hard exudates, and the macular star. The presence of severe arteriolar disease in accelerated hypertension distinguishes it from optic neuroretinitis.

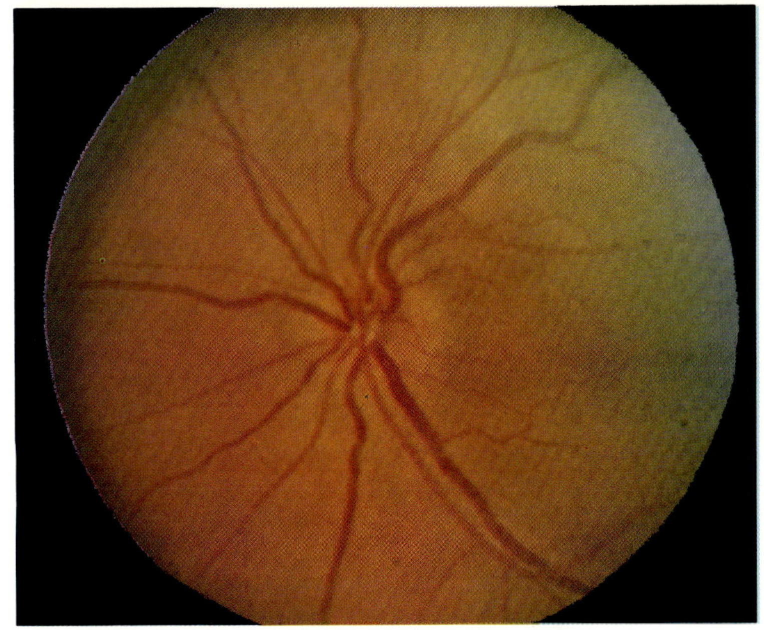

Plate 199. O.S. Central. Optic neuritis. Note the hyperemia of an indistinctly outlined optic disc.

Plate 200. O.D. Central. Normal disc of the same patient as Plate 199. The disc is clearly outlined and normal in color. Did you notice the venous tortuosity in Plates 199 and 200?

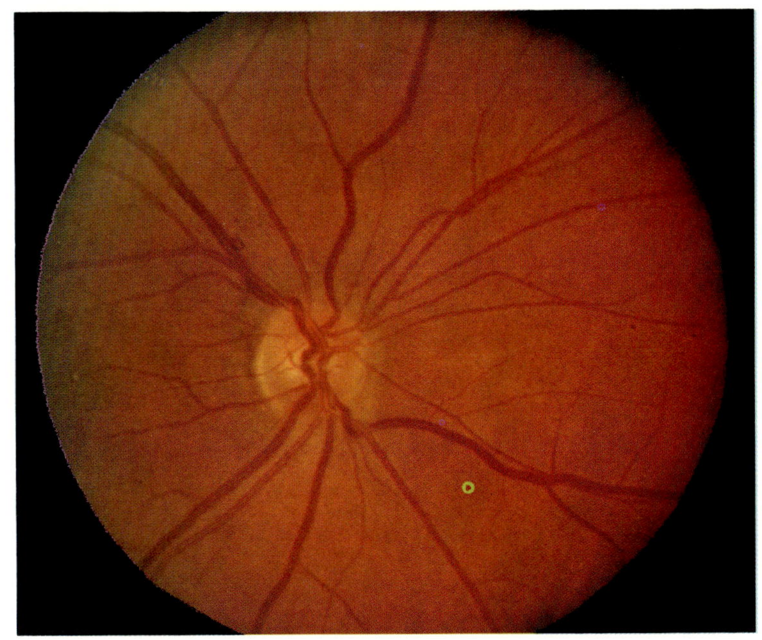

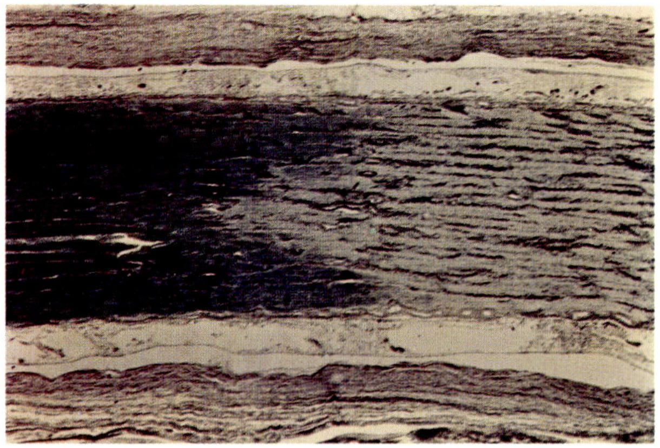

Plate 201. Longitudinal section of intraorbital portion of the optic nerve of patient with multiple sclerosis. The characteristic changes of demyelination are present. Note the abrupt loss of myelin (normally stained dark blue) in the center of the section. The loss of myelin is reflected by the reduction to absence of the intense blue color (myelin stain, × 12).

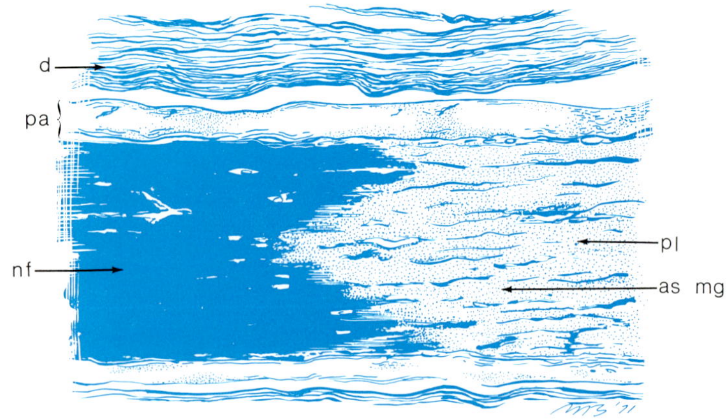

Drawing 201. Plate 201 (pa. pia-arachnoid; d, dura; nf, myelinated nerve fibers; pl, plaque of demyelinated fibers; as and mg, astrocytes and microglia).

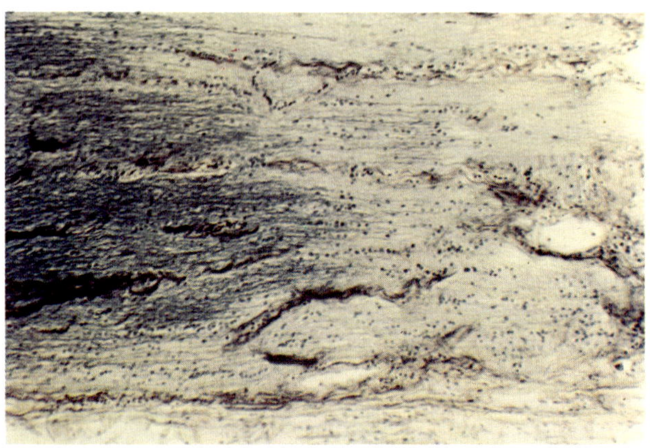

Plate 202. Higher magnification of the center of Plate 201. Within the plaque, axis cylinders are reduced in number, their myelin is absent, and many astrocytes and microglia are present (myelin stain, × 80).

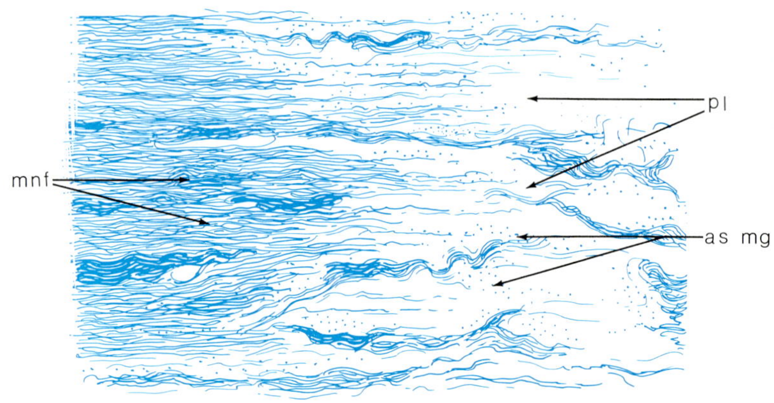

Drawing 202. Plate 202 (mnf, myelinated nerve fibers; pl, plaque of demyelinated nerve fibers; as and mg, astrocytes and microglia).

PATHOGENESIS AND PATHOLOGY

The major causes of optic neuritis may be classified under the following general headings.[263]

1. Infection
2. Degeneration
3. Nutritional deficiency and metabolic disorders
4. Drugs, poisons
5. Vascular disease

Infection

Generally infection of the optic nerve results from direct extension of infection from adjacent structures (intraocular, intraorbital, and paranasal sinus). Hematogenous spread of infection is believed to be a less common cause of optic neuritis. The inflammatory response within the nerve consists of hyperemia, edema, perivascular cuffs of lymphocytes, and proliferation of astrocytes. Degeneration of nerve fibers, gliosis, and fibrosis follow persistence of the inflammatory response. Fulminant infection leads to diffuse infiltration of polymorphonuclear leukocytes, suppuration, and hemorrhagic infarction. In perineuritis, the pia and arachnoid are involved by direct extension of infection of the correspondng membranes of the brain. Inflammatory cells are found in the subarachnoid space which envelops the optic nerve.

Degeneration

Demyelination is the most common degenerative change observed in the optic nerve. Multiple sclerosis is the prime example of that pathologic alteration. The destruction of myelin sheaths is accompanied by degenerative changes in the oligodendroglia. The liberated lipid of the disintegrated myelin is phagocytized by macrophages. Astrocytic response follows, forming plaques of glial tissue (Plate 201 and Drawing 201). In the plaques, the axis cylinders may be normal or reduced in number, the myelin disappears, and the astrocytes and microglia are prominent (Plate 202 and Drawing 202).

The lesions tend to assume a perivenous distribution and collections of chronic inflammatory cells are observed around the blood vessels. The pathogenesis of this form of demyelinating disease has not been established.

Nutritional Deficiency and Metabolic Disorders

Metabolic disorders[264-268] which include "tobacco–alcohol" amblyopia[269, 270] are forms of retrobulbar neuritis which follow severe dietary restriction, particularly of B vitamins. Severe and prolonged malnutrition may be associated with optic atrophy (see p. 195). Loss of myelinated fibers of the optic nerve, particularly of the papillomacular bundle, is the major pathologic change.[267, 270] A loss of ganglion cells of the macula occurs, but it is not known whether this is primary or secondary to the changes in the optic nerve.[271] This type of degenerative change has been described in the visual pathway of the rat after prolonged, experimentally induced thiamin deficiency,[272] but comparable lesions may occur in relation to deficiency of vitamin B_{12} and perhaps of other B vitamins as well.

Drugs, Poisons

Retrobulbar neuritis, often followed by optic atrophy, is known to occur after the ingestion of methyl alcohol. Usually the scotomas which follow methyl alcohol ingestion are very large and the visual loss is complete. The pathologic changes consist of degeneration of retinal ganglion cells, distortion of the nerve fiber layer of the retina, and accumulation of cellular debris in the region of the optic nerve.[273] Lead and quinine intoxication are other alleged causes of optic neuritis.

Vascular Disease

The ischemic optic neuropathy of central retinal artery occlusion is characterized by the presence of edema of the inner retinal layers and necrosis of retinal ganglion cells and their axons (see pp. 33–34). Ultimately, optic atrophy develops (see p. 193).

OPTIC NEURITIS AND CLINICAL STATES

Optic neuritis may follow such intraocular diseases as anterior uveitis, chorioretinitis, neoplasm, and vitreous hemorrhage.[245 (pp. 567-641)] Orbital infection and meningitis are other important causes.[245 (pp. 567-641)] Extension of infection from the paranasal sinuses is an uncommon cause of optic neuritis.[274]

Multiple sclerosis is the most common cause of optic neuritis. Defective vision is frequently an early manifestation of this disorder.[275, 276] The optic neuritis is usually monocular, evolving rapidly as a rule, and associated with a central or paracentral scotoma. Generally, in the early stages of the disease, the disc appears to be normal. If the pathologic change is situated just behind the lamina cribrosa, there are ophthalmoscopic signs such as venous engorgement and blurring of the disc margins with only slight elevation.[275] Generally the process subsides within several weeks, but recovery may not be complete and temporal pallor of the disc may follow. In a small proportion of patients, the optic neuritis may be bilateral. A certain portion of these patients eventually develop classical multiple sclerosis. Neuromyelitis optica, also called Devic's disease, is simply a form of multiple sclerosis in which optic nerve and spinal cord lesions are combined. Encephalitis periaxialis diffusa (Schilder's disease) is another demyelinative disease which is occasionally associated with optic neuritis; the visual loss in this disorder is usually due to cerebral disease, that is, interruption of the geniculocalcarine pathway. Acute disseminated encephalomyelitis, which follows an acute exanthematous disease (measles or chickenpox) or vaccination,[2 (p.599)] is rarely associated with optic neuritis.

Metabolic disorders associated with optic neuritis include malnutrition accompanied by manifestations of pellagra,[277, 278] neuritic beriberi in prisoners of war,[264, 268] and alcoholism.[270, 279] So-called "tobacco–alcohol" amblyopia[269, 270, 280] is probably due to nutritional deficiency rather than the toxic effects of alcohol and/or tobacco. This form of optic neuritis, at least in its early stages, can be reversed by the administration of vitamin B complex and particularly thiamin chloride.[268-270]

Optic neuritis is a rare complication of diabetes mellitus,[281, 282] hyperthyroidism,[283-285] and pernicious anemia.[286]

Various poisons which include methyl alcohol,[273] lead,[4 (p. 666)] and carbon disulphide[4 (p. 666)] may be the cause of optic neuritis and subsequent optic atrophy. Commonly used drugs which may produce optic neuritis include quinine,[287, 288] chloramphenicol,[289-291] and isoniazid.[292-294]

The ischemic optic neuropathy associated with central retinal artery occlusion occurs most commonly in elderly patients who have hypertension and diabetes mellitus.[53] Embolic occlusion of the central retinal artery is most frequently associated with atheromatous–thrombotic disease of the internal carotid arteries.[37] Aortic[44] and mitral valve disease,[53]

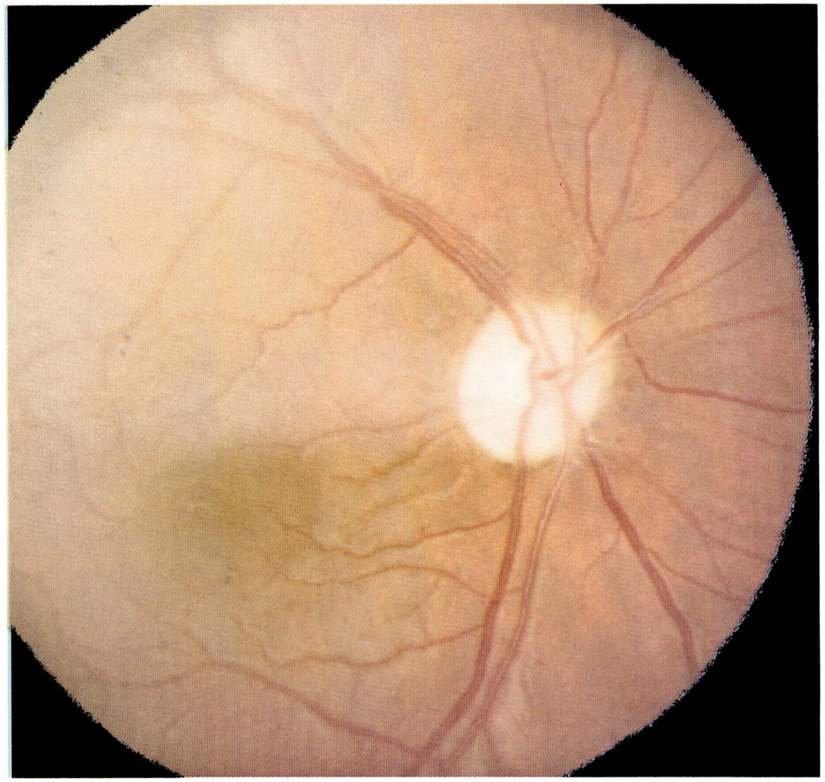

Plate 203. O.D. Central and temporal. Optic atrophy. Note the pale and sharply outlined optic disc. Very few small blood vessels cross its borders.

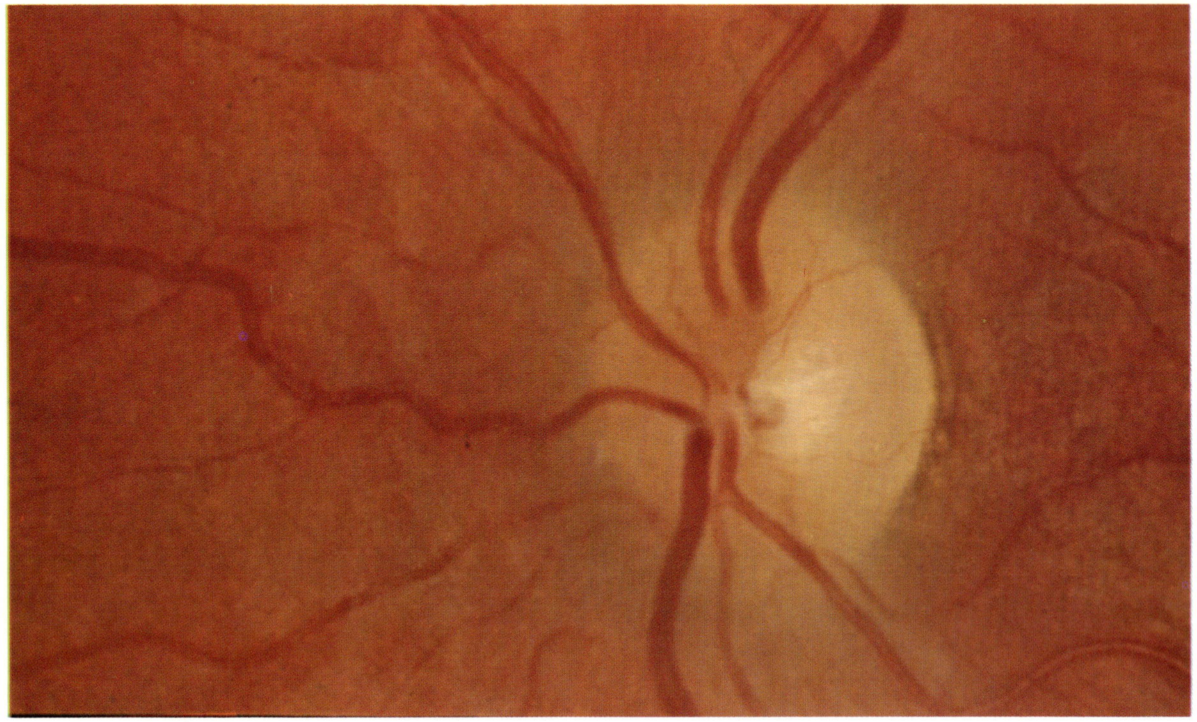

Plate 204. Magnified view O.S. Patient with multiple sclerosis. Note the indistinct, nasal, superior, and inferior borders of the optic disc. The nerve head color is normal and its temporal margin is distinct.

myocardial infarction,[42] and subacute bacterial endocarditis are less common sources of emboli. Temporal arteritis is the most common form of systemic vasculitis which is responsible for central retinal artery occlusion.[37] (See pp. 29–36 for a detailed presentation of central retinal artery occlusion.)

Optic Atrophy

The term optic atrophy is applied to the clinical triad of *pallor of the optic disc, reduced visual acuity, and defects in the visual field.*

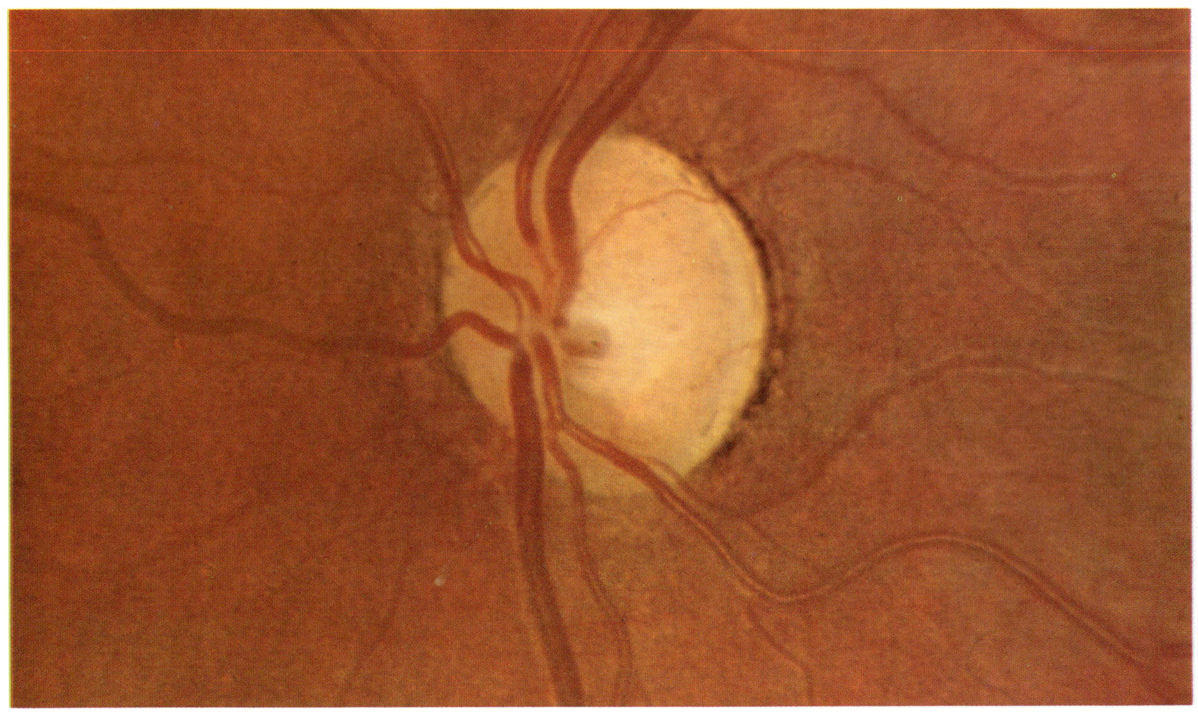

Plate 205. O.S. In same patient as Plate 204 observed 10 months later. Pallor of the disc is present, particularly the temporal portion. All the margins are now very distinct and few blood vessels cross over them.

CLINICAL FINDINGS

In optic atrophy the disc is pale, white or gray in color, and its margins are generally sharp (Plate 203). When the papillomacular bundle alone is affected, the pallor may involve only the temporal portion of the disc (Plates 204 and 205). Comparison of Plates 204 and 205 with Plate 206 (the normal optic disc of the other eye of the same patient) demonstrates that temporal pallor may be subtle and difficult to recognize. An associated sign of optic atrophy consists of a reduction of the number of small blood vessels which cross the borders of the disc.[295, 296] Kestenbaum[295] identified three types of blood vessels which cross the disc, namely arteries, veins, and "small vessels" which cannot be recognized as either arteries or veins. Normally about ten "small vessels" can be counted. With optic atrophy, that number is reduced to five or less. Marked depression of the nerve head, referred to as cupping, may be an additional manifestation of optic atrophy.

The term primary optic atrophy is applied when the disc margins are distinctly outlined and the normal sievelike lamina cribrosa is visible (retinal photography often fails to show the lamina cribrosa in a normal disc). These abnormalities are observed when disease is confined to the portion of the optic nerve proximal to the lamina cribrosa, as in tabes dorsalis, retrobulbar neuritis, and trauma. In contrast, the secondary optic atrophy which follows optic neuritis, papilledema, and central retinal artery occlusion is followed by glial and fibrotic tissue response. As a result the nerve head is gray; its margins are indistinct (Plate 207), and the lamina cribrosa is obscured. Although such differences can be detected clinically, they do not provide a totally reliable means of classifica-

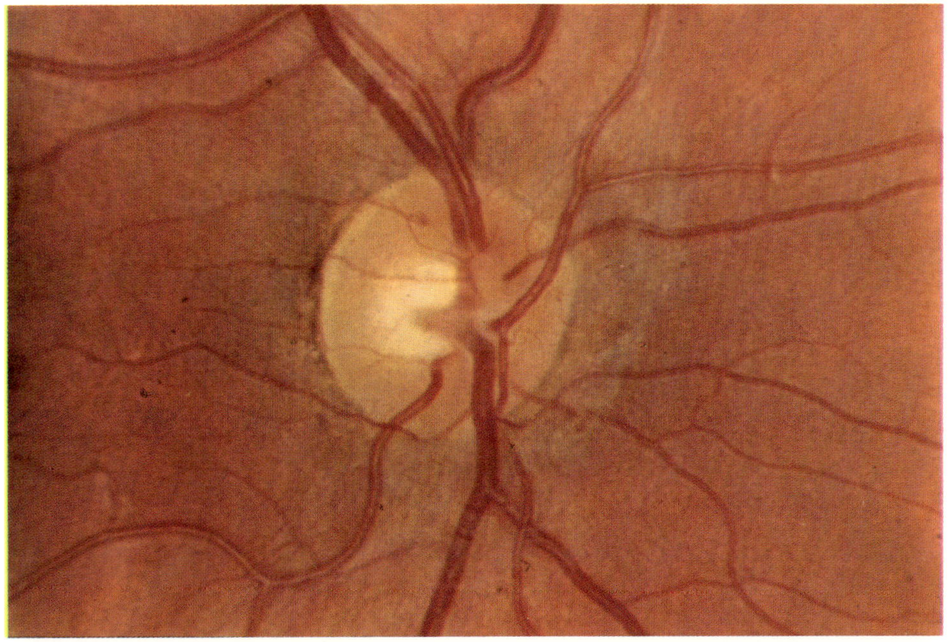

Plate 206. O.D. The normal disc has distinct margins. The temporal margin is sharper than the nasal one. It is flat. It is pink except for the white physiologic cup. A sunburst effect is created by the retinal fibers as they enter the nerve head.

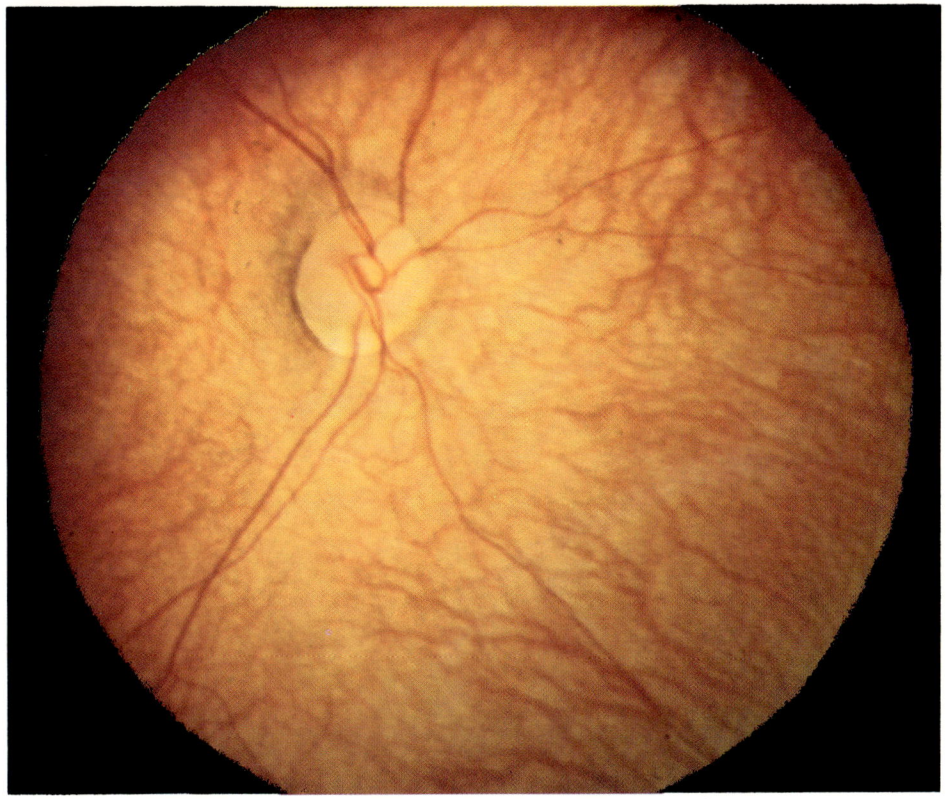

Plate 207. O.D. The patient, a blond infant, is blind. Disc is pale and gray in color. The margins are indistinct. Note inferior scleral crescent (see p. 187). Many broad choroidal blood vessels lie behind the retinal vessels. Note how the inferior crescent is sharply outlined and can be mistaken for the disc margin. Careful examination discloses the true disc margin and the difference in color between the scleral ring and the nerve head.

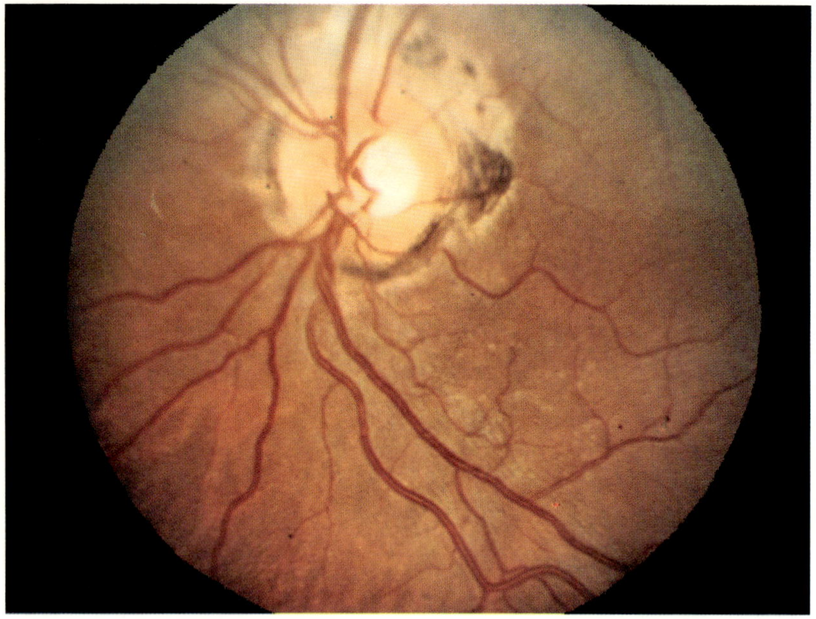

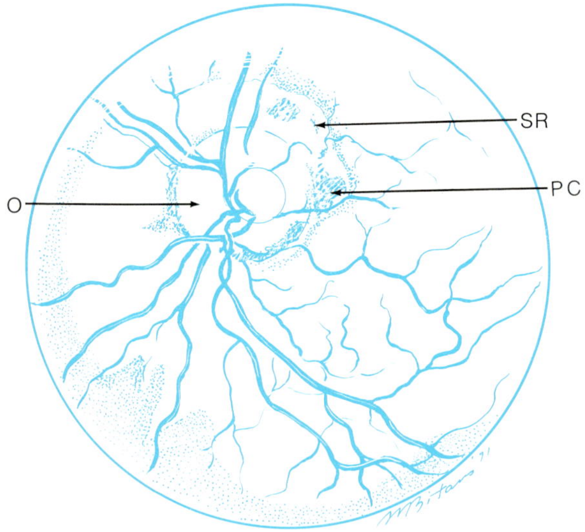

Plate 208. O.S. Superior and temporal scleral ring containing patches of pigment. Disc margin can be outlined easily.

Drawing 208. Plate 208 (O, optic nerve; SR, scleral ring; PC, pigmented crescent).

Plate 209. Temporal, white crescent outlines a normal optic disc. A choroidal vessel, visible as a broad orange band, lies behind the inferior temporal vein. Patient was markedly myopic.

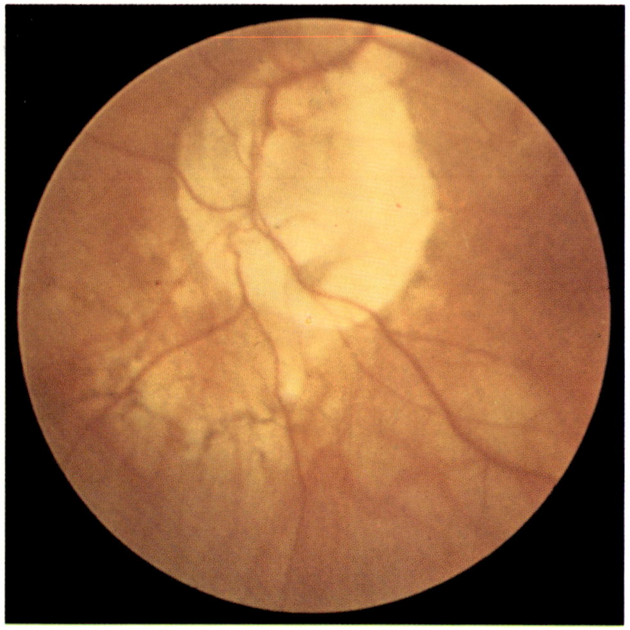

Drawing 209. Plate 209 (O, optic nerve; SR, scleral ring; ChV, choroidal vessel).

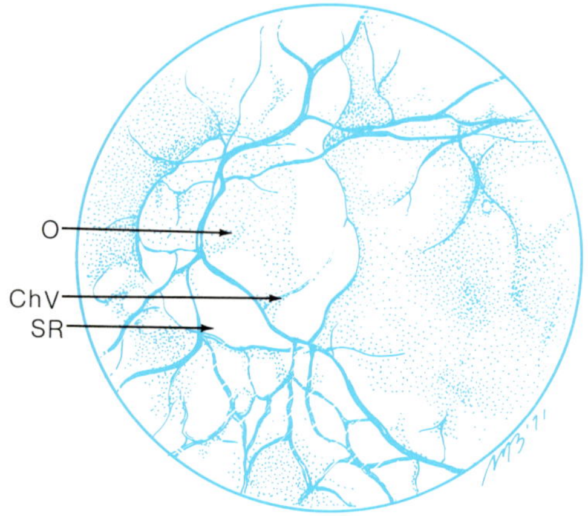

tion since the location of the lesion is as important as the nature of the disease in the production of the type of optic atrophy. Generally, when optic atrophy develops after either the loss of retinal ganglion cells or disease of the papilla of the nerve, the secondary form is observed. In contrast, when the optic nerve disease is located proximal to the intraocular portion, primary optic atrophy develops.

The visual loss of optic atrophy is usually gradual and eventually leads to blindness. The initial visual field loss is for color; ultimately the scotoma also develops for white. Since the optic nerve is the afferent limb of the light reflex, abnormalities of the pupillary response occur in optic atrophy. If the optic atrophy is bilateral, neither pupil will constrict when stimulated directly with light. If optic atrophy is unilateral, the direct pupillary response to light will be lost in the affected eye; in addition, when light is directed to the blind eye, no consensual pupillary response will be elicited in the normal opposite eye. In contrast, when light is directed to the normal eye, which still has a normal afferent limb, a consensual constriction of the pupil will occur in the eye with optic atrophy.

As noted earlier, the diagnosis of optic atrophy is dependent upon a triad of abnormalities, namely, pallor of the disc, reduced visual acuity, and the demonstration of a visual field defect. That diagnosis should not be made on the basis of only the ophthalmoscopic appearance of the optic disc. It is essential to perform the following diagnostic studies when optic atrophy is suspected:

1. Perimetry to detect visual field defects.
2. Test of visual acuity (particularly for color).
3. Observation of the pupillary response of direct and consensual light stimulation.
4. Funduscopic examination.

Pallor of the disc may have causes other than optic atrophy. The normal pink blush of the optic disc has its origin in the number and caliber of the capillaries within the nerve head, and the color of the blood within those vessels. Hence, as might be expected, the disc may be pale in severe anemia. The pale gray disc of the infant probably is the result of incomplete myelinization of the nerve proximal to the lamina cribrosa. Care must be taken to avoid mistaking this normal finding for optic atrophy.

The white scleral ring or crescent, which may either completely surround the disc or be limited to either the temporal or inferior border, may be mistaken for a pale disc margin (Plates 207–209 and Drawings 208 and 209).

In severe myopia the scleral crescent may be wide and extend in all directions. As a result the entire disc may be surrounded by a broad, irregular white ring through which choroidal pigment and vessels may be visible (Plate 209 and Drawing 209). In myopia the elongation of the eyeball pulls the choroid and pigment cell layer of the retina away from the optic nerve and exposes the underlying sclera (Drawing 4 demonstrates the normal relationship of the choroid and sclera to the optic nerve).

In glaucoma, the deep and broad physiologic cup may be mistaken for optic atrophy (Plate 210 and Drawing 210). Characteristically, in glaucoma, the retinal vessels are displaced nasally (Plate 210 and Drawing 210) and the disc margins are normal.

Although the clinical findings of glaucoma can generally be differentiated from optic atrophy, it can eventually lead to severe degeneration of the optic nerve (see pp. 191–93).

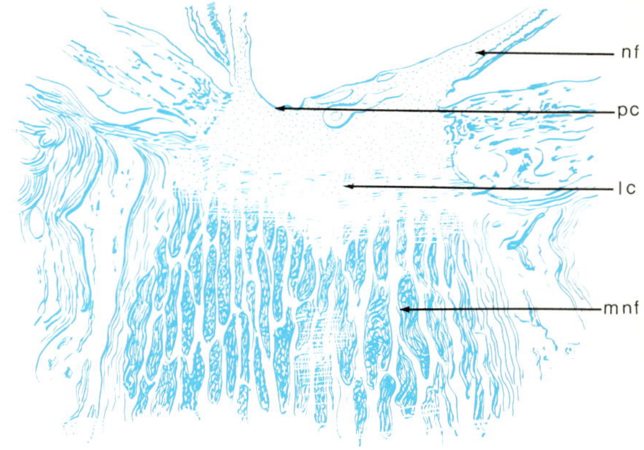

Drawing 4. Plate 4 (nf, nerve fiber layer; pc, physiologic cup; lc, lamina cribrosa; mnf, myelinated nerve fibers).

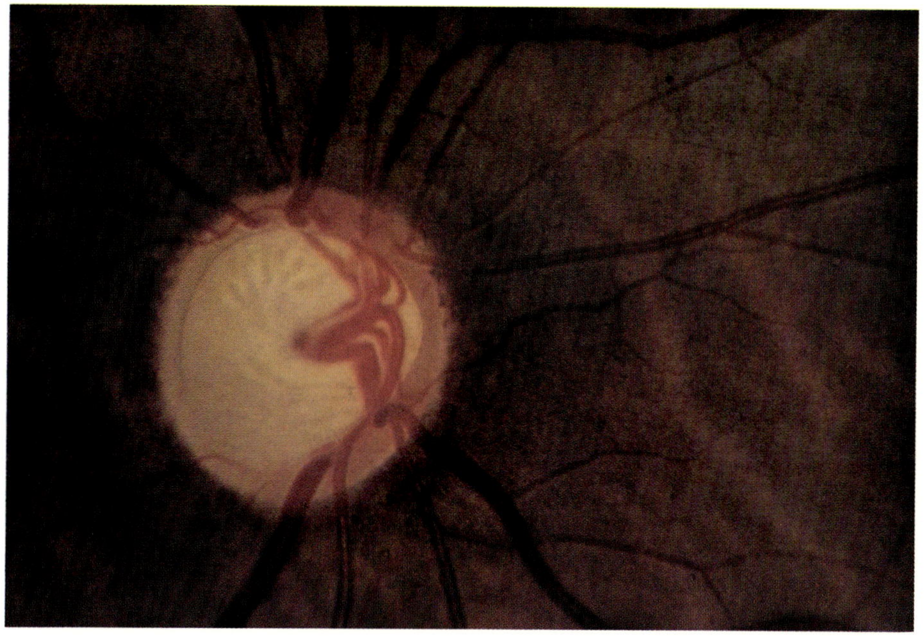

Plate 210. O.D. Note the broad physiologic cup and the nasal displacement of the retinal blood vessels. The disc is not pale and its margins are no more distinct than one finds normally. The lamina cribrosa is visible as a grid within the broad physiologic cup.

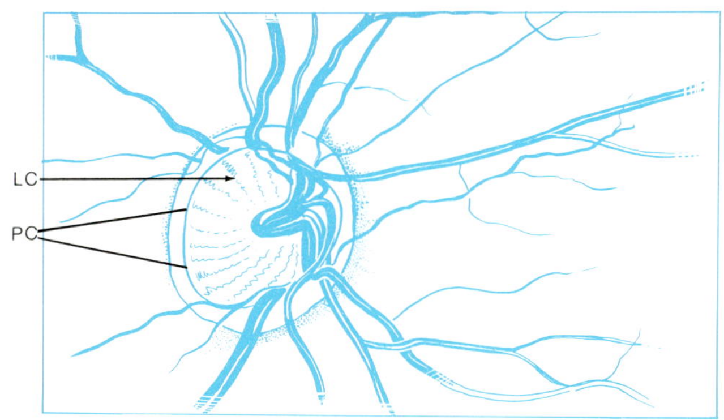

Drawing 210. Plate 210 (PC, physiologic cup; LC, lamina cribrosa).

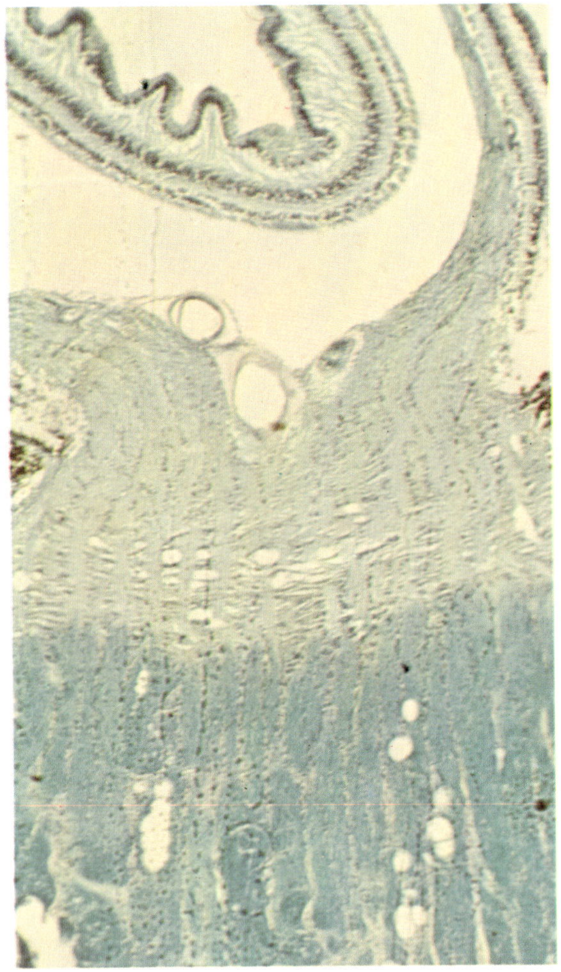

Plate 211. Section of normal optic nerve and retina. Note the orderly arrangement of the well-stained myelinated fibers (LFB, × 20).

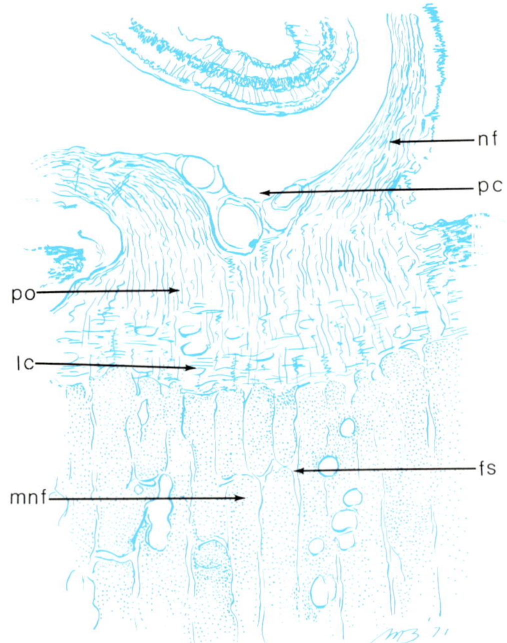

Drawing 211. Plate 211 (ps, physiologic cup; nf, nerve fiber layer; po, papilla of optic nerve; lc, lamina cribrosa; mnf, myelinated nerve fibers; fs, fibrous septa).

Plate 212. Note the decreased size of the optic nerve, the sparse myelinated fibers, the increase in septal fibrous tissue (stained blue) (LFB, × 16).

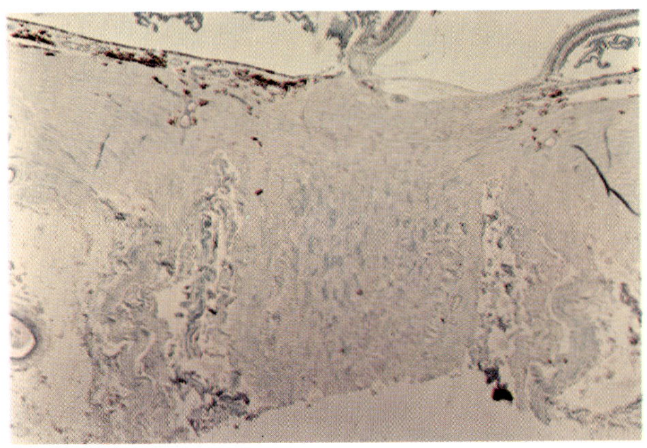

Drawing 212. Plate 212 (nfo, loss of nerve fibers in optic nerve; fs, increased fibrous septal tissue; as, astrocytes; mg, microglia).

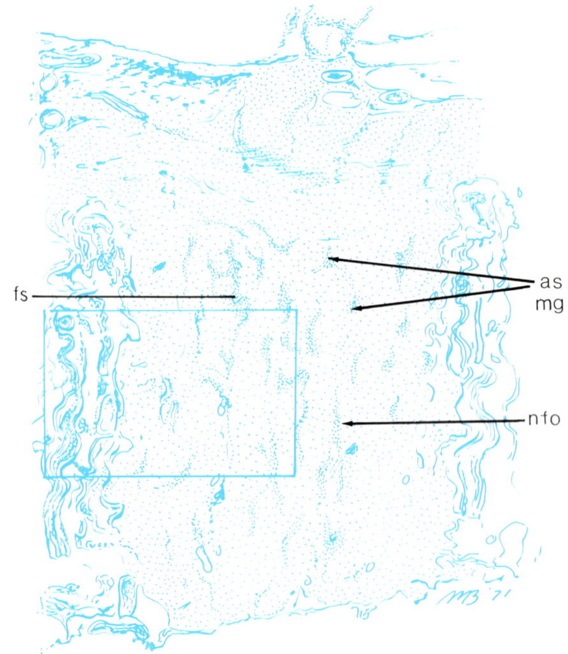

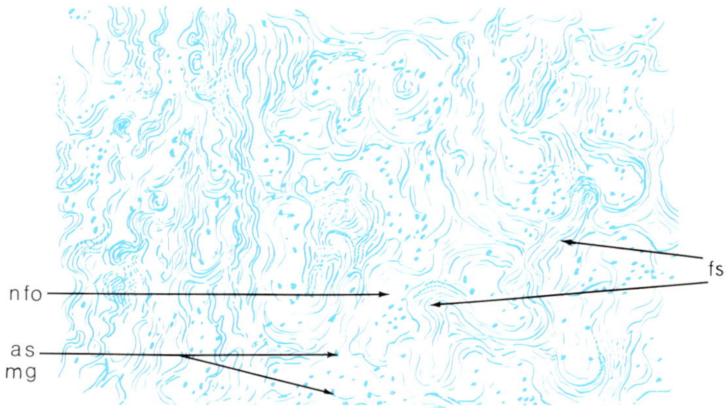

Drawing 213. Plate 213 (nfo, loss of nerve fibers in optic nerve; fs, increased fibrous septal tissue; as and mg, proliferation of astrocytes and microglia).

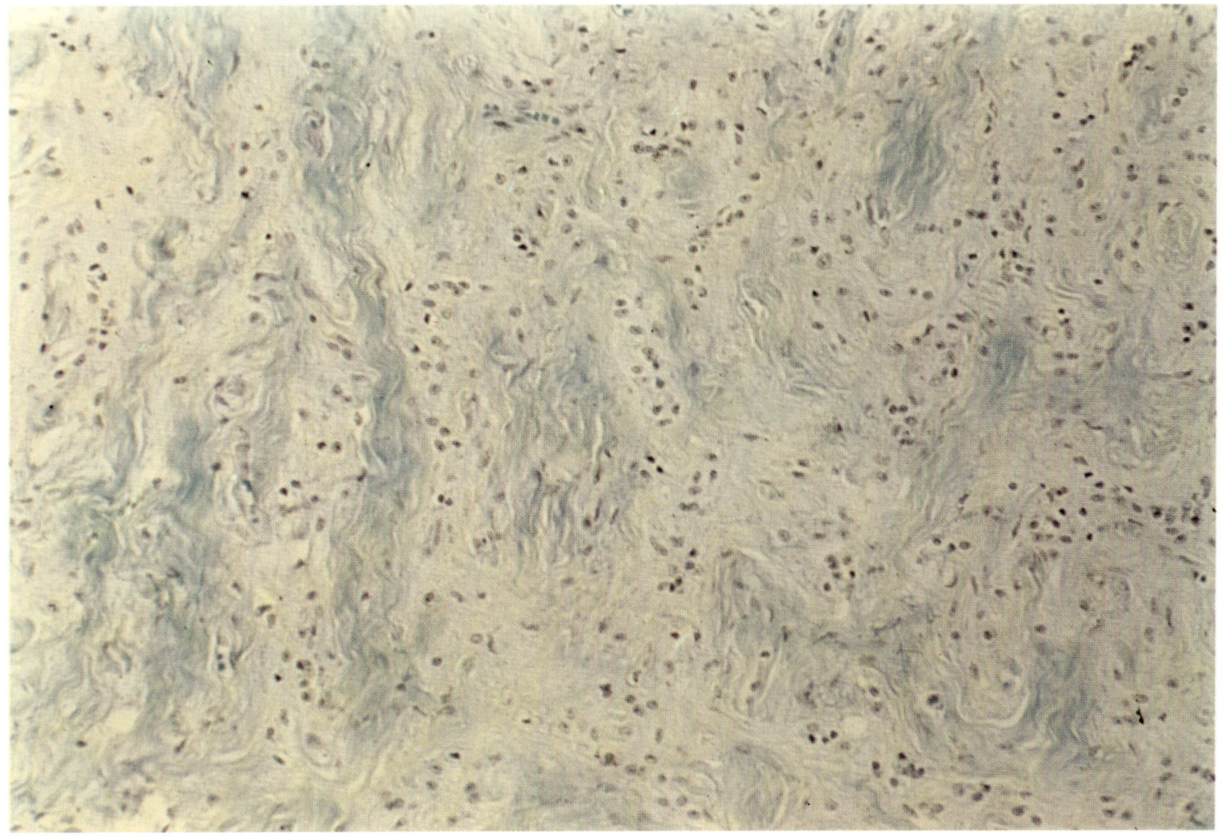

Plate 213. Enlarged view of abnormal segment of Plate 212. Note increased fibrous tissue (broad blue masses), the increased cellularity (astrocytes and microglia), and absence of nerve fibers (LFB, × 100).

PATHOLOGY AND PATHOGENESIS

The morphologic changes of optic atrophy consist of loss of axons with replacement gliosis, and fibrosis. When many axons are destroyed, there may be a decrease in the size of the nerve. The reduced number of axons is accompanied by an increase in the number of astrocytes, the invasion of microglia, and marked increase in the fibrous tissue of the septa (Plates 211–213 and Drawings 211–213; compare Plates 211 and 212).

The axonal degeneration which leads to optic atrophy may be the result of ascending degeneration (ascending optic atrophy), or descending degeneration (descending optic atrophy).

Plate 214. O.S. Magnified view of the optic disc demonstrating the development of optic atrophy following papilledema. The disc margins are indistinct and partially obscured by a white membrane. At 3 o'clock there is a sharply defined white patch. The above changes probably represent the gliosis which follows long standing papilledema. Did you notice the concentric rings (halos) around the disc and the venous sheathing at 6 o'clock?

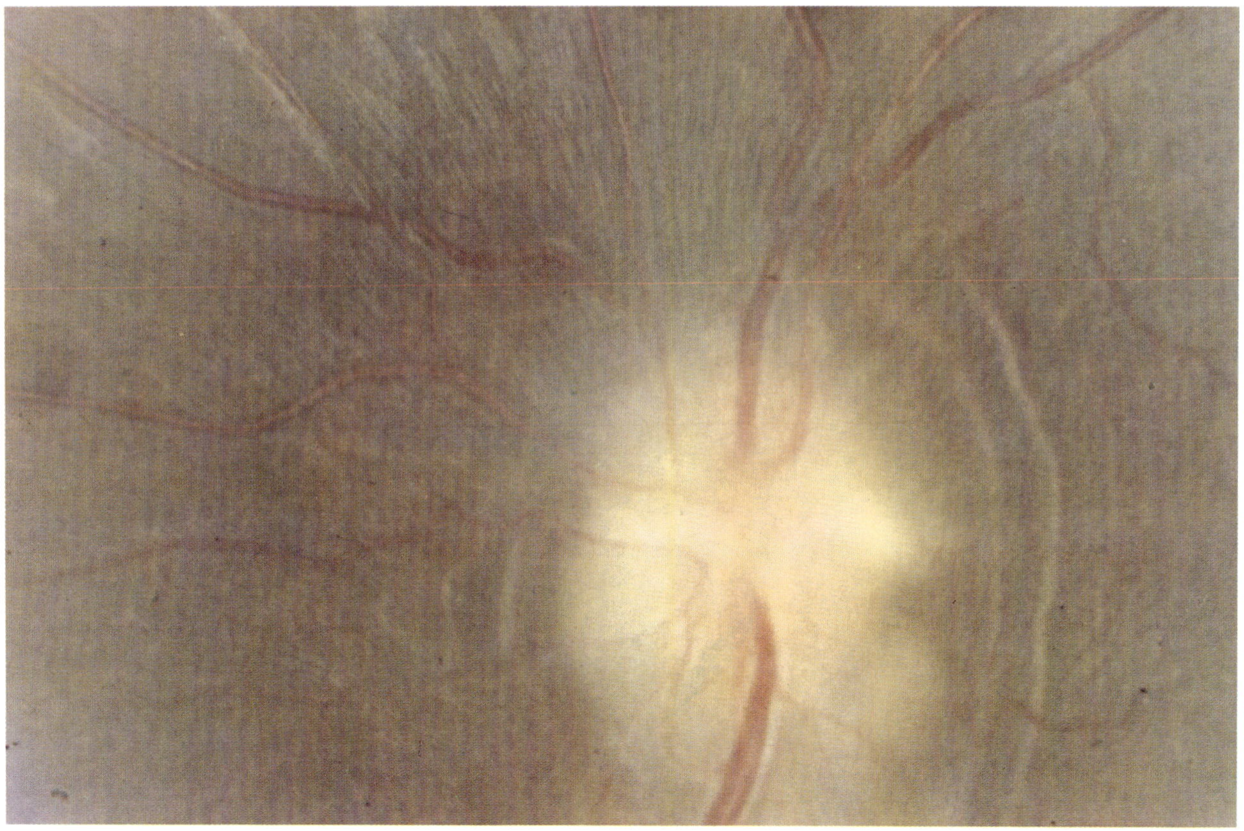

Ascending Degeneration of Axons of the Optic Nerve (Ascending Optic Atrophy)

Ascending optic atrophy is secondary to retinal diseases which lead to destruction of ganglion cells and the nerve fiber layer of the retina. When the ganglion cells are damaged the ascending axons of the optic nerve are interrupted and undergo Wallerian degeneration. The myelin and axis cylinders are fragmented. The myelin fragments fuse and envelop the axons in an ellipsoid structure called a digestion chamber. The liberated products of myelin and axoplasm are phagocytized by macrophages. The inflammatory response is generally minimal and is determined by the nature and extent of the original injury. As nerve fibers disintegrate and disappear, shrinkage of the optic nerve occurs. Glial and fibrocytic response is rapid and haphazard. The resultant gliosis and fibrosis may cover a good portion of the optic papilla and obscure normal landmarks. The clinical findings associated with secondary optic atrophy result.

Ascending optic atrophy has multiple causes, as outlined below:

Post–inflammatory

Optic neuritis which involves the papilla is frequently associated with suppurative endophthalmitis and panophthalmitis, chorioretinitis, intraocular neoplasms, and vitreous hemorrhage. Such changes often lead to degeneration of nerve fibers and ganglion cells. Gliosis and fibrosis of the papilla, and ascending degeneration of the axons of the optic nerve follow.

Post–papilledema

In our previous discussion of papilledema (pp. 174–81) reference was made to the development of degenerative changes in the papilla. Such changes included the formation of cytoid bodies, chromatolysis of retinal ganglion cells, and subsequent ascending Wallerian degeneration of optic nerve fibers. Microglia proliferate and phagocytize the degenerative products. The process continues with proliferation of astrocytes and subsequent gliosis. Perivascular infiltration of inflammatory cells may be observed. The central vessels of the papilla may become hyalinized and thickened and the smaller vessels occluded. The transformation of papilledema to optic atrophy generally takes place in 6 to 12 months[245 (p. 583)] (Plate 214).

Degenerative

1. **Retinitis pigmentosa.** The morphologic changes of retinitis pigmentosa are initiated by degeneration of rods, cones, and cells of the pigment layer.[297] Pigment migration follows, ultimately localizing around blood vessels and in the inner layers of the retina. The destruction of neural elements and pigmentary changes lead to gliosis throughout the retina (Plate 215 and Drawing 215). The degenerative process may distort ganglion cells, produce degeneration of axons, and optic atrophy (see p. 199).

2. **Lipid storage diseases.** Amaurotic familial idiocy (Tay–Sach's disease) and essential lipoid histiocytosis (Niemann–Pick's disease) are hereditary lipid storage disorders. Degeneration of ganglion cells of the retina is a prominent morphologic change in both diseases.[298, 299] The destruction of ganglion cells leads to degeneration of their axons and accounts for the optic atrophy of Tay–Sach's and Niemann–Pick's diseases.[298-302] The nerve cells of the inner nuclear layer, rods, cones, and the pigment cells may also be destroyed.

3. **Glaucoma.** Long standing glaucoma produces degeneration of ganglion cells and their nerve fibers. Some gliosis follows those degenerative changes.[2 (p. 714)] A characteristic histological change, known as cavernous optic atrophy, occurs frequently (Plate 216 and Drawing 216). The changes consist of severe degeneration of the optic nerve with connective tissue replacement. The disc is excavated to various depths. The nerve fibers of the papilla are compressed, fused, atrophied, and replaced by connective tissue. The lamina cribrosa is depressed, at times well below the level of the sclera (Plate 216 and Drawing 216). These findings may be associated with either the cavernous form of optic atrophy or

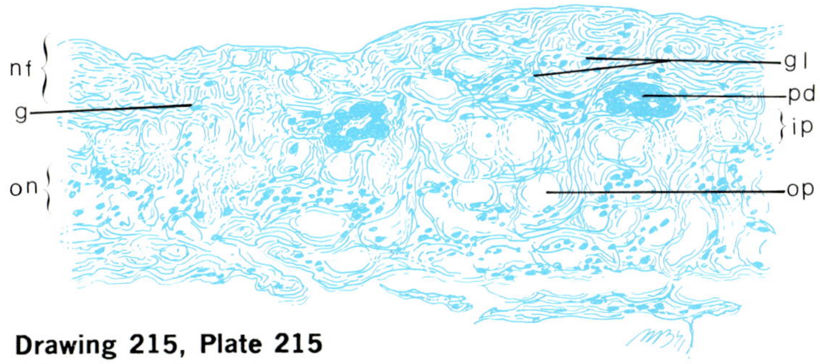

Drawing 215, Plate 215 (nf, nerve fiber layer; gl, gliosis; g, ganglion cells; ip, inner plexiform layer; op, outer plexiform layer (loss of axons); on, outer nuclear layer (disrupted); pd, perivascular pigment deposit).

Plate 215. Section of retina from patient with retinitis pigmentosa which demonstrates perivascular infiltration of melanin, a decrease in the normal number of ganglion cells, and gliosis in the nerve fiber layer. There is loss of inner nuclear cells, loss of axons of the outer plexiform layer, and disruption of the nuclei of the rods and cones. The absence of rods and cones may be either artefactual or the result of the disease process (LFB, × 70).

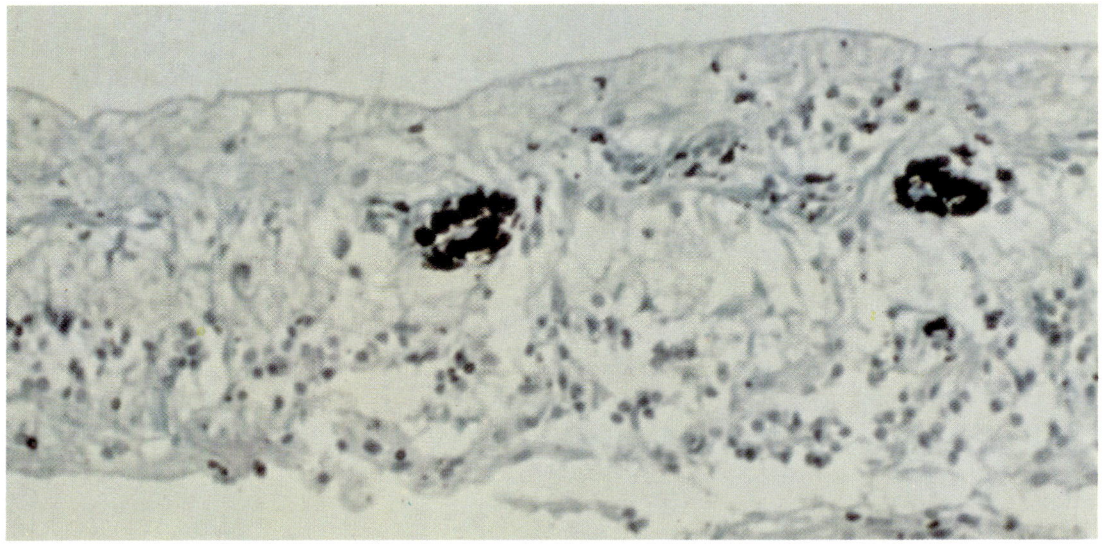

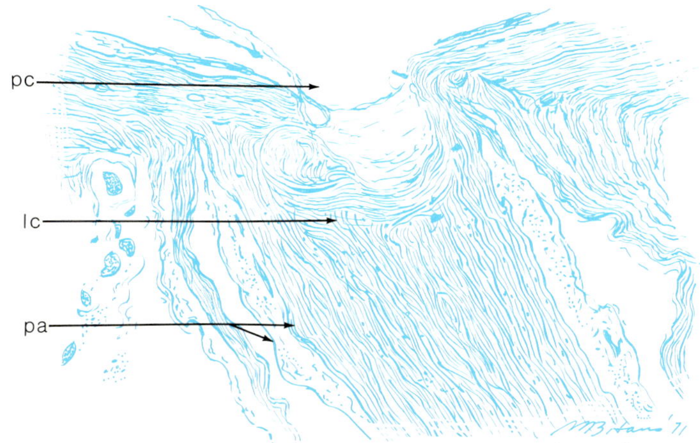

Drawing 216. Plate 216 (pc, fibrosis in a depressed optic cup; lc, lamina cribrosa; pa, pia–arachnoid).

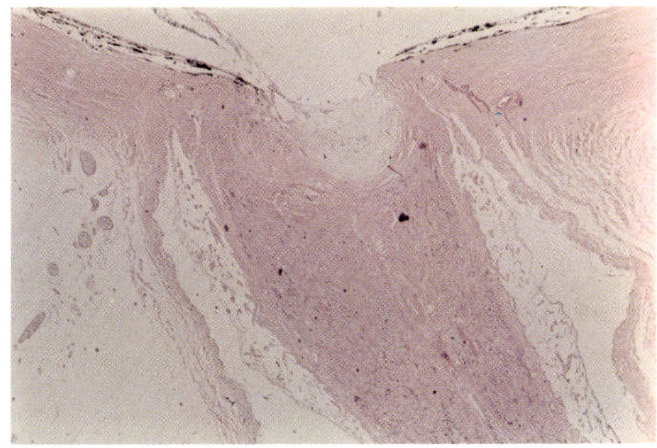

Plate 216. Optic atrophy in glaucoma. Note the deep excavation of the disc, the pale–staining connective tissue in the excavated area, the depression of the lamina cribrosa, the decreased size of the entire optic nerve (H&E, × 12).

Plate 217. Section of retina and optic nerve. Note the embolic occlusion of a thick–walled artery, the markedly swollen nerve fibers of the optic nerve and its papilla, and the glial response. Very few retinal ganglion cells are visible (PTAH, × 50).

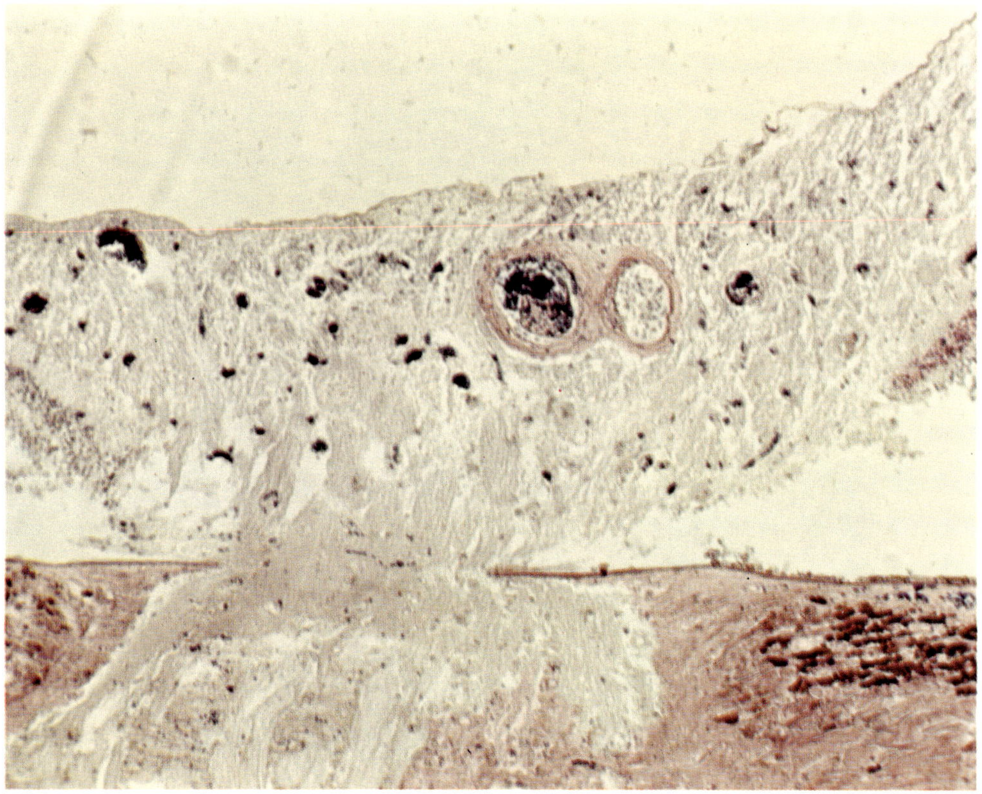

Drawing 217. Plate 217 (po, swollen nerve fibers in papilla of optic nerve; a, fibrin–occluded arteriole; ch, choroid).

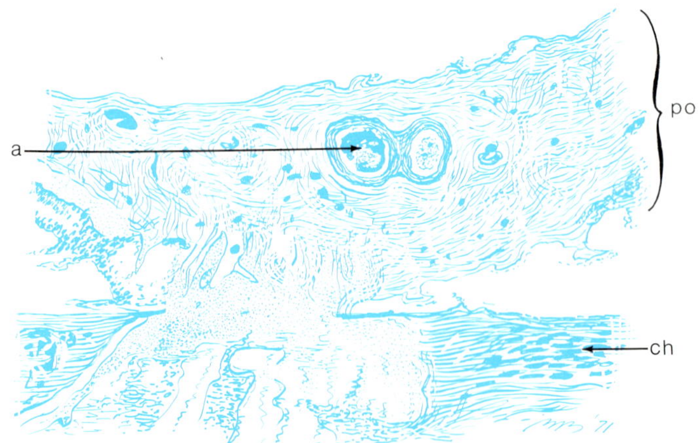

with fibrosis in some forms of secondary glaucoma.[2 (pp. 714-716)] Gliosis of the papilla, generalized atrophy of the nerve, and disorganization of the columns of nuclei may also be observed.[303 (p. 147)]

Increased intraocular tension and diminished blood supply have been offered as the cause of optic atrophy observed in glaucoma.[304] Hayreh[305] believes that the nerve fiber lesions in glaucoma are the result of impairment of choroidal blood supply and are located primarily in the optic disc, rather than in the retina. Through the use of fluorescein angiograms, he[305] has demonstrated that the optic disc normally receives part of its blood supply from the peripapillary choroidal vessels. He[306] postulates that an imbalance develops in glaucoma between intraocular and choroidal artery pressures. This, in turn, impairs the choroidal blood supply to the disc and accounts for the optic nerve involvement.[306, 307]

Circulatory — Ischemic Neuropathy

Either obstruction or reduction of blood flow through the central retinal artery leads to destruction of ganglion cells and their axons in the nerve fiber layer of the retina (Plate 217 and Drawing 217). Glial proliferation in the papilla and ascending degeneration of the fibers of the optic nerve are the subsequent pathologic changes which account for the optic atrophy of ischemic neuropathy. The causes of ischemic neuropathy include occlusion of the central retinal artery which results from atherosclerosis and thrombosis, embolization, and temporal arteritis. Occlusive disease of the common carotid arteries in pulseless disease may impair retinal blood flow enough to produce the above changes in the retina and optic nerve.[50]

Toxic

Methyl alcohol ingestion may produce degenerative changes in the retina (as described on p. 183). Presumably ascending degeneration of optic nerve fibers results from the ganglion cell loss after methyl alcohol ingestion. The histologic changes of quinine intoxication consist of destruction of retinal ganglion cells and nerve fibers, thickened vessel walls, narrowed lumens, and thrombosis.[308] Presumably such changes precede the degeneration of optic nerve fibers and the optic atrophy which may rarely occur after ingestion of quinine. Histologic studies of the optic atrophy associated with chloramphenicol toxicity include destruction of ganglion cells of the retina and loss of myelin of the optic nerves extending to the chiasm.[291] Lead intoxication may produce papilledema followed by optic atrophy.

Hereditary Optic Atrophy

A form of hereditary optic atrophy, known as Leber's disease, is generally observed after puberty.[309] Its pattern of inheritance may be either sex–linked recessive[309] or autosomal recessive.[310]

A study of the visual pathway of a patient with Leber's disease[311] disclosed extensive atrophy of retinal ganglion cells. The optic nerve was atrophic and gliosis and fibrosis of the papilla were present. Atrophy of cells of the inner nuclear layer was also observed.

Other forms of hereditary optic atrophy are noted at birth or in early childhood. The types include one with a dominant mode of inheritance from either an affected male or female[312-315] and a less common form of early onset or congenital optic atrophy which is transmitted as a recessive.[296] The pathology of either of the above disorders is not known.

Descending (Retrograde) Degeneration

Retrograde degeneration results from lesions of the axons of the intraorbital, intracanalicular, and intracranial portions of the optic nerve. The reaction of the ganglion cell, known as chromatolysis, begins within 48 hours. The ganglion cell swells and the Nissl granules disappear. The nucleus enlarges and becomes eccentric. Ultimately the ganglion cells degenerate and disappear. The glial and fibrocytic response is gradual and orderly. The glial tissue replaces the axon bundles and the process is called columnar gliosis. This type of axonal reaction is observed in primary optic atrophy.

Descending optic atrophy has multiple causes, as outlined below:

Retrobulbar Neuritis

1. **Inflammation**

   (a) Meningitis — direct extension of infection with pyogenic meningitis may lead to perineuritis. The infection may extend into the substance of the optic nerve by way of the pial fibrous septa and blood vessels.

   (b) Orbital infection may be followed by infection of the fibers of the optic nerve. The ensuing invasion of inflammatory cells, suppuration, and hemorrhagic infarction can cause destruction of axons of the nerve.

   (c) Syphilis of the central nervous system. Optic atrophy is often associated with tabes dorsalis. It is less commonly observed in general paresis and meningovascular syphilis. The initial lesion consists of an inflammation of the pia. Lymphocytes

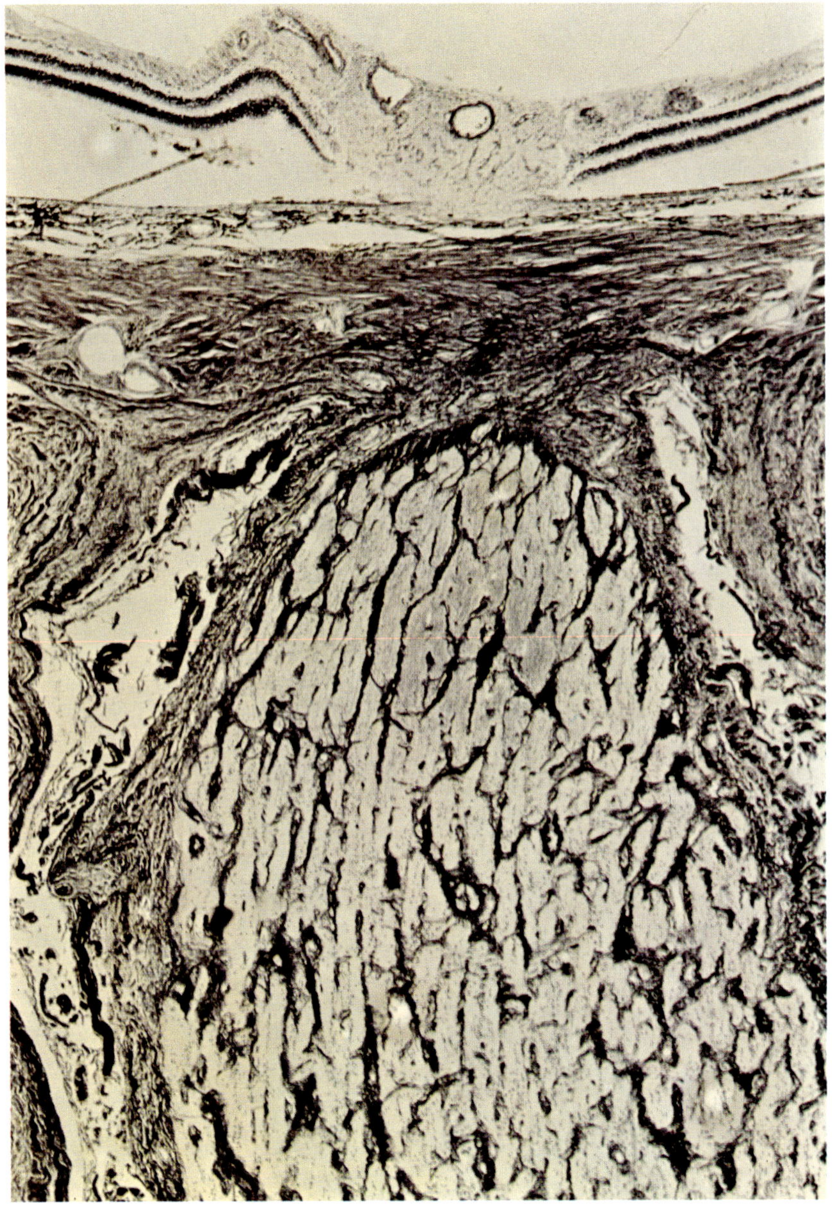

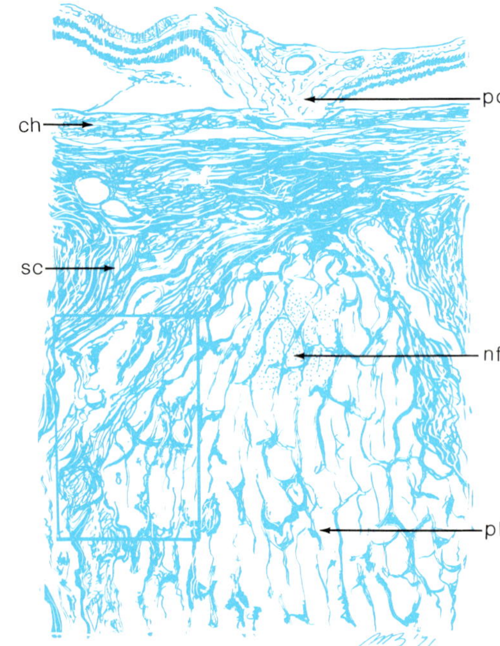

Drawing 218. Plate 218 (po, papilla of optic nerve; ch, choroid; sc, sclera; pl, plaque (demyelinated fibers); nf, myelinated nerve fibers).

Plate 218. The optic nerve does not penetrate the sclera in this section. Note that few of the optic nerve fibers stain blue–black (indicating the presence of myelin). The remaining fibers have lost their myelin. The fibrous septa of the optic nerve are prominent (myelin stain, × 20).

and plasma cells form perivascular cuffs in that membrane. The inflammatory process extends into the substance of the nerve by way of pial septa. Fibrous thickening of the pia and its extensions into the nerve accompanies the degeneration of its axons.

2. **Demyelinative diseases.** Multiple sclerosis is the most common cause of optic arophy in this type of disease. (see p. 197).

   The histologic changes associated with the destruction of myelin and subsequent gliosis have already been described (see pp. 182–83 and Plates 218–220 and Drawings 218–220).

3. **Nutritional disorders.** Avitaminosis B, generally accompanied by clinical evidence of pellagra, beriberi, and peripheral neuropathy, occur in severe malnutrition, alcoholism, and so-called "tobacco-alcohol" amblyopia, and may lead to optic atrophy. The few available histologic studies of the optic nerve associated with those disorders consistently demonstrated loss of myelin in the optic nerves, particularly in the papillomacular bundles.[267, 270]

Pressure Atrophy

1. Tumors of the optic nerve, such as the optic glioma, will destroy all elements in its path and diffusely enlarge the optic nerve. Tumors of the sheath and adjacent dura, such as meningioma and neurofibroma, may produce compression atrophy of the optic nerve. Compression of the optic nerves at the chiasm by pituitary tumors and craniopharyngiomas often results in bilateral optic atrophy.[316]

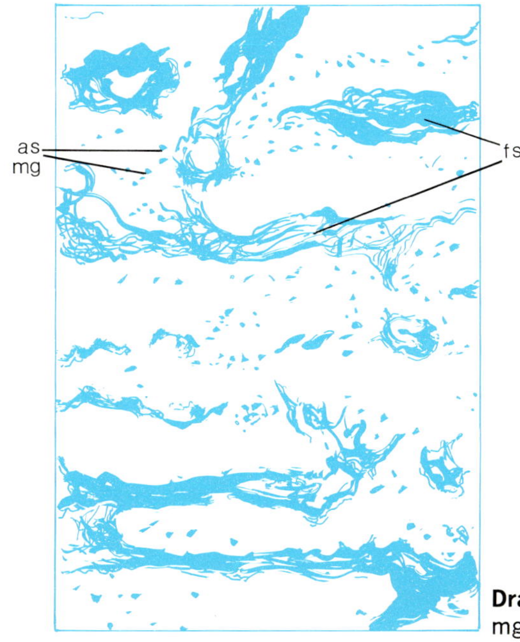

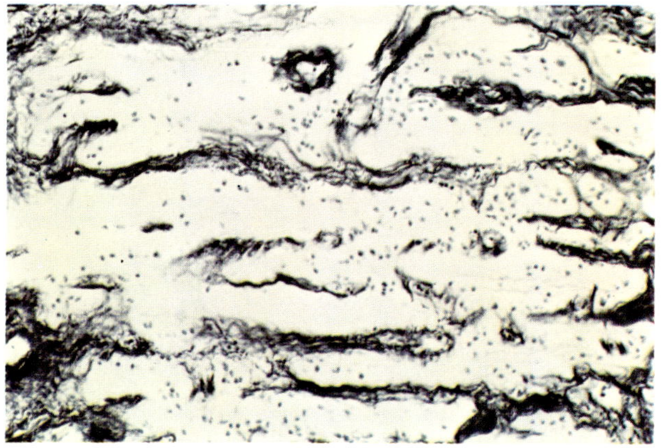

Plate 219. Note the absence of nerve fibers and myelin sheaths. Increased size of fibrous septa and marked cellularity are prominent features (myelin stain, × 100).

Drawing 219. Plate 219 (fs, fibrous septa; as and mg, astrocytes and microglia).

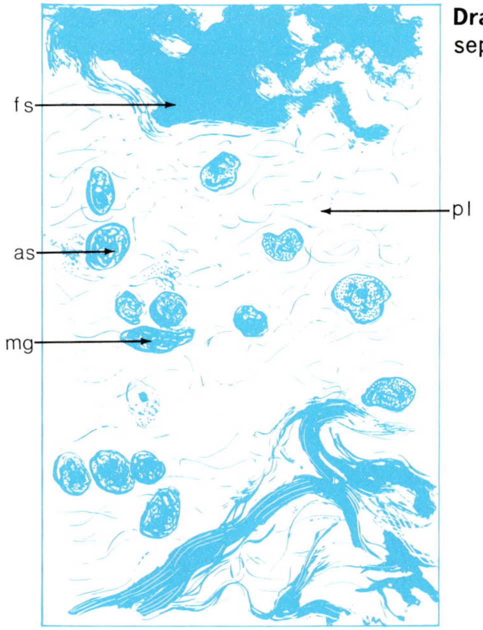

Drawing 220. Plate 220 (pl, plaque; fs, fibrous septa; as, astrocytes; mg, microglia).

Plate 220. Note loss of myelin, few poorly stained nerve fibers, increased number of astrocytes, and prominent fibrous septa. Few microglia are present (myelin stain, × 480).

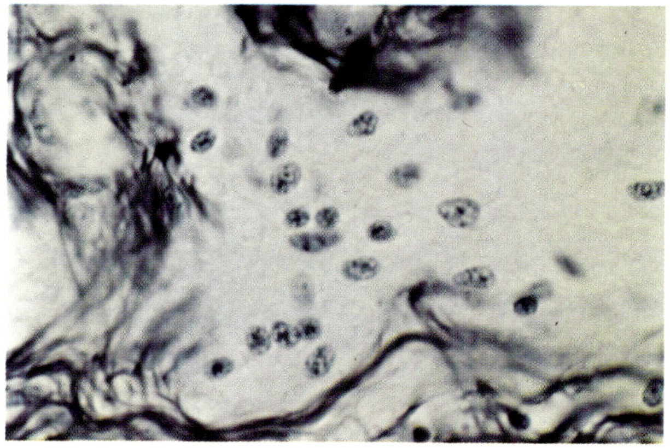

2. Saccular aneurysms which arise from the internal carotid, anterior cerebral, and anterior communicating arteries may compress the optic nerves.
3. Opticochiasmic arachnoiditis is described as a localized inflammatory process at the base of the brain.[316] The involved arachnoid responds with fibrosis which may encase and compress the optic nerves and the optic chiasm.[317] Invasion of the optic nerve by the inflammatory process may add another mechanism for degeneration of its nerve fibers.[317] The etiology of this entity is often obscure although it may follow meningitis and head injury.[317]
4. Hydrocephalous and cerebral neoplasms may produce degeneration of the optic nerves without antecedent papilledema.[2 (p. 625)] The chiasmal syndrome of bilateral optic atrophy and bitemporal hemianopia has been described with a suprasellar meningioma.[316] Foster Kennedy recognized the association of ipsilateral primary optic atrophy and contralateral papilledema with either frontal lobe tumor or abscess.[318]

Trauma

Head injury may produce optic atrophy by avulsion of the nerve from the eyeball and either laceration or transection of the nerve.[2 (p. 601)] Hemorrhage into its sheath with subsequent compression[4 (p. 678)] and interference with the blood supply of the nerve are other causes.[319] The above alterations of the optic nerve are usually accompanied by skull fracture.

THE CLINICAL PATHOLOGICAL CORRELATION OF OPTIC ATROPHY

The pallor of the optic disc can be related to the destruction of nerve fibers and their replacement by glial tissue. Loss of nerve fibers and a general decrease in size of the optic nerve accounts for the cupping. When atrophy follows either papillitis or papilledema, the papilla is filled with proliferating glial and fibrous tissue. As a result, the lamina cribrosa is obscured, the disc is gray, and cupping is not observed. The glial proliferation may extend beyond the confines of the nerve head and distort its margins, thus providing the mechanism for the irregular edges of the disc. Such changes produce the clinical finding classified as secondary optic atrophy. In primary optic atrophy, the disc is white, the lamina cribrosa is visible, and the disc margins are sharp. In that form of optic atrophy which results from degeneration of the optic nerve proximal to the globe there is no distortion of the papilla by gliosis or fibrosis. Vascular occlusion accounts for the decreased number of small vessels which cross the disc margins.

OPTIC ATROPHY AND CLINICAL STATES

Disease of the central nervous system is the most frequent cause of optic atrophy. The long standing papilledema associated with expanding intracranial lesions, such as tumor, eventually lead to degenerative changes in the optic papilla and subsequent atrophy of the nerve.[249] Cushing[316] recognized the association of optic atrophy and bitemporal visual field defects with lesions at the optic chiasm.[320]* The specific lesions include suprasellar meningioma, pituitary adenoma, suprasellar craniopharyngioma, glioma of the optic chiasm, and suprasellar aneurysms. Cogan[3 (p. 210)] emphasizes that optic atrophy and blindness in one eye, associated with partial atrophy and temporal hemianopsia in the other eye, are diagnostic of a parachiasmal lesion. In fact, he believes that such a clinical picture is as characteristic of chiasmal lesions as bitemporal hemianopsia. Kennedy[318] described the presence of ipsilateral optic atrophy and contralateral papilledema in the presence of either tumor or abscess of the frontal lobe (the Foster–Kennedy syndrome). He[321] subsequently demonstrated the same syndrome in association with an aneurysm of the internal carotid artery. Yashin and Schlezinger[322] confirmed its presence in a patient with an enlarged tortuous and sclerotic anterior cerebral artery which compressed the optic nerves.

In children, Cordes[323] pointed out that congenital hydrocephalus, craniopharyngioma, and cerebral neoplasms were common causes of optic atrophy. In children, secondary optic atrophy following papilledema is likely to result from cerebellar tumors, pinealomas, and craniopharyngiomas in the region of the aqueduct. Tumors of the optic nerve within the orbit, such as glioma, produce unilateral optic atrophy, exophthalmos, and radiologic evidence of an enlarged optic foramen.[3 (p. 136)]

In the original description of the chiasmal syndrome of optic atrophy and bitemporal hemianopia, Cushing[316] also noted that chronic local arachnoiditis and syphilitic meningitis were offending agents. The arachnoiditis, referred to as optocochiasmic arachnoiditis, of unknown etiology, has been described by others as a cause of the chiasmal syndrome.[317, 324, 325] It is not surprising that this peculiar form of arachnoiditis has also been described as a cause of the Foster–Kennedy syndrome.[326]

Head injury may be associated with optic atrophy and different types of visual field de-

*See reference 320 for a review of field defects.

fects. These include bitemporal hemianopsia with injury to the chiasm.[319] Homonymous hemianopia, at times with central scotoma, is reported with trauma involving the occipital lobes.[327, 328, 320*] Direct injury to the optic nerve[2 (p. 601)] and hemorrhage into its sheath with subsequent compression[4 (p. 678)] may be followed by atrophy. Subdural hematoma and birth injury[323] are other causes.

Retrobulbar neuritis followed by optic atrophy is a common finding in multiple sclerosis. Visual disturbance may be the first symptom of that disease.[276, 329-331] Although initially transient in many instances, ultimately visual loss becomes progressive and clinical evidence of optic atrophy, particularly temporal pallor, becomes evident. Some of the other manifestations of the disease such as nystagmus, slurred speech, ataxia, and pyramidal tract signs are usually present when optic atrophy is evident. Optic atrophy is less common in the other demyelinative diseases (see p. 183).

Extremely rare causes of optic atrophy include Charcot–Marie–Tooth disease,[332] metachromatic leukoencephalopathy,[333] subacute sclerosing panencephalitis,[334] cerebral aplasia,[323] and cerebral birth injuries.[323, 335] Craniosynostosis, early closure of the sutures of the skull with resulting scaphocephalopathy, oxycephaly, brachycephaly, and phagiocephaly may be associated with optic atrophy.[323, 336]

Metabolic disorders associated with optic atrophy in children include osteopetrosis,[337, 338] Morquio's disease,[323] Tay–Sach's disease,[298, 300-302, 334, 339-340] and Niemann–Pick's disease.[299, 341] The classic retinal abnormality in both of the lipidoses is the cherry–red spot (Plate 221; see p. 191). This abnormality is the result of degeneration of the ganglion

Plate 221. The cherry–red spot of a child with Tay–Sach's disease. Note the red fovea which is surrounded by a gray ring.

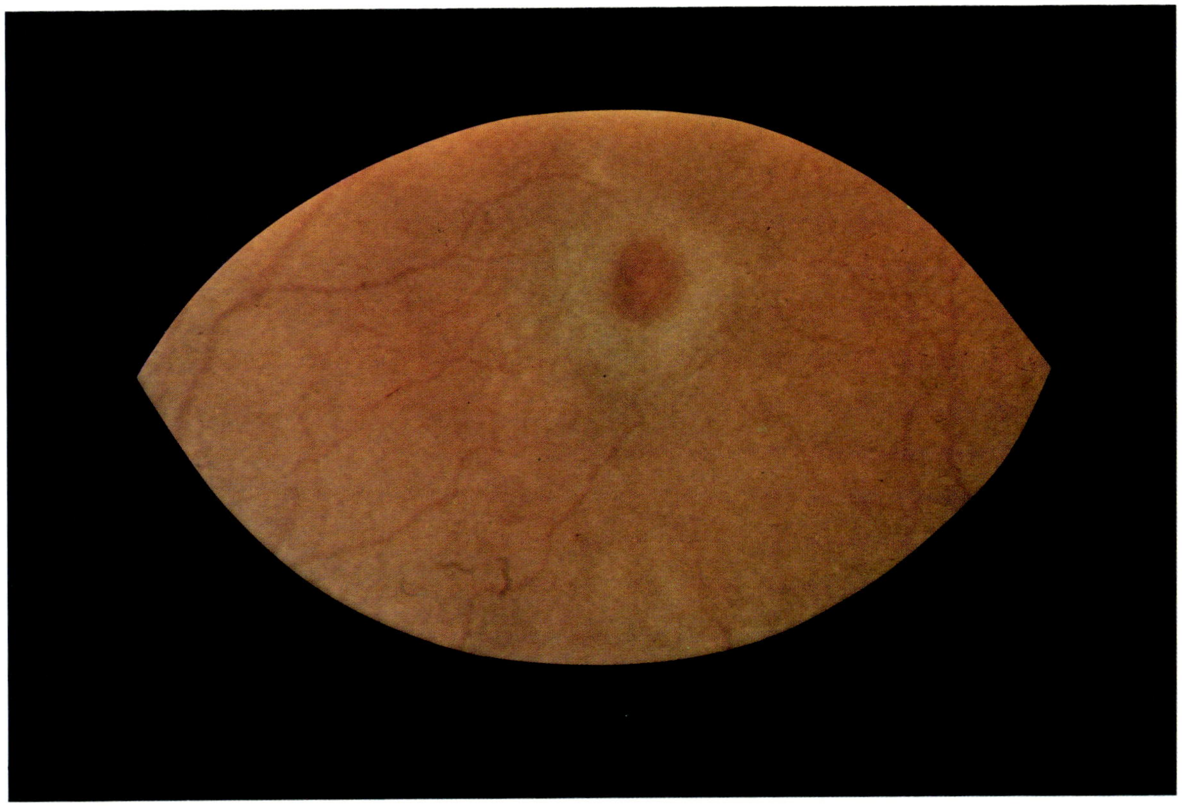

cells which surround the macula and provide a gray ring around the uninvolved fovea.

In adults, pernicious anemia[286, 342] and diabetes mellitus[281, 343-345] are infrequently associated with optic atrophy. In hyperthyroidism the development of optic atrophy may follow either retrobulbar neuritis or, more frequently, papilledema,[346, 347] and is generally accompanied by marked exophthalmos.[284] Hyperparathyroidism and Paget's disease of bone are extremely rare causes of optic atrophy.[3 (p. 173)]

The nutritional deficiencies associated with severe dietary restriction in prisoners of war,[264-268] alcoholism,[270] and "tobacco–alcohol" amblyopia[270, 271, 280] may cause optic atrophy.

A variety of toxic substances and drugs such as lead,[4 (pp. 664-666)] methyl alcohol,[273, 348] chloramphenicol,[291] isoniazid,[294] and tryparsemide[4 (p. 674)] are known to produce optic atrophy.

Leber's optic atrophy is the most common form of hereditary disease affecting the optic nerve. It is more common in men and generally has its onset as an acute retrobulbar neuritis between the ages of 20 to 30 years.[309] It is frequently bilateral from the onset. A rapid decline of central vision is accompanied by swelling and hyperemia of the disc.[309] Gradually the disc becomes pale and its margins are noted to be sharp. A central scotoma becomes evident. Although some improvement of vision may occur, progressive visual loss is more likely.[309] Nystagmus, keratoglobus (a globular protrusion of the cornea) cataract, and abnormal pigment deposits[349] in the retina may accompany the optic atrophy.[310] Olivopontocerebellar atrophy and Fredreich's ataxia are also described with Leber's optic atrophy.[350] The inheritance pattern is believed to be either autosomal or sex-linked recessive.[309]

Other forms of hereditary optic atrophy are manifested early in life and may have either a dominant[312-315, 351] or recessive[309, 314, 351] mode of transmission. The dominant form may be either congenital[314] or it may become manifest during infancy.[313, 314] The congenital form[314] is associated with severe visual impairment. Nystagmus is frequently present. The optic atrophy is complete and the visual fields are severely constricted. The infantile form[312, 315] generally has its onset at about 3 years of age and affects the sexes equally. The visual loss is gradual and the disc is generally white with a deep cup and sharp margins. The recessive type, which may be either congenital or may develop soon after birth, is less common than the dominant form.[314] The optic atrophy is severe and there may be complete loss of vision.[309] Nystagmus is frequently present.[309, 314]

Behr's hereditary optic atrophy has been described as a syndrome which consists of bilateral optic atrophy, pyramidal tract signs, ataxia, spastic gait, muscular hypertonia, clubfoot, weakness of vesical sphincters, mental deficiency, and nystagmus.[309, 351] The optic atrophy is generally temporal and rarely complete. The disease, after some progression, becomes static. It involves both sexes equally and it is generally transmitted as a recessive.[309] Less commonly it may have a dominant mode of transmission.[309]

Vascular disease may affect the optic nerve through compression by an intracranial aneurysm[316, 321, 352-358] and by ischemia from interference with its blood supply.[4 (pp. 680-684), 37, 47,]

Intracranial aneurysms represent a tumor mass which produces symptoms by compression of brain substance and/or the cranial nerves. In addition, the aneurysms may rupture and produce subarachnoid hemorrhage. When hemorrhage develops, funduscopy may disclose a subhyaloid hemorrhage[354, 359, 360] and/or rapidly developing papilledema.[354, 359] The intracranial aneurysms may be saccular, fusiform, or arteriovenous.[354]

The saccular form is the most common. Such aneurysms often arise from a vessel of the circle of Willis and compress the optic nerves. The sites of origin include the internal carotid, the anterior cerebral, and the anterior communicating arteries. Less frequently the aneurysms arise from the ophthalmic artery. Jefferson[352] noted that supraclinoid aneurysms, which originate from the carotid artery at the origin of the ophthalmic or posterior communicating arteries, and at the bifurcation of the main trunk, are likely to produce visual changes. The supraclinoid aneurysms are situated in the region of the chiasm above the cavernous sinus.[353] As aneurysms expand, they are associated with headache, varying degrees of visual loss, visual field defects, and in some instances complete blindness associated with optic atrophy. Optic atrophy may be an isolated sign of a carotid aneurysm.[361] The initial optic nerve change may be manifest as papilledema or retrobulbar neuritis. The subclinoid aneurysms, according to Jefferson,[352] arise within the cavernous sinus and rarely produce visual symptoms. When subclinoid aneurysms affect the optic nerve, the associated involvement of the third, fourth, and sixth cranial nerves produces ptosis, ophthalmoplegia, and diplopia.[352, 355] Since the fifth cranial nerve may also be involved, pain, varying degrees of hypesthesia, and weakness of the mastication muscles may also be present.[352, 357]

Arteriovenous fistulae between the internal carotid artery and cavernous sinus may cause unilateral optic nerve compression and loss of visual acuity.[355] These vascular abnormalities may follow a skull fracture and can be recognized by the presence of pulsating exophthalmos and a bruit over the eye.

Although the sudden onset of headache, definitive visual field defects, and cranial nerve involvement may lead one to suspect an intracranial aneurysm (saccular or fusiform), cerebral arteriography provides the most accurate method of diagnosis.

Ischemic optic neuropathy, when associated with occlusion of the central retinal artery, results in sudden visual loss. The pale retina, narrow arterioles, the "boxcar" change in the venules, and the cherry–red fovea are the classic findings. Initially the optic nerve may appear to be normal. However, in some instances papilledema may develop. Within a period of several days, pallor of the disc may be observed. Optic atrophy occurs within a period of 1 year.

Occlusion of the central retinal artery occurs most frequently after age 50 in patients with hypertension and diabetes mellitus.[53] The common causes of obstruction of the central retinal artery include atherosclerosis with local thrombosis,[2 (pp. 64-66)] embolism,[30, 37] and temporal arteritis.[47, 48] Polyarteritis nodosa[49] and sickle cell disease[76] are less frequent causes. In pulseless disease, the retinal ischemia is the result of occlusion of the common carotid arteries.[50] Migraine[4 (p. 196)] and the untoward response to oral contraceptives[51, 52] are additional causes.

The visual loss following massive extraocular hemorrhage is usually transient.[362] It may, however, be accompanied by the development of optic atrophy, at times preceded by papilledema.[362] This sequence of events, along with the development of cotton wool patches with massive extraocular hemorrhage,[109] suggests that hypoxia may be the causative factor.

Optic atrophy develops with the progression of pigmentary changes in retinitis pigmentosa[4 (p. 684), 297] (see p. 191). This familial, degenerative disease often manifests itself in early childhood with diminished night vision. Decreased visual acuity during the day follows. Funduscopy discloses irregular pigment deposits which generally envelop the retinal veins. The pigment deposits in the retina increase in number. Arterioles and venules are attenuated and eventually appear as white threads (Plate 222). Optic atrophy and blindness may be the end result.

Chorioretinitis, if extensive, may be followed by atrophy of the optic nerve.

Glaucoma[2 (pp. 627, 714-716), 303 (p. 147), 304] may be followed by optic atrophy (see pp. 191–93).

Plate 222. O.S. Nasal. Retinitis pigmentosa. The green fundus color is a photographic artefact. The disc is normal. The retinal vessels are narrowed. Several of them appear as white threads. Irregular and round masses of pigment are visible. Many clumps surround the retinal vessels. Choroidal vessels (orange bands) are visible behind the retinal blood vessels.

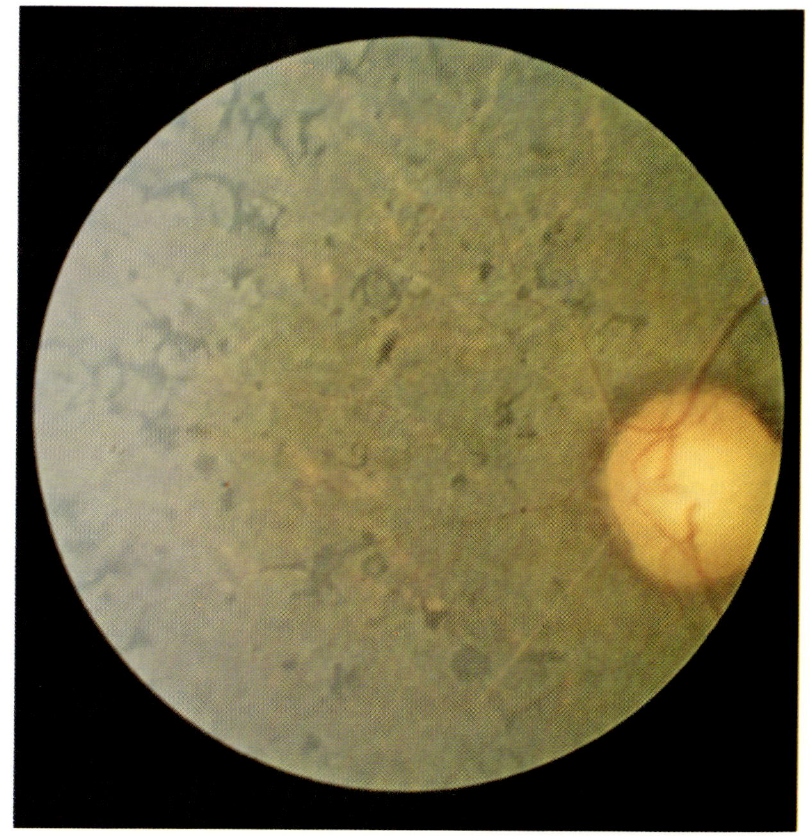

ANNOTATED BIBLIOGRAPHY

Anatomy of the Optic Nerve

Adler, F. H.: *Physiology of the Eye; Clinical Application*, 4th ed., pp. 652–705, Mosby, St. Louis, 1965. A good presentation of the visual pathway.

Francois, J. and Neetens, A.: *Vascularization of the Optic Pathway. Part I, Lamina Cribrosa and Optic Nerve*, Br. J. Ophthalmol., **38:** 472, 1954.

Francois, J. and Neetens, A.: *Central Retinal Artery and Central Optic Nerve Artery*, Br. J. Ophthalmol., **47:** 21, 1963. The two articles by Francois and Neetens present the complex blood supply of the optic nerve in detail.

Wolff, E.: *Anatomy of the Eye and Orbit, Including the Central Connections, Development, and Comparative Anatomy of the Visual Apparatus*, 5th ed., revised by R. J. Last, pp. 295–317, Saunders, Philadelphia, 1961. A detailed presentation of the anatomy of the optic nerve.

Papilledema

Hayreh, S. S.: *Pathogenesis of Oedema of the Optic Disc (Papilloedema)*, Br. J. Ophthalmol., **48:** 522, 1964. Experimental production of papilledema.

Hogan, M. J. and Zimmerman, L. E. (eds.): *Ophthalmic Pathology. An Atlas and Textbook*, 2nd ed., pp. 587–589, Saunders, Philadelphia, 1962. A clear, concise presentation of the pathology and pathogenesis of papilledema.

Paton, L. and Holmes, G.: *The Pathology of Papilledema. A Histologic Study of Sixty Eyes*, Brain, **33:** 389, 1911. An excellent description of the pathologic changes of papilledema and a good discussion of its pathogenesis.

Optic Neuritis — General Review

Hogan, M. J. and Zimmerman, L. E. (eds.): *Ophthalmic Pathology. An Atlas and Textbook*, 2nd ed., pp. 590–600, Saunders, Philadelphia, 1962. A good review of the pathologic changes and causes of optic neuritis.

Malnutrition, Alcoholism and Tobacco-Alcohol Amblyopia

Carroll, F. D.: *The Etiology and Treatment of Tobacco–Alcohol Amblyopia*, Am. J. Ophthalmol., **27:** 713, 847, 1944.

Fisher, M.: *Residual Neuropathological Changes in Canadians Held Prisoners of War by the Japanese, (Strachan's Disease)*, Can. Serv. Med. J., **11:** 157, 1955.

Victor, M., Mancall, E. L. and Dreyfus, P. M.: *Deficiency Amblyopia in the Alcoholic Patient. A Clinicopathologic Study*, Arch. Ophthalmol., **64:** 1, 1960. The articles by Fisher, Carroll, and Victor *et al.* are excellent presentations of the optic neuritis and optic atrophy associated with malnutrition.

Demyelinative Diseases

Berliner, M. L.: *Acute Optic Neuritis in Demyelinating Diseases of the Nervous System*, Arch. Ophthalmol., **13:** 83, 1935.

Optic Atrophy

Ballantyne, A. J. and Michaelson, I. C.: *Textbook of the Fundus of the Eye*, 2nd ed., pp. 671–687, Williams & Wilkins, Baltimore, 1970. A good presentation of the clinical findings in optic atrophy.

Cogan, D. G.: *Neurology of the Visual System*, pp. 133–149, Charles C Thomas, Springfield, Ill., 1966. A very good discussion of the clinical and pathological alterations of optic atrophy and papilledema.

Papilledema, Optic Neuritis, and Optic Atrophy

Hogan, M. J. and Zimmerman, L. E. (eds.): *Ophthalmic Pathology. An Atlas and Textbook*, 2nd ed., pp. 623–627, Saunders, Philadelphia, 1962. A good general discussion of the pathology of optic atrophy.

Walsh, F. B. and Hoyt, W. F.: *Clinical Neuro–Ophthalmology*, 3rd ed., Vol. I, pp. 567–641, Williams & Wilkins, Baltimore, 1969. An excellent comprehensive discussion of all the above abnormalities of the optic nerve.

Test Plates (unlabeled retinal photographs)

Questions and Answers D1–D10

Plate D1

Clinical findings: A 21–year–old female with recurrent urinary tract infection. A severe constant generalized headache has been present for one month. Intravenous and retrograde pyelograms disclosed congenital absence of the right kidney and marked dilatation of the left renal pelvis and calyces. Bl. P. 180/130 mmHg, BUN 74 mg/100 ml creatinine 7.4 mg/100 ml, Hct. 32%, Hb 10 gms/100 ml. Plate D1 — O.S. — central and temporal.

QUESTIONS — D1

Question 1. Note abnormalities (see answer, this page).

Question 2. The abnormalities are indicative of either optic neuritis or papilledema. What clinical information would you try to obtain in order to differentiate those two entities?

Question 3. Examination disclosed that the disc abnormality was bilateral. The pupils were equal in size and responded readily to light. The patient had no pain with either movement or palpation of the eye. There was no visual disturbance and visual fields revealed only a slightly enlarged blind spot. What is your diagnosis?

ANSWERS — D1

Answer 1. The optic disc is slightly hyperemic and its margins are indistinct. The nerve fibers entering the superior temporal portion of the nerve head are separated. The vessels leaving the disc are elevated and dip over the edges. Venular tortuosity is marked. The arterioles are narrow. The macula is normal. There is a flame–shaped hemorrhage which contains a central white spot at 2 o'clock, 3 disc diameters from the nerve head.

Answer 2. Observe:

a. Whether the disc abnormality is bilateral.
b. Difference in size of the pupils.
c. Pupillary response to direct light stimulation.
d. Whether pain is elicited by movement or palpation of the eye.
e. The presence or absence of visual loss.
f. Whether visual field abnormalities can be detected.

Answer 3. Papilledema.

References

Walsh, F. B. and Hoyt, W. F.: *Clinical Neuro–Ophthalmology,* 3rd ed., Vol. I, pp. 567–641, Williams & Wilkins, Baltimore, 1969.

PLATE D1

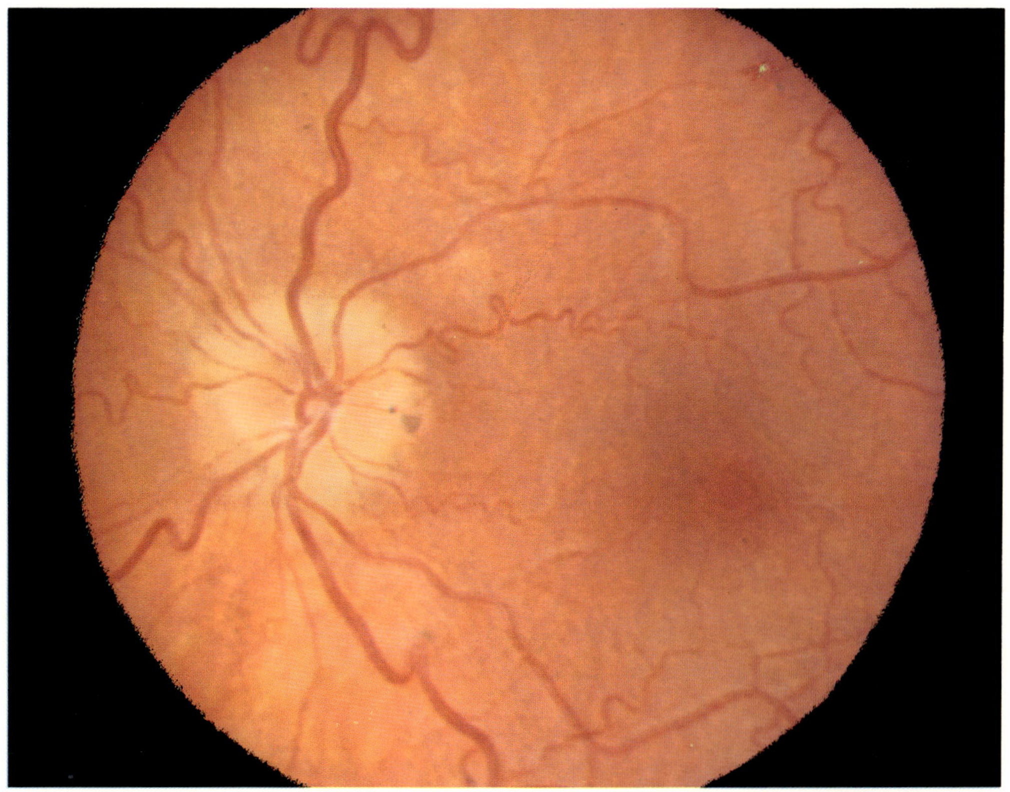

Plate D2

Clinical findings: A 40–year–old male admitted to the hospital with the classic clinical picture of delirium tremens. Physical examination, including neurologic examination, disclosed no abnormalities except for the bilateral funduscopic changes as noted in Plate D2. Bl. P. 130/80 mmHg. Plate D2 — O.D. — central.

QUESTIONS — D2

Question 1. Note the abnormalities (see answer, p. 203).

Question 2. What is your differential diagnosis?

Question 3. In view of the clinical findings what further studies are indicated?

Question 4. Based upon the data presented which of the possibilities can be excluded? State reasons.

Question 5. In view of the lack of neurologic signs, normal cerebrospinal fluid and electroencephalogram, the patient was discharged. He was carefully observed for 6 months. During that time, he had neither headache nor neurologic localizing signs. The findings noted in the optic nerve remained unchanged. The disc elevation remained at one diopter. Do you think that the disc findings represent papilledema?

Question 6. What are the pathologic changes of drusen bodies of the optic nerve?

Question 7. How do they differ from the other variety of drusen or colloid bodies?

PLATE D2

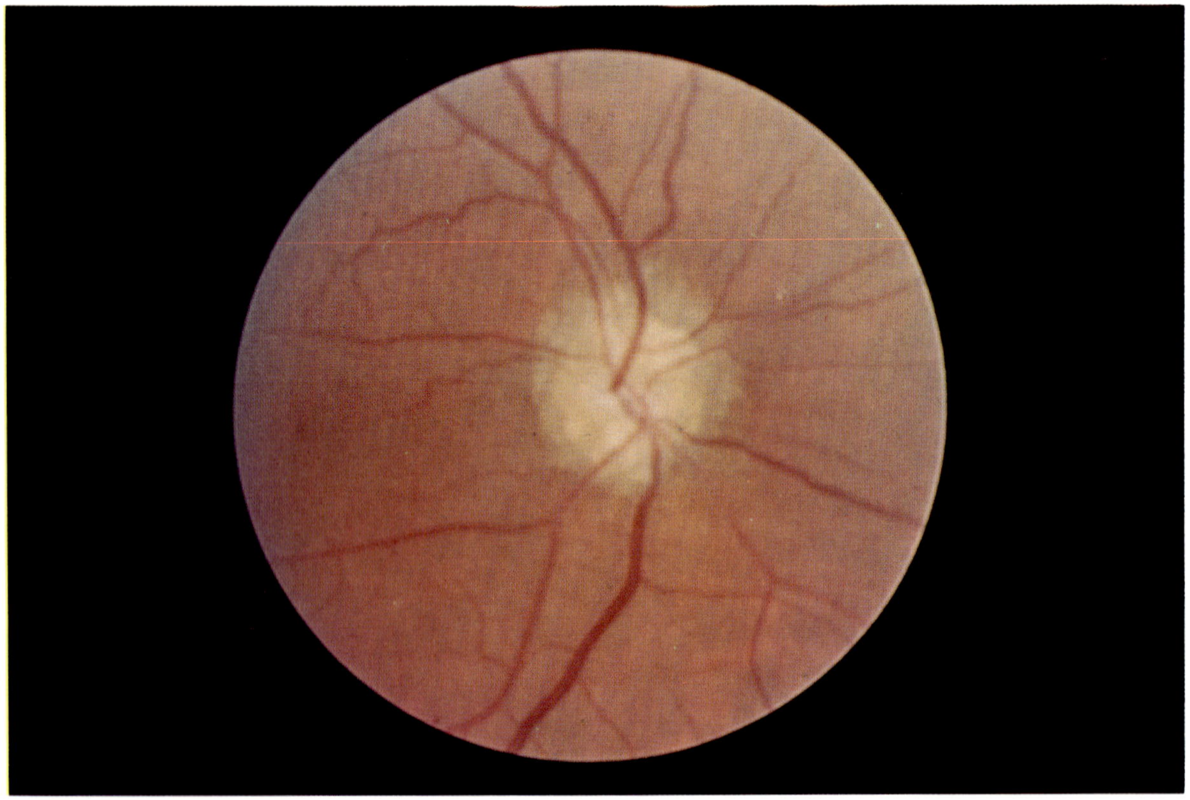

ANSWERS — D2

Answer 1. The disc margins are indistinct. The vessels emerging from it appear to be slightly elevated. There are numerous small, white, oval lesions on the disc, some of which extend over its edges. The arterioles and venules are normal. There are no extravascular lesions.

Answer 2.
- a. Optic neuritis
- b. Papilledema
- c. Hypermetropia
- d. Drusen bodies of the optic disc

Answer 3.
- a. Skull films disclose no bony defects; the pineal body is calcified and is midline. The sella turcica is normal.
- b. Lumbar puncture — normal pressure, normal protein, and no cells.
- c. Visual acuity 20/20 — O.U.
- d. Visual fields — normal except for slight enlargement of blind spot of both eyes.
- e. Electroencephalogram — normal.

Answer 4.
- a. Optic neuritis — normal vision and absence of scotoma.
- b. Hypermetropia normal visual acuity.

Answer 5. In view of the lack of progressive change in the optic nerve and clinical findings papilledema is most unlikely. The changes are consistent with drusen bodies of the optic nerve.

Answer 6. See p. 177.

Answer 7. See pp. 76–78.

References

Duke–Elder, W. S.: *Textbook of Ophthalmology,* Vol. III, *Diseases of the Inner Eye,* pp. 3062–3064, Mosby, St. Louis, 1940.

Duke–Elder, W. S. and Dobree, J. H.: *Diseases of the Retina,* in: Duke–Elder, W. S. (ed.): *System of Ophthalmology,* Vol. X, pp. 645–652, Mosby, St. Louis, 1967.

PLATE D3

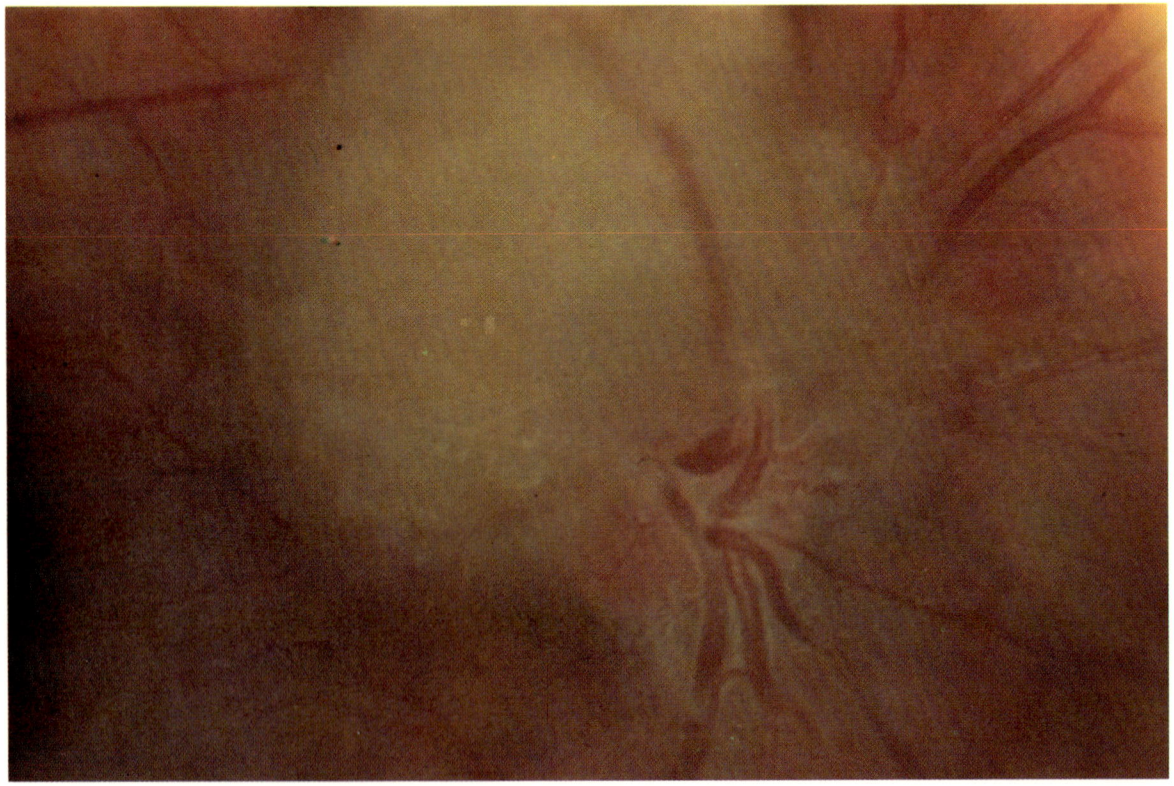

Plate D3

Clinical findings: A 14–year–old boy who was thought to be normal except that he was a slower learner than his siblings. I.Q. at 7 was 65; it decreased to 47 at age 11. Vision and hearing were normal. There were no convulsive episodes. Examination disclosed the presence of numerous red–brown papules over the face, forehead, and malar areas. Vitiligo was noted over the trunk and extremities. Vision was normal; pupils reacted to light and in accommodation. Neurologic examination was normal. X-ray of skull demonstrated calcification in the basal ganglia and superior walls of the ventricles. Plate D3 — O.D.

QUESTIONS — D3

Question 1. Note abnormalities (see answer, this page).

Question 2. Based on the clinical history, the physical and laboratory findings, what is your diagnosis?

Question 3. What is the nature of the lesion noted on funduscopy?

ANSWERS — D3

Answer 1. There is a large, white mass extending upward from the superior portion of the disc. It seems to elevate the superior nasal vein.

Answer 2. Tuberous sclerosis.

Answer 3. Hamartoma.

References

Ballantyne, A. J. and Michaelson, I. C.: *Textbook of the Fundus of the Eye,* 2nd ed., pp. 436–439, Williams & Wilkins, Baltimore, 1970.

Reese, A. B.: *Relation of Drusen of the Optic Nerve to Tuberous Sclerosis,* Arch. Ophthalmol., **24:** 187, 1940.

Plate D4

Clinical findings: A 48–year–old male who has been nearsighted since early childhood. He has worn glasses to correct the refractive error since age 4. Two years ago, he was found to have diabetes mellitus. Glycosuria has been minimal since a regimen of an isocaloric diet and a daily dose of 45 units of NPH insulin was instituted. Bl. P. 180/125 mmHg. Retinal photograph D4 — O.D. During the funduscopic examination, the examiner noted that the retina and optic nerve could not be seen distinctly even with the use of a minus 20 lens of the ophthalmoscope. When the examination was performed while the patient wore his glasses, the view of the fundus became sharp. Plate D4 corresponds to the view obtained during the second examination.

PLATE D4

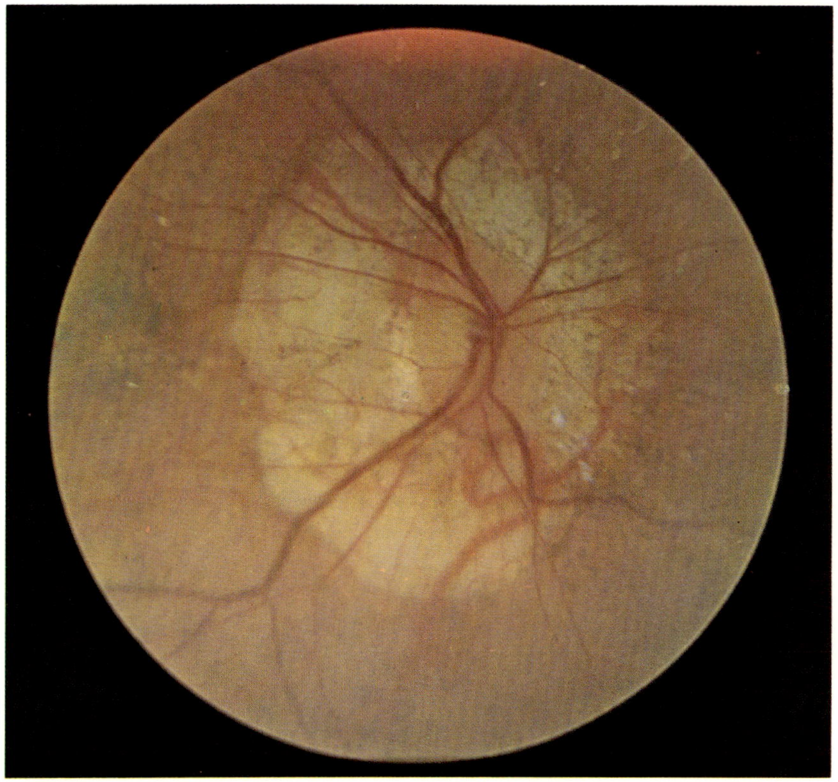

QUESTIONS — D4

Question 1. Describe findings (see answer, this page).

Question 2. What explanation can you offer for the patient's visual impairment and the funduscopic changes?

ANSWERS — D4

Answer 1. A normal optic disc is completely surrounded by a broad, irregular, white scleral ring. Within that peripapillary scleral ring, there are several small deposits of pigment. In addition, choroidal vessels are visible as broad, orange–red bands beneath the retinal vessels at the 4–to–6 and 11 o'clock areas of the ring about the disc. The pigment of macular area is irregularly placed.

Answer 2. The history and funduscopic changes are consistent with the diagnosis of severe myopia. In a patient with severe myopia the entire optic fundus may be hazy even when the examiner uses a −20 lens (red) of his ophthalmoscope. If the examination is performed with the patient wearing his corrective lenses the image becomes sharp. The scattered pigment of the macula is a common occurrence in malignant or severe myopia. Macular hemorrhage is another complication of myopia.

References

Ballantyne, A. J. and Michaelson, I. C.: *Textbook of the Fundus of the Eye*, 2nd ed., pp. 473–482, Williams and Wilkins, Baltimore, 1970.

Hogan, M. J. and Zimmerman, L. E. (eds.): *Ophthalmic Pathology. An Atlas and Textbook*, 2nd ed., pp. 113–117, Saunders, Philadelphia, 1962.

Plate D5

Clinical findings: A 28–year–old man who has had insulin dependent diabetes mellitus for 16 years. Section of the pituitary stalk was performed 4 years ago for progressive bilateral retinopathy. Visual acuity, which had been severely impaired prior to the operative procedure, improved considerably for 1 year. Three weeks before retinal photograph D5 was taken, the patient noted a large area of haziness in his left lateral visual field. Plate D5 — O.S. — central and temporal.

QUESTIONS — D5

Question 1. Describe changes (see answer, this page).

PLATE D5

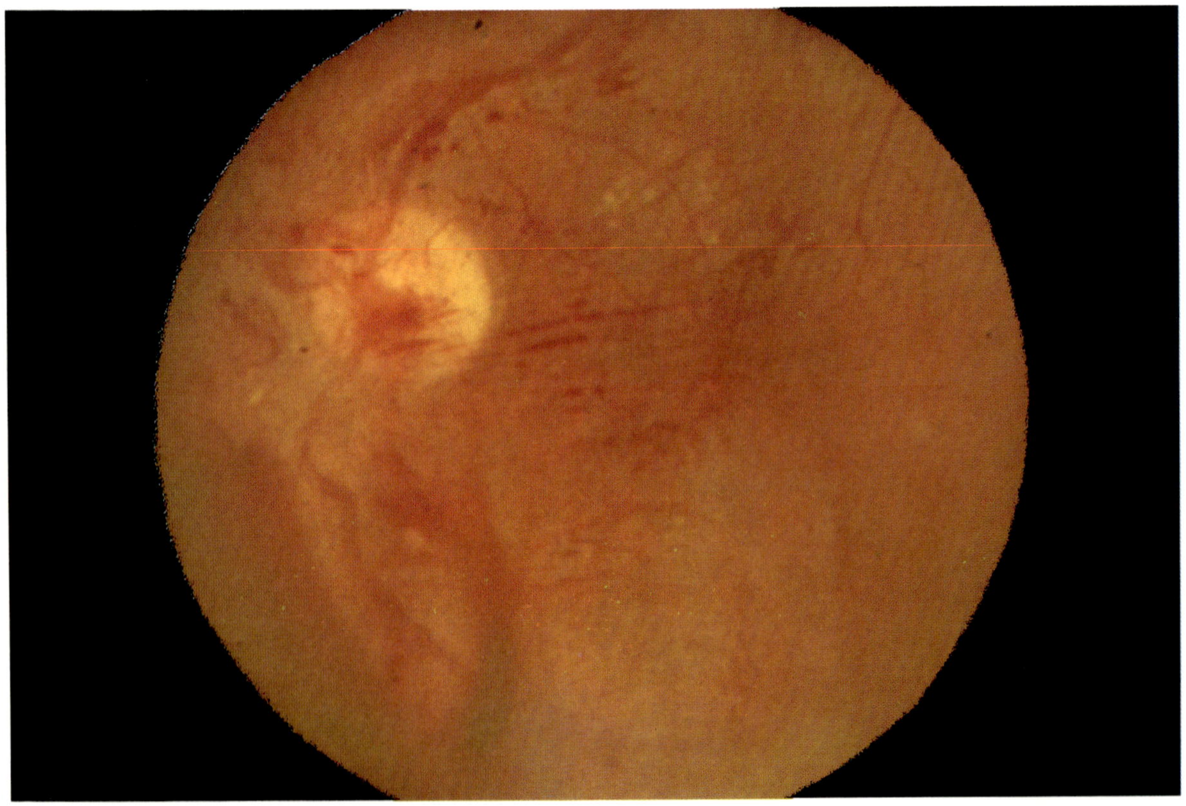

ANSWERS — D5

Answer 1. A large, preretinal hemorrhage is visible nasal and inferior to the disc. It is brown–black in color and overlies the retinal vessels. The nerve head margins are distinct. There are many linear hemorrhages in the optic nerve and retina extending toward the macula. There is neovascularization of the optic disc. Several hard exudates are present above the macula. Venous engorgement and tortuosity are noted. Several microaneurysms can be seen above the disc.

References

Ballantyne, A. J. and Michaelson, I. C.: *Textbook of the Fundus of the Eye,* 2nd ed., pp. 122–139, *Williams & Wilkins,* Baltimore, 1970.

Ballantyne, A. J.: *New–Formed Vessels in the Fundus Oculi,* Ophthalmologica, **118:** 611, 1949.

Plate D6

Clinical findings: A 40–year–old male suddenly became blind in the left eye 2 years ago. Along with permanent total visual loss of the left eye, the patient noted persistent, throbbing, temporal headache, and weakness since the onset of the present illness. Examination disclosed Bl. P. 160/100 mmHg, and tenderness over the left temporal artery. Temperature during the first week ranged between 38 and 38.5°C. The leukocyte count was 15,000 mm³ with a predominance of polymorphonuclear leukocytes. Plate D6 represents the funduscopic findings on the day of admission. Plate D6 — O.S. — temporal.

QUESTIONS — D6

Question 1. Describe the findings of the left fundus D6 (see answer, this page).

Question 2. What is the nature of the optic nerve abnormality?

Question 3. Based upon the history and physical findings, what produced the optic atrophy?

Question 4. What diagnostic study is indicated to establish the etiology of the central retinal artery obstruction? What disease would you try to find?

PLATE D6

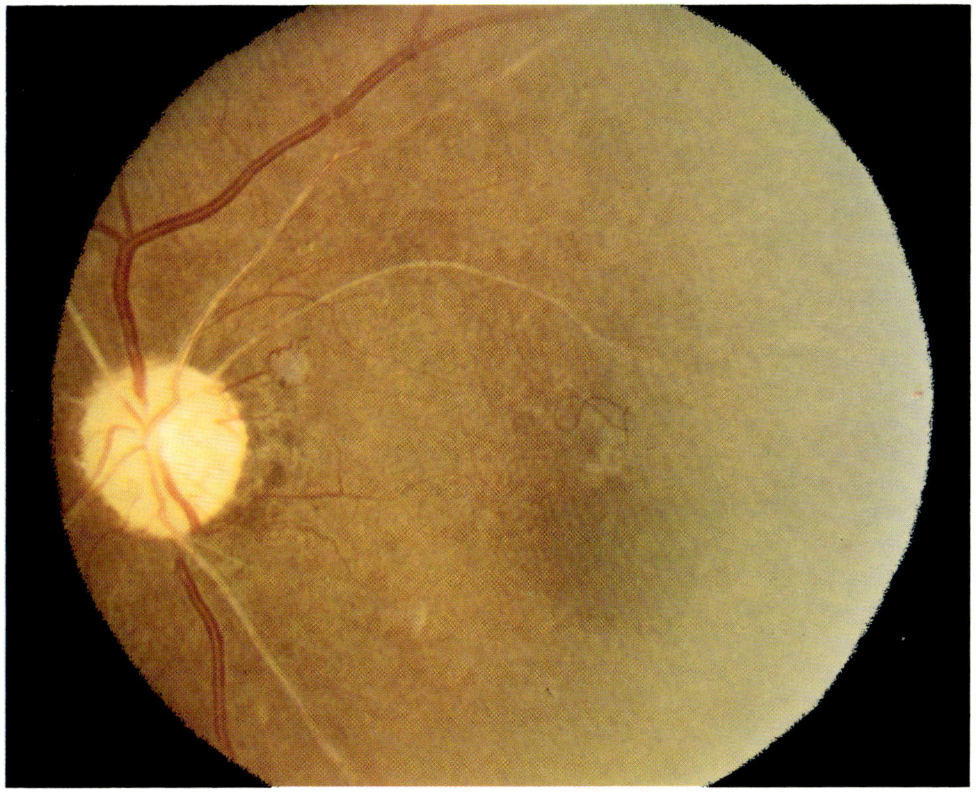

ANSWERS — D6

Answer 1. The optic disc is pale and its borders are irregular. The normally visible lamina cribrosa is not seen. Few small blood vessels cross the disc margins. The arterioles demonstrate "copper and silver wire" change. Hard exudates are present at 2 and 5 o'clock.

Answer 2. Optic atrophy (secondary) (see pp. 190, 193).

Answer 3. Central retinal artery occlusion (see pp. 30–36).

Answer 4. Biopsy of the tender temporal artery to look for the histologic changes of temporal arteritis.

References

Crosby, R. C. and Wadsworth, R. C.: *Temporal Arteritis. Review of the Literature and Report of Five Additional Cases,* Arch. Intern. Med., **81:** 431, 1948.

Henkind, P., Charles, N. C., and Pearson, J.: *Histopathology of Ischemic Optic Neuropathy,* Am. J. Ophthalmol., **68:** 78, 1970.

Plate D7

Clinical findings: A 33–year–old female who was admitted to the hospital with a story of severe and constant headache. Examination disclosed a blood pressure of 280/170 mmHg and moderate left ventricular hypertrophy. At ages 25 and 31, while pregnant, her diastolic blood pressures ranged between 110–130 mmHg and generalized convulsions developed. During the current admission, the BUN was 65 mg/100 ml and the creatinine 5 mg/100 ml. Funduscopy disclosed bilateral changes as noted in Plate D7. Plate D7 — O. D. — central and nasal.

QUESTIONS — D7

Question 1. Describe the funduscopic changes in D7 (see answer, this page).

Question 2. Identify the abnormality of the optic nerve. What pathologic changes of the nerve account for the clinical findings?

Question 3. What beneficial changes might be observed in this patient's fundi with successful antihypertensive therapy?

PLATE D7

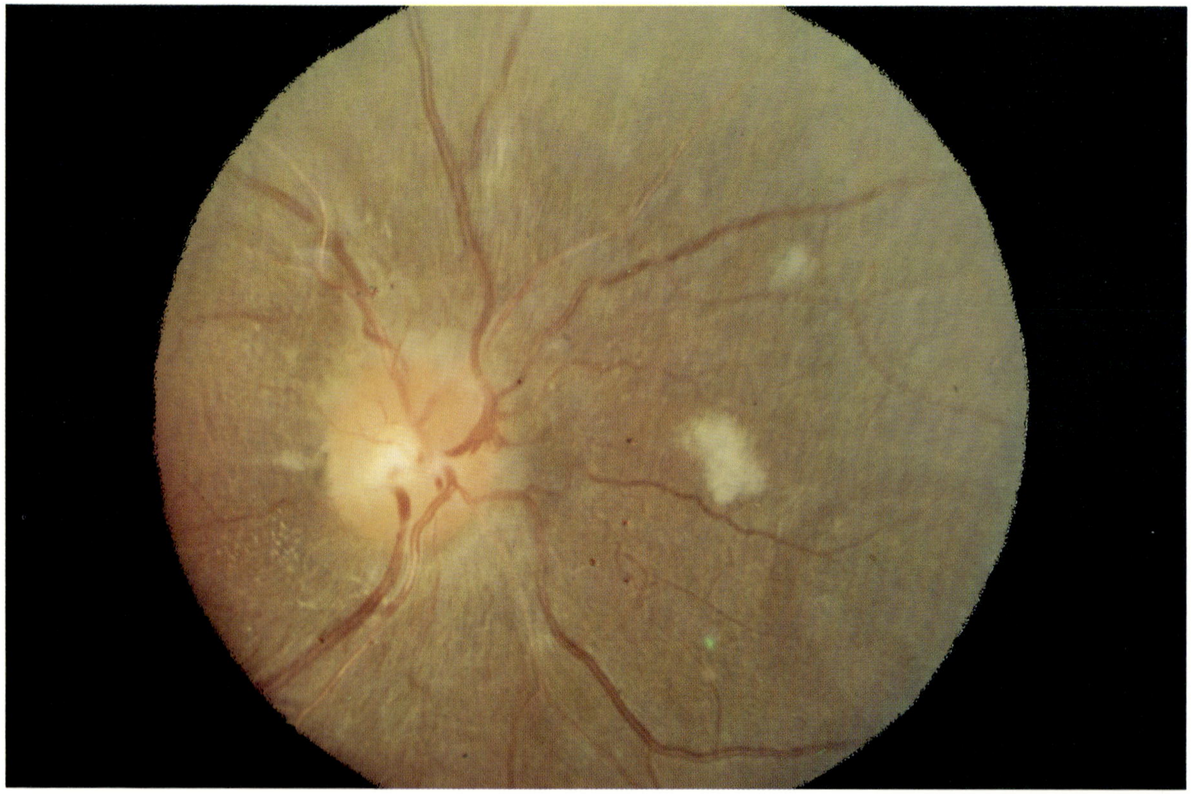

ANSWERS — D7

Answer 1. The optic disc is hyperemic and its margins are indistinct. Separation of nerve fibers is noted at the superior and inferior borders of the optic nerve. A halo surrounds the nasal margin of the disc. The superior nasal and inferior temporal veins are elevated at the disc margins. "Copper wire" arterioles and arteriovenous compression are noted. Several cotton patches are present. The peculiar, dark semicircle noted inferior and nasal to the large cotton wool patch is noted. Its significance is not apparent.

Answer 2. Papilledema associated with malignant or accelerated hypertension (see pp. 179–80).

Answer 3. Regression of papilledema and cotton wool patches.

References

Lockhart, G., Von Noorden, G., Duston, H. P., Corcoran, A. C., and Page, I. H.: *The Course of Retinopathy in Treated Malignant Hypertension*, Arch. Intern. Med. **106:** 205, 1960.

Paton, L. and Holmes, G.: *The Pathology of the Papilledema. A Histological Study of Sixty Eyes*, Brain, **33:** 289, 1911.

Plate D8

Clinical findings: A 48–year–old black male who noted periodic, severe, knifelike pains in both legs, clumsiness of gait, and failing vision for the past 2 years. Examination disclosed unequal pupils, L>R. The pupils failed to respond to light. They did respond in accommodation. Perception of pain, temperature and vibratory sense was markedly decreased in both legs. Deep tendon reflexes were absent at the knees and ankles. The plantar reflexes were flexor. Retinal photograph D8 (O.D.) was taken on admission. O.S. showed the same changes. Plate D8 — O.D. — central and temporal.

QUESTIONS — D8

Question 1. Describe findings (see answer, this page).

Question 2. What is the nature of the disc abnormality?

Question 3. What diagnostic procedures would be most likely to establish an etiologic diagnosis?

PLATE D8

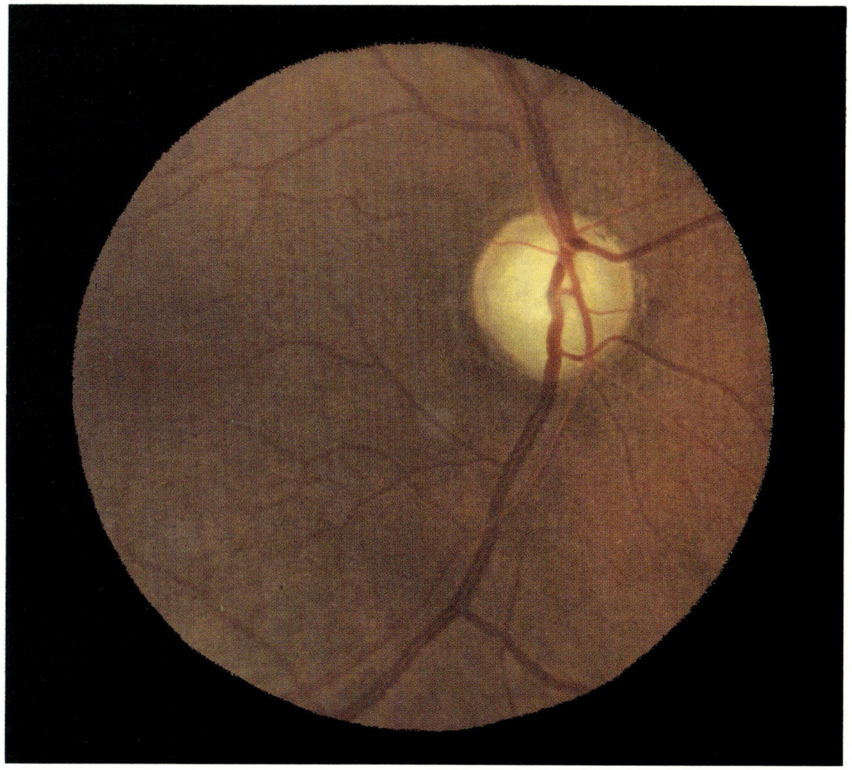

ANSWERS — D8

Answer 1. The disc is pale; its margins are sharp and the lamina cribrosa is visible as a sievelike structure within the physiologic cup. Few small vessels cross the disc margins. The retinal arterioles and venules are normal.

Answer 2. Optic atrophy (primary) (see pp. 193–96).

Answer 3. Serologic tests for syphilis of the blood and spinal fluid.

Reference

Woods, A. C.: *Optic Neuropathies: A Simplified Classification and Outline for Etiologic Diagnosis,* Am. J. Ophthalmol., **31:** 1053, 1948.

Plate D9

Clinical findings: A 55–year–old obese female was admitted to the hospital having had a moderately severe generalized headache for 2 weeks. In addition, she complained of dyspnea with moderate physical activity and a cough producing clear sputum for the past 6 years. Bl. P. 250/110 mmHg. The heart was normal in size; the rhythm was regular and there were no murmurs. The configuration of the thorax was normal and the lateral costal excursion was decreased slightly bilaterally. The percussion note was resonant and scattered inspiratory and expiratory rhonchi were audible over both legs. Pulmonary function studies, arterial blood gases, and pH were normal. Neurologic examination disclosed no abnormalities. Cerebrospinal fluid pressure was 220 mm of water; the protein was 30 mg/100 ml. There were no cells. Skull films, electroencephalogram, pneumoencephalogram, and visual fields were normal. Hct. 50%, Hb 16 gm/100 ml, WBC 9,800 mm³. Retinal photograph D9 — O.D. was taken the day of admission. The funduscopic changes were present in both eyes and remained the same throughout the 2 weeks of hospitalization. Plate D9 — O.D. — central.

QUESTIONS — D9

Question 1. List abnormalities (see answer, this page).

Question 2. In view of the lack of neurologic abnormalities, as determined by physical examination and laboratory studies, it was reasonable to exclude a brain tumor. In view of the other findings, what other possibilities exist in this patient to explain the papilledema?

Question 3. Can you exclude any of the possibilities mentioned?

ANSWERS — D9

Answer 1. Optic disc is hyperemic and poorly marginated. The tortuous and engorged veins are elevated over the disc. Nerve fiber separation is present at the superior nasal border of the nerve head. A halo is present around the superior and nasal aspect of the disc. A scleral ring is present. The arterioles are narrow.

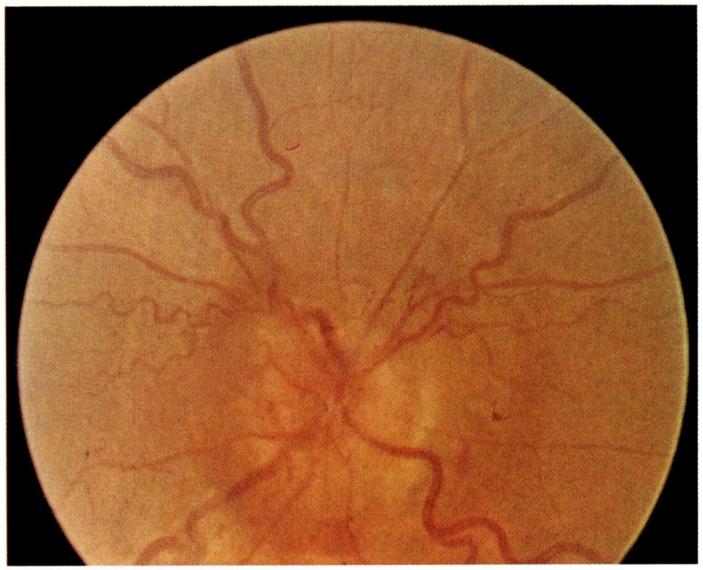

PLATE D9

Answer 2.

a. Hypertension
b. Chronic obstructive pulmonary disease with hypercapnia
c. Pseudo–tumor cerebri

Answer 3. a. Hypertension. The papilledema of hypertension is generally associated with a higher diastolic blood pressure, ranging over 130 mmHg. In addition one would expect more striking vascular disease (arteriovenous compression and possibly "silver wire" change) and such extravascular lesions as hemorrhage, cotton wool patches, and hard exudates.

b. The papilledema of respiratory failure is generally accompanied by hypercapnia and acidosis.

The working clinical diagnosis was pseudo–tumor cerebri (benign intracranial hypertension). This syndrome consists of prolonged, increased intracranial pressure in the absence of ventricular abnormalities and focal neurologic signs. Headache, blurred vision, and papilledema are the most common findings. The composition of the spinal fluid is normal despite the elevated pressure. The etiology is not apparent and the prognosis is favorable. Within several months, all the manifestations generally disappear.

References

Foley, J.: *Benign Forms of Intracranial Hypertension — "Toxic" and "Otitic" Hydrocephalus,* Brain, **78:** 1, 1955.

Miller, A., Bader, R. A., and Bader, M. E.: *The Neurologic Syndrome Due to Marked Hypercapnia, with Papilledema,* Am. J. Med., **33:** 309, 1962.

Plate D10

Clinical findings: A 26–year–old obese female who was admitted for study because of a frontal headache for two weeks. General physical and neurologic examinations revealed no abnormalities. Visual fields, skull films, and electroencephalograms were normal. Spinal fluid pressure was elevated; spinal fluid protein was 25 mg/100 ml and there were no cells. Bl. P. 120/84 mmHg. Plate D10 — O.D.

QUESTIONS — D10

Question 1. List abnormalities (see answer, this page).

Question 2. How do you interpret the changes observed in the optic disc?

Question 3. Is there reason to be concerned about persistent papilledema?

Question 4. What explanation is offered for the development of the halo of papilledema?

Question 5. Are the anomalous hyaloid vessels likely to produce any ill effects?

PLATE D10

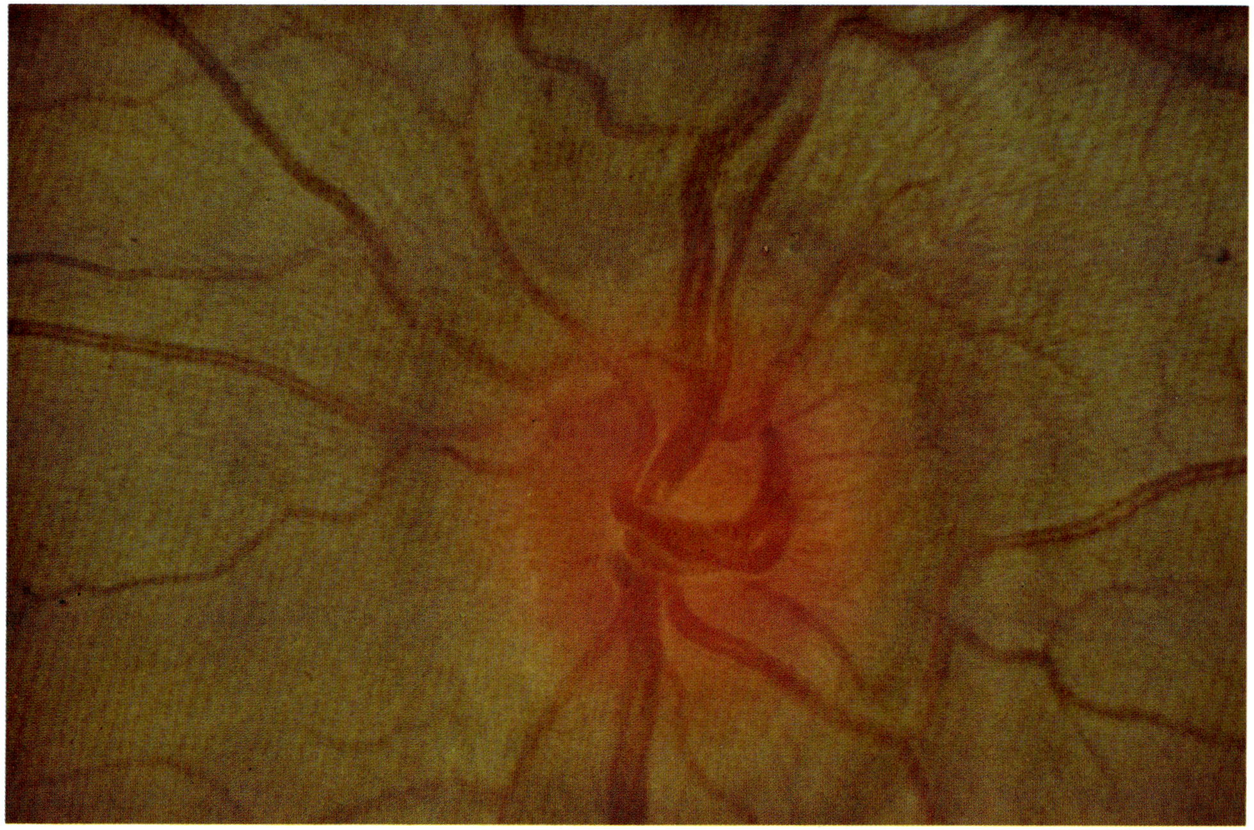

ANSWERS — D10

Answer 1. The margins of the hyperemic nerve head are indistinct and surrounded by a dark halo. The vessels extending from the disc do not appear to be elevated. The nerve fibers are separated as they enter the inferior nasal part of the disc. A large blood vessel extends forward from the disc.

Answer 2. a. Papilledema.
b. Persistent hyaloid blood vessel.

No adequate explanation for the papilledema could be found. Within a period of two weeks, the patient's headache decreased in intensity. The papilledema persisted. The plan called for further observation.

Answer 3. Yes. Prolonged papilledema may be followed by optic atrophy.

Answer 4. The halo is believed to be the result of folding of the retina adjacent to the papilla. It is thought that such folds result from the pressure applied laterally by the edematous optic disc.

Answer 5. No. They rarely produce symptoms or any other complications.

References

Cogan, D. G.: *Neurology of the Visual System,* pp. 137–149, Charles C Thomas, Springfield, Ill., 1966.

Duke–Elder, W. S.: *Normal and Abnormal Development. Part II, Congenital Deformities,* in: Duke–Elder, W. S. (ed.): *System of Ophthalmology,* Vol. III, pp. 764–793, Mosby, St. Louis, 1963.

Chapter VIII
THE CLINICAL APPLICATION OF FUNDUSCOPY

THE CLINICAL APPLICATION OF FUNDUSCOPY: A PERSONAL VIEW

It is important to recognize that the retina and optic nerve have a limited number of responses to disease. As a result, similar clinical findings are observed in a wide variety of diseases. For example, the extravascular lesions of the retina are common denominators of many different disorders, i.e., accelerated hypertension, scleroderma, polyarteritis nodosa, disseminated lupus erythematosus, diabetes mellitus, leukemia, multiple myeloma, and anemia (see Chapter III). A comparable uniform response can be demonstrated in the abnormalities of the optic nerve. For example, papilledema may either be produced by increased intracranial pressure or associated with such diverse disorders as hypoparathyroidism, respiratory acidosis, and leukemia. The relationship of optic neuritis and atrophy to a wide variety of diseases of the nervous system, particularly multiple sclerosis, as well as avitaminosis B and drug intoxication, is equally obvious (see Chapter VII).

In view of these stereotyped responses of the retina and optic nerve to disease, one may ask how the examiner distinguishes the various forms of retinopathy. The answer rests first with the assessment of all the changes observed during funduscopy and secondly through the correlation of these changes with all the available clinical and laboratory data. In broad terms the specific retinopathies may

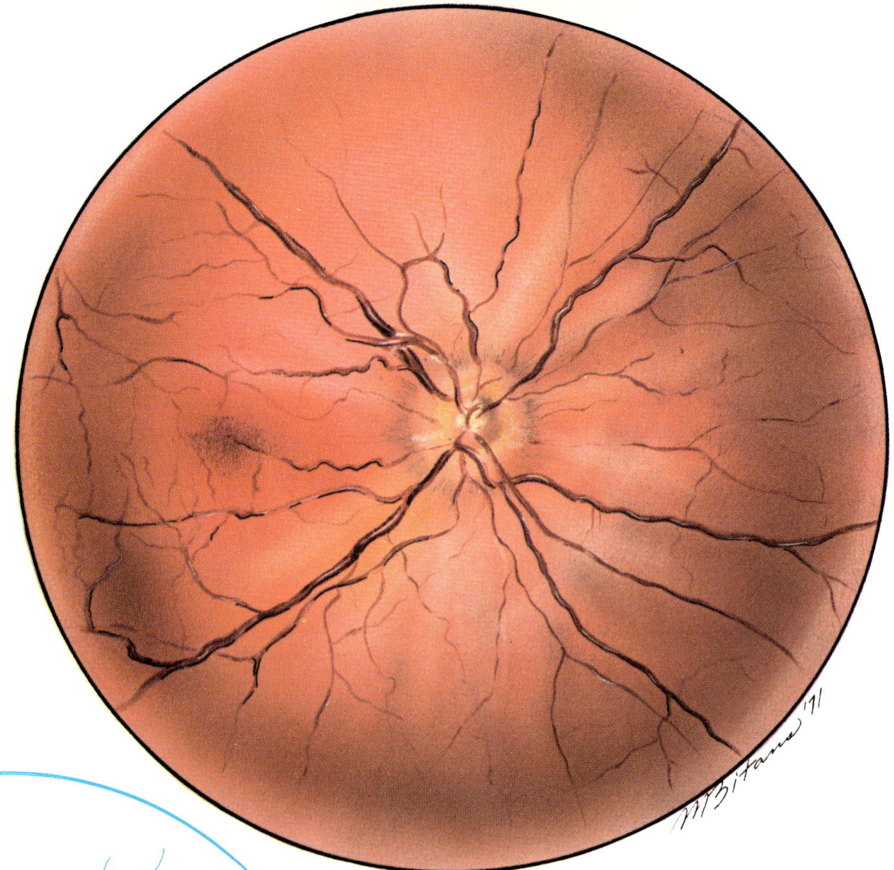

Plate 223 and Drawing 223. O.D. Diffuse and focal arteriolar narrowing are pronounced. The arteriovenous compression which involves the superior temporal arteriole and venule may not be significant since it occurs within a disc diameter of the nerve head. Several small hard exudates are present in the macula. Slight venular tortuosity is present.

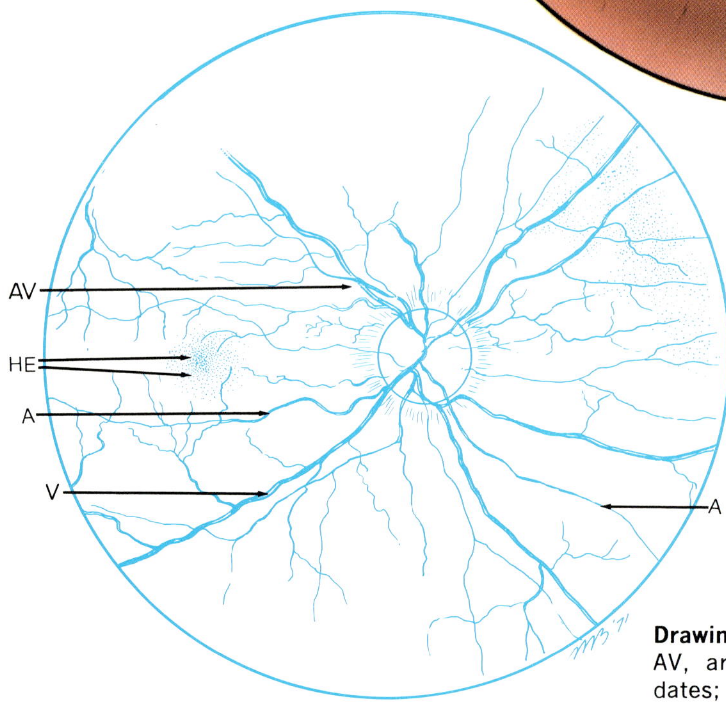

Drawing 223. Plate 223 (A, arteriolar narrowing; AV, arteriovenous compression; HE, hard exudates; V, venular tortuosity).

be divided into two major groups depending upon the dominance of either *artierolar or venular* disease.

Hypertension provides the classic form of arteriolar disease (Plates 223–227 and Drawings 223–227). The arteriolar changes include diffuse and focal narrowing (Plates 223–227 and Drawings 223–227), significant arteriovenous compression (Plates 224, 225 and Drawings 224, 225), and "silver wire" change (Plate 225 and Drawing 225). Cotton wool patches and hard exudates are present in Plates 225–227 and Drawings 225–227. Additional abnormalities include hemorrhage and microaneurysm (Plate 226 and Drawing 226), papilledema (Plates 225, 227 and Drawings 225, 227), and a macular star (Plate 227 and Drawing 227).

The prime form of venular disease is exemplified by diabetic retinopathy (Plates 228–231 and Drawings 228–231). The venular changes include engorgement, tortuosity (Plates 228–231 and Drawings 228–231), and sheathing (Plate 230 and Drawing 230). The number of visible microaneurysms ranges from a few (Plates 228, 229 and Drawings 228, 229) to many (Plates 230, 231 and Drawings 230, 231). Extravascular lesions include hemorrhage, cotton wool patches, and hard exudates (Plates 230, 231 and Drawings 230, 231). Neovascularization is prominent in Plate 231 and Drawing 231.

Although the extravascular lesions and microaneurysms are observed in the retinopathy associated with both the arteriolar disease of hypertension and the venular abnormalities of diabetes mellitus, certain additional major differences are apparent:

1. The microaneurysm is common in patients with diabetes mellitus and rare in those with hypertension.

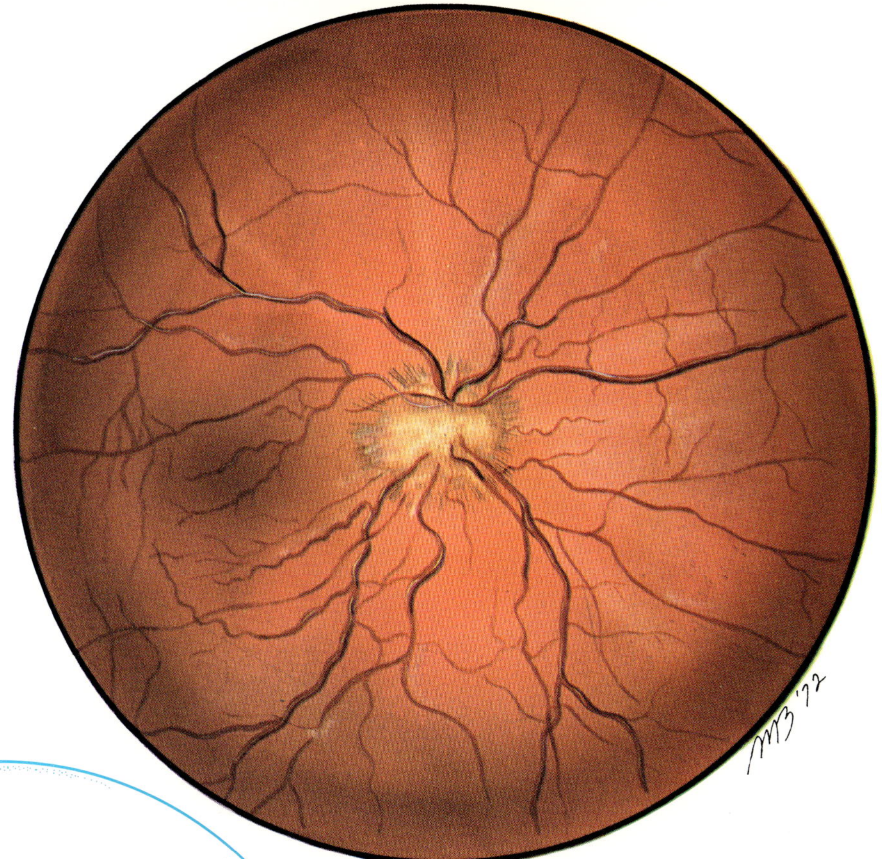

Plate 224 and Drawing 224. Diffuse arteriolar narrowing is present. Arteriovenous compression and displacement are observed to involve the superior temporal and inferior nasal arterioles and venules. The superior temporal arteriole is tortuous.

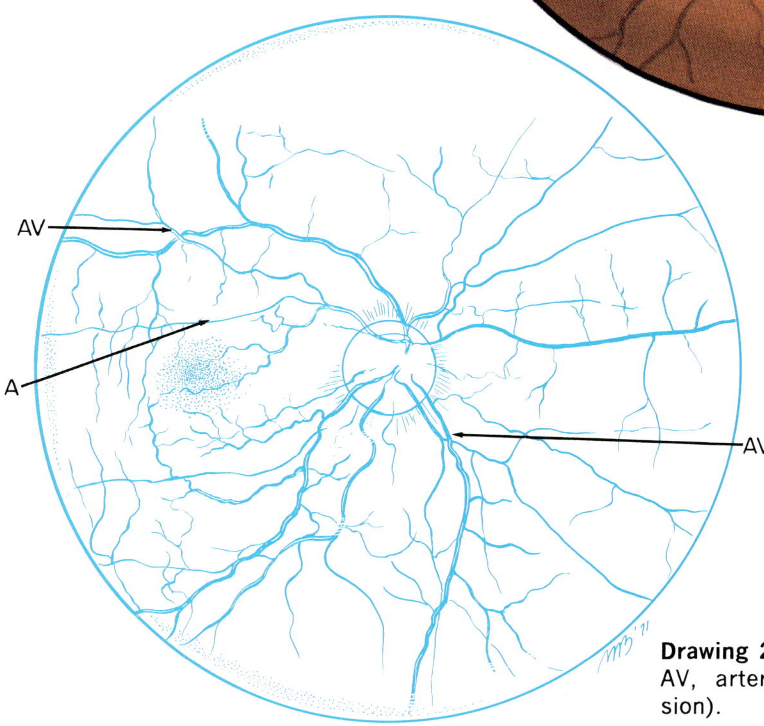

Drawing 224. Plate 224 (A, arteriolar narrowing; AV, arteriovenous displacement and compression).

2. Neovascularization and proliferative retinopathy are observed frequently in diabetes, but rarely in hypertension.

3. Papilledema may be a manifestation of accelerated hypertension. The optic nerve is rarely involved in diabetes mellitus and appears as either optic neuritis or optic atrophy.

Based upon the concept that the retinopathies may be separated into those with predominantly either arteriolar or venular disease, the division of disorders shown in the following classifications seems appropriate.

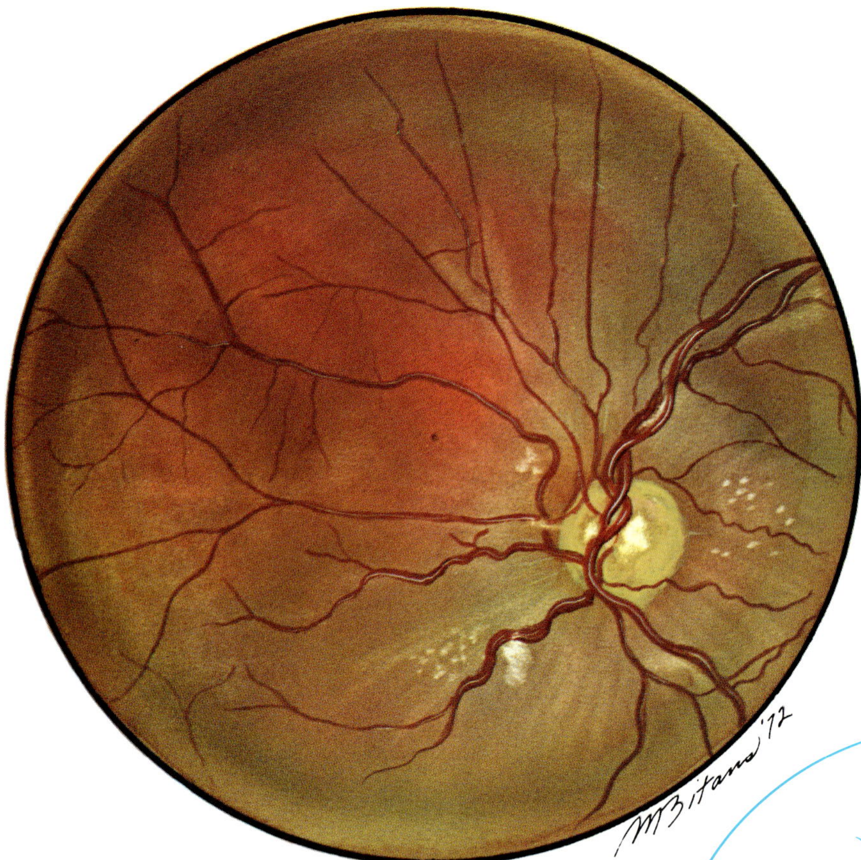

Plate 225 and Drawing 225. O.S. Arteriolar narrowing is present. Arteriovenous compressions are observed at the second crossing of the superior temporal and at the first crossing of the superior nasal vessels. Engorgement and tortuosity of venules occur distal to the sites of compression. The portion of the superior nasal arteriole immediately adjacent to the disc has become a broad "silver wire." A cotton wool patch is present at 7 o'clock, 1 disc diameter from the optic disc. Numerous hard exudates are present. The nasal, superior, and inferior disc borders are indistinct. Nerve fiber separation is observed around all of the nerve head margins except for the midtemporal borders.

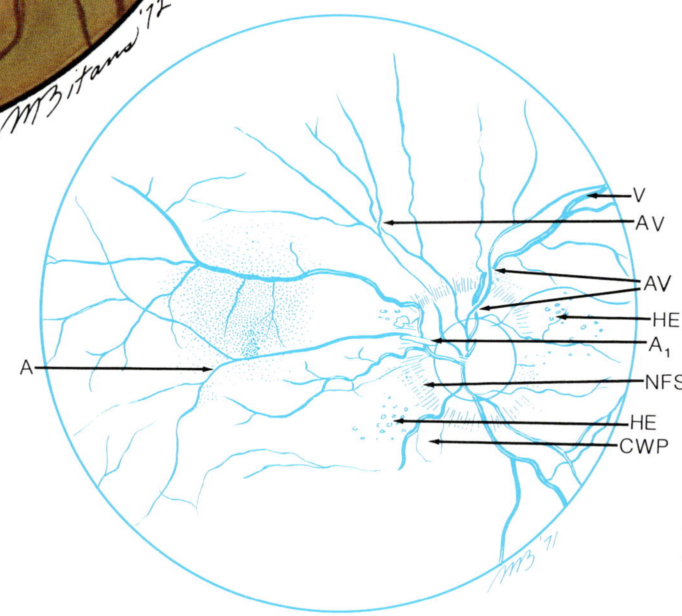

Drawing 225. Plate 225 (A, arteriolar narrowing; AV, arteriovenous compression; V, venous engorgement and tortuosity distal to A–V compression; A_1, "silver wire" arteriole; CWP, cotton wool patch; HE, hard exudate; NFS, nerve fiber separation).

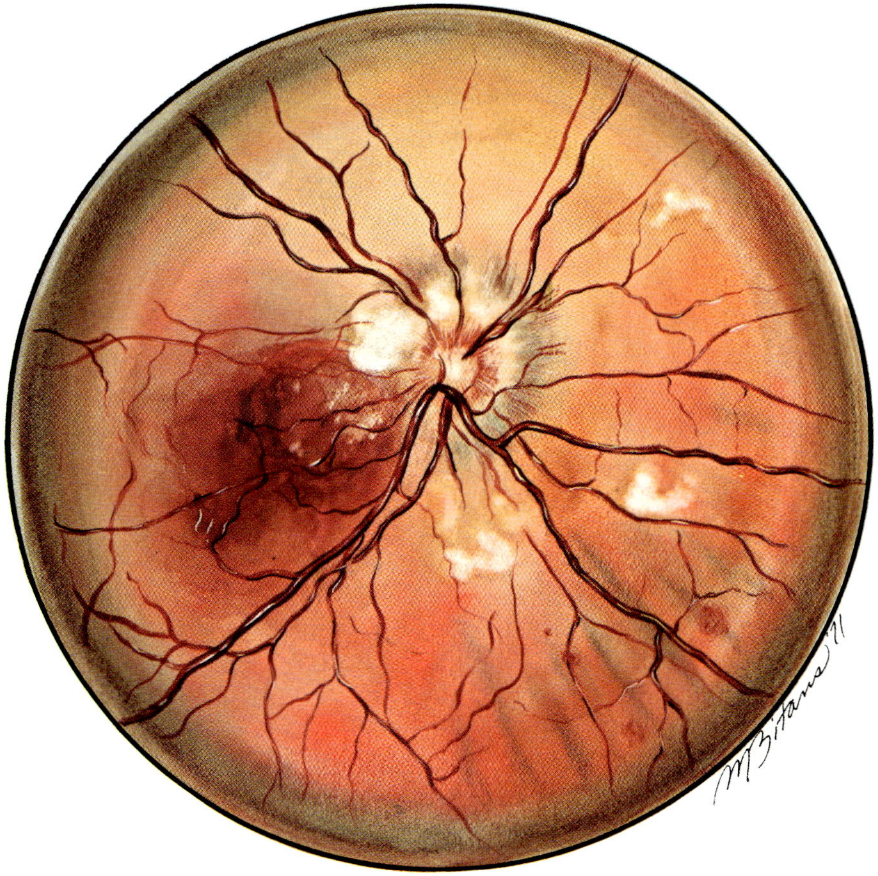

Plate 226 and Drawing 226. O.D. Diffuse arteriolar narrowing is present. Cotton wool patches surround an indistinctly marginated disc, and at 1, 5, and 6 o'clock, 1–2 disc diameters away from the optic nerve. Hard exudates are present temporal to the disc. A solitary microaneurysm is present at 5 o'clock, 3 disc diameters from the disc. Several hemorrhages are present in the same area.

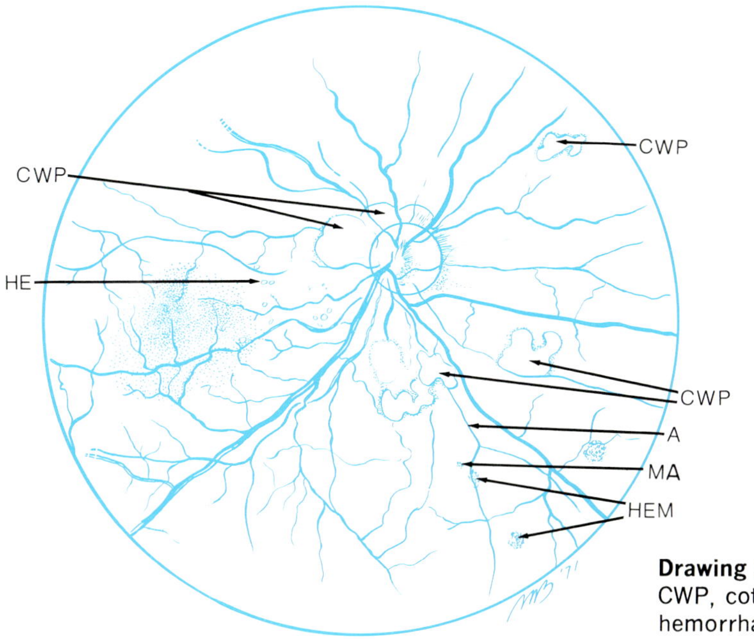

Drawing 226. Plate 226 (A, arteriolar narrowing; CWP, cotton wool patch; HE, hard exudate; HEM, hemorrhage; MA, microaneurysm).

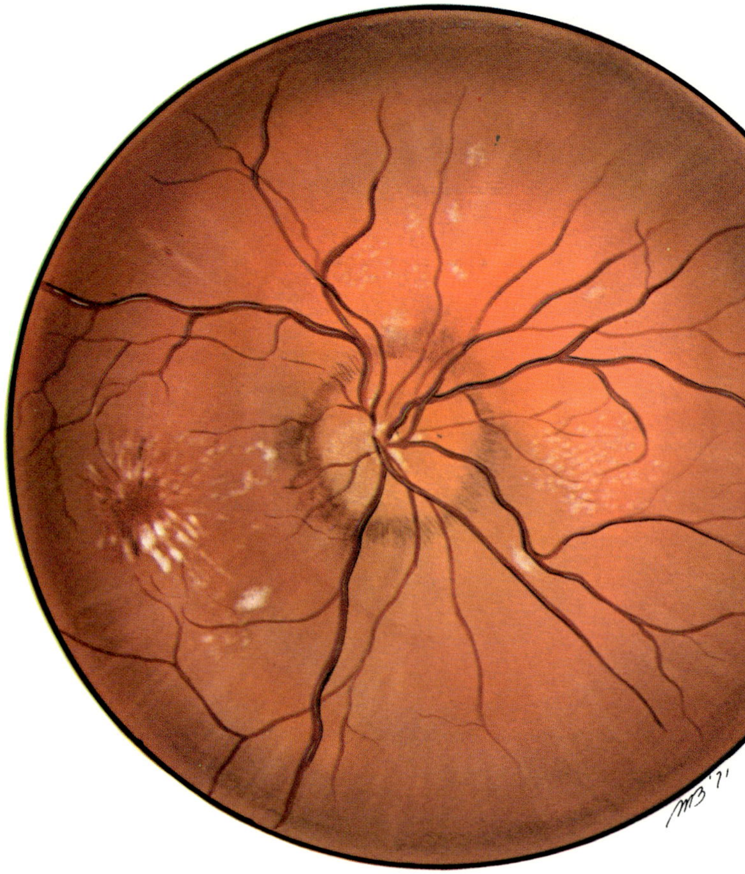

Plate 227 and Drawing 227. O.D. The optic disc is markedly elevated and its indistinct margins are surrounded by a halo. Engorged and slightly tortuous veins dip over the protuberant nerve head. The arterioles are narrow. Arteriovenous displacement is noted inferiorly and temporally, at 7 o'clock, 2 disc diameters below the optic nerve. The inferior temporal arteriole shows parallel sheathing. Arteriovenous compression is present, at the first crossing, at 11 o'clock. Numerous hard exudates are present around almost the entire disc. A macular star is present. Numerous cotton wool patches are also present.

Drawing 227. Plate 227 (O, elevated and edematous optic disc; CWP, cotton wool patch; HE, hard exudate; MS, macular star; ASH, arteriolar sheathing; AV, AV compression).

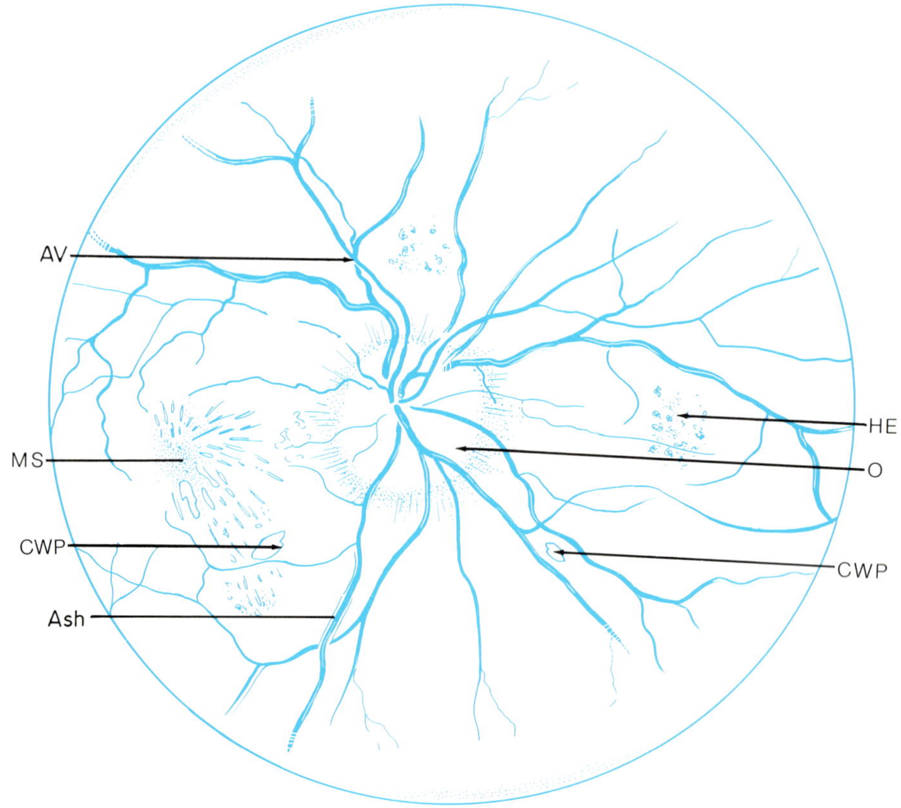

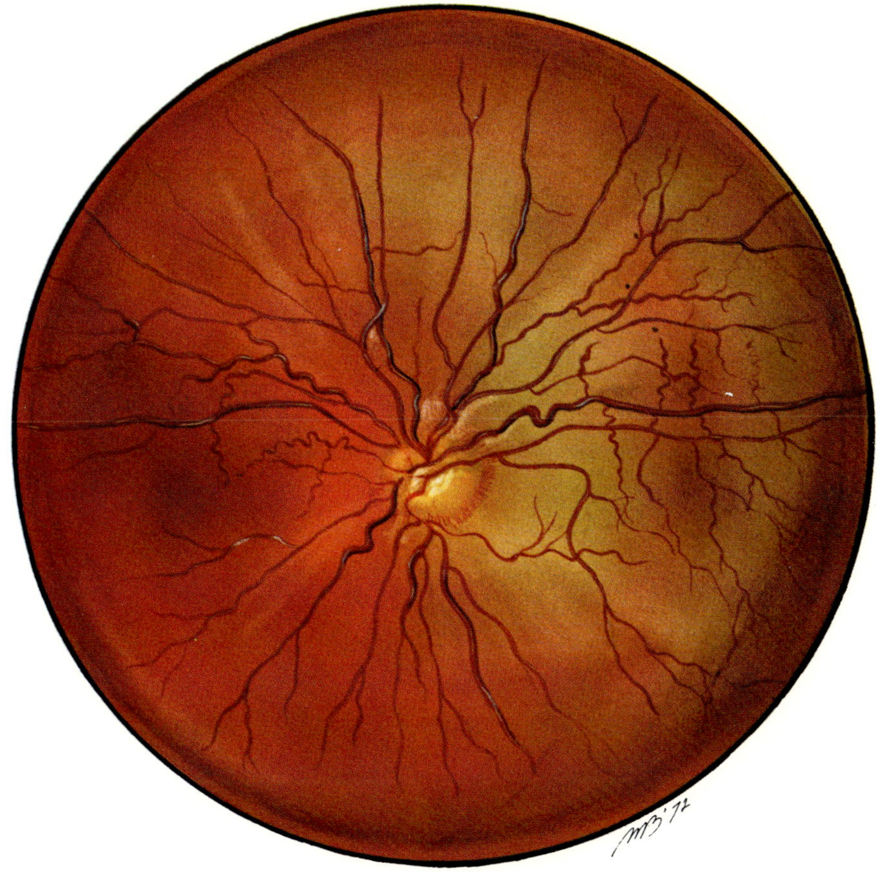

Plate 228 and Drawing 228. O.S. Venular engorgement and tortuosity are marked. Several microaneurysms are observed above the macula.

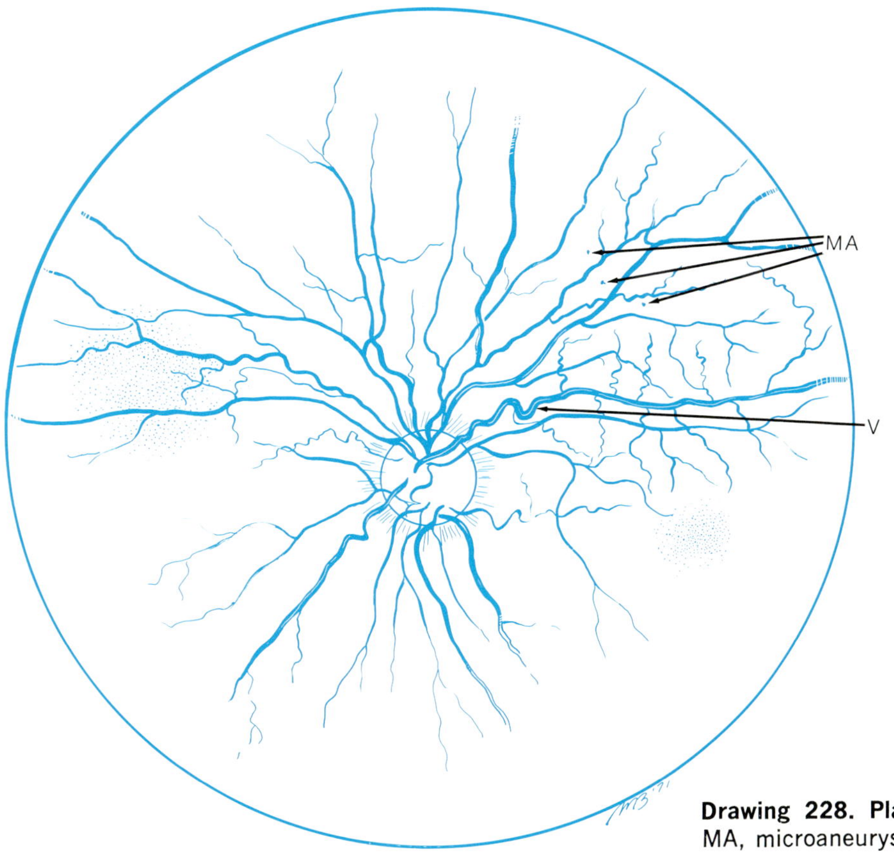

Drawing 228. Plate 228 (V, venular tortuosity; MA, microaneurysm).

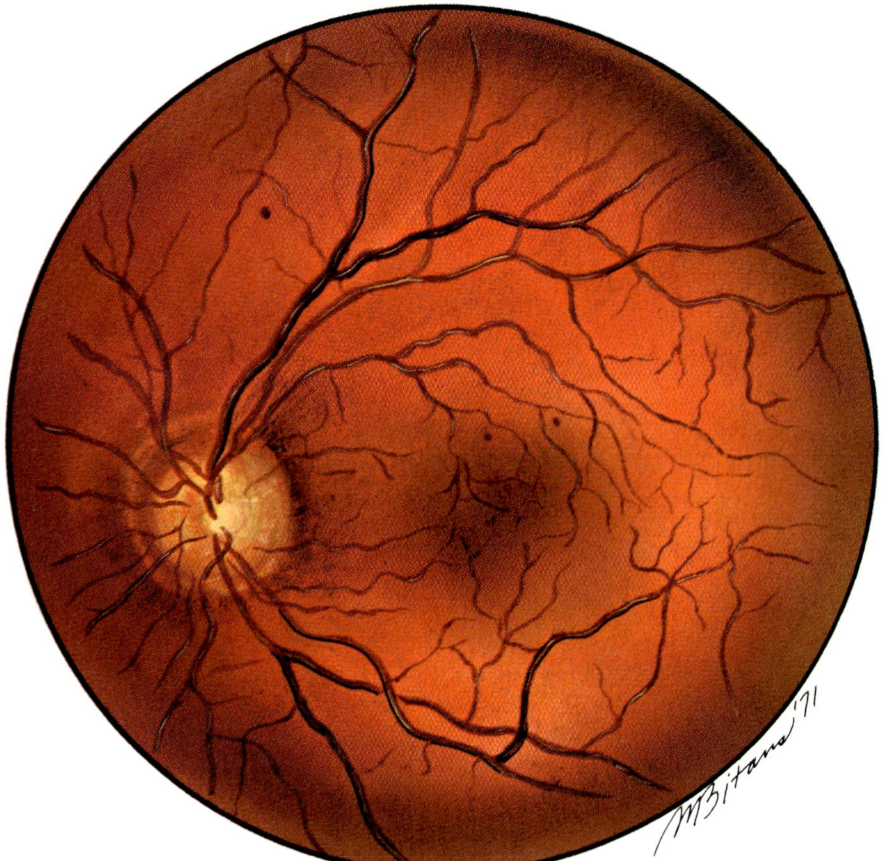

Plate 229 and Drawing 229. O.S. Venular engorgement and slight tortuosity are present. Several microaneurysms are observed in the macular area. A round hemorrhage is present 2 disc diameters above the disc, at 1 o'clock.

Drawing 229. Plate 229 (V, venular tortuosity; HEM, hemorrhage; MA, microaneurysm).

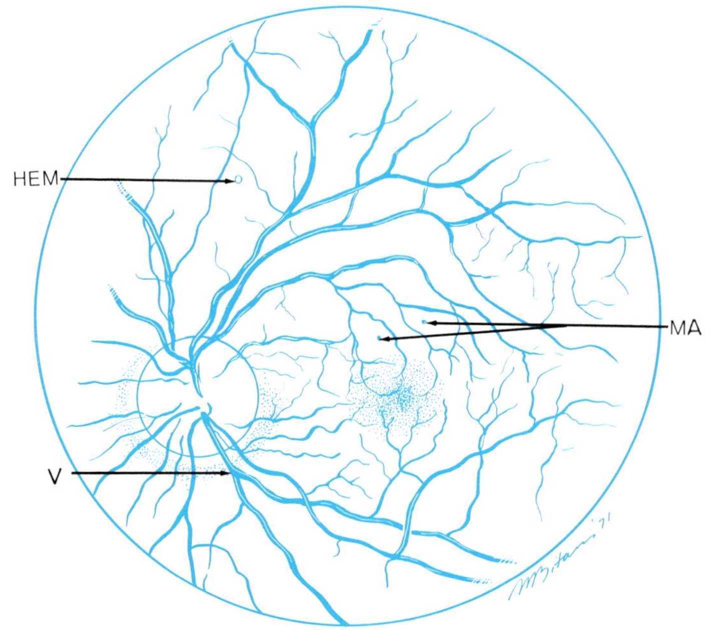

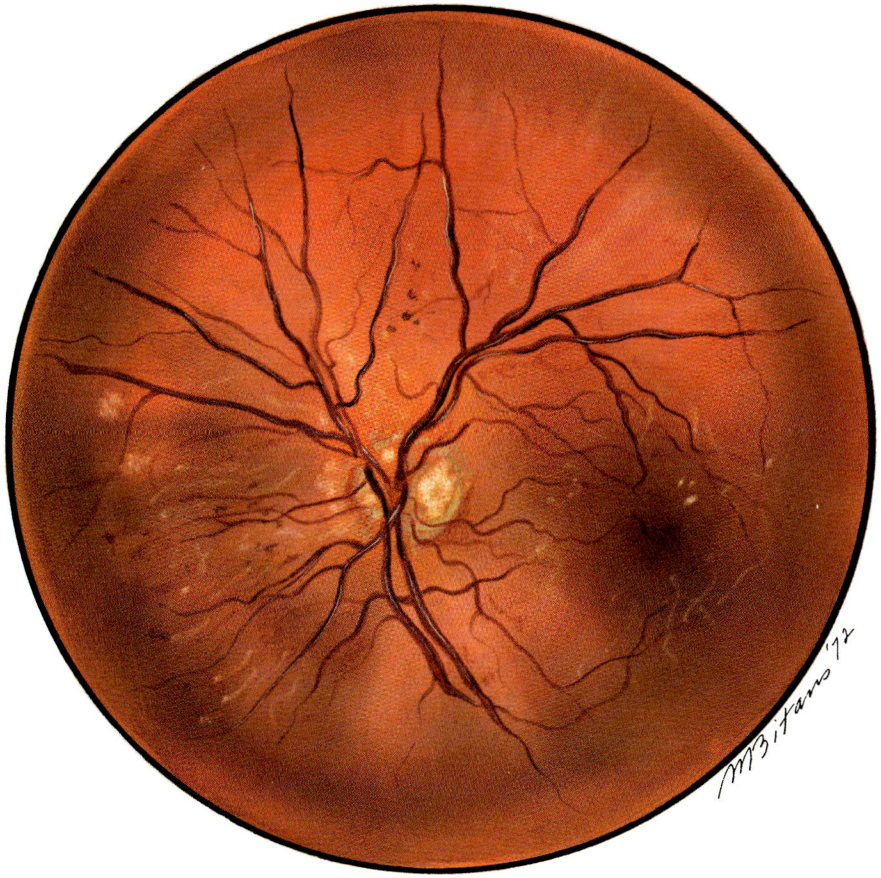

Plate 230 and Drawing 230. O.S. Venular engorgement is present. Parallel sheathing is noted along the superior branch of the superior temporal venule. A cotton wool patch is present at 10 o'clock, 3 disc diameters nasal to the nerve head. Hard exudates are present in the macular and nasal areas. Multiple hemorrhages and microaneurysms are present over the nasal and superior retinal segments.

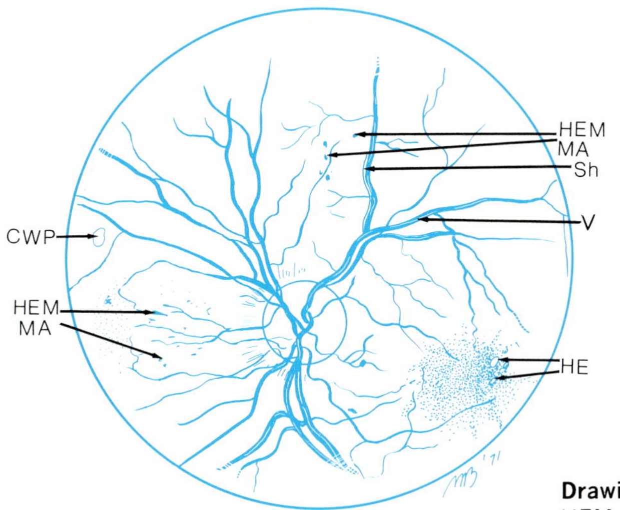

Drawing 230. Plate 230 (V, venular engorgement; HEM, hemorrhage; MA, microaneurysm; CWP, cotton wool patch; HE, hard exudate; SH, sheathing).

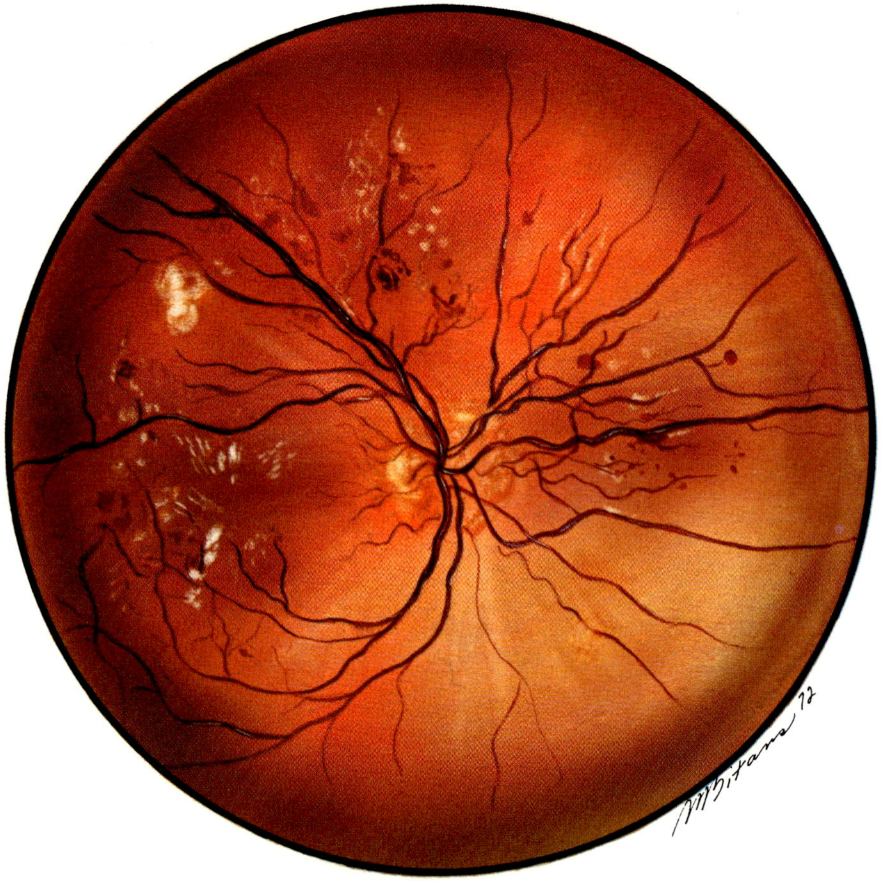

Plate 231 and Drawing 231 O.D. Venular engorgement and slight tortuosity are present. Numerous round and linear hemorrhages are present over the superior, nasal, and temporal portions of the retina. Microaneurysms are observed in the same areas. A cotton wool patch is present at 11 o'clock, 3 disc diameters from the nerve head. Hard exudates are present in the macula and in the superior temporal portion of the retina. Fine, tortuous, small vessels extend from the disc and form irregular networks well out into the nasal portion of the retina. Hemorrhage and microaneurysms are in the immediate vicinity of these areas of neovascularization.

Drawing 231. Plate 231 (V, venous engorgement and tortuosity; NV, neovascularization; HEM, hemorrhage; MA, microaneurysm; CWP, cotton wool patch; HE, hard exudate).

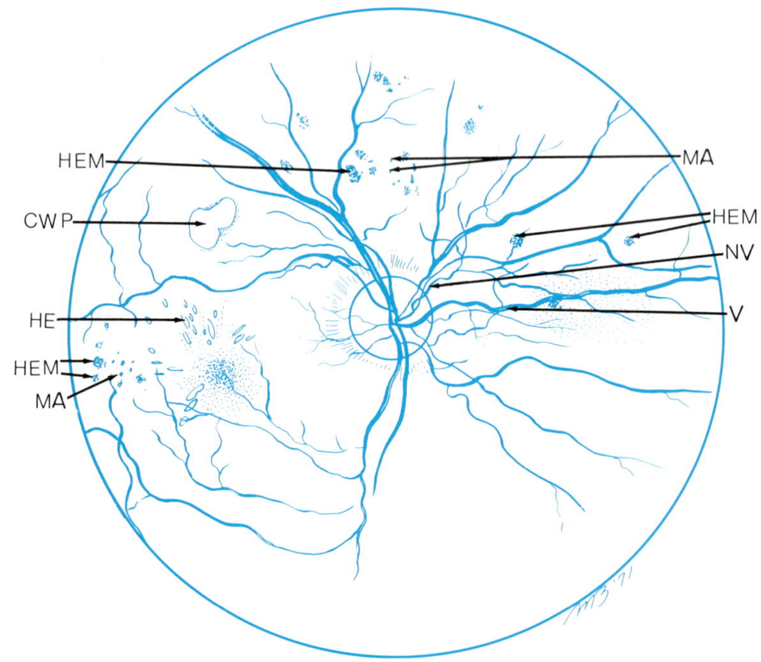

CLASSIFICATION OF RETINOPATHY

ARTERIOLAR DISEASE	VENULAR DISEASE
Hypertension	Diabetes mellitus
a. Essential	Sickle cell disease
b. Renal vascular disease	Polycythemia vera
c. Pheochromocytoma	Multiple myeloma
d. Hyperaldosteronism	Macroglobulinemia
e. Toxemia of pregnancy	Leukemia
f. Coarctation of the aorta	Anemia
Polyarteritis nodosa	a. Iron deficiency
Lupus erythematosus	b. Pernicious anemia
Scleroderma	c. Hereditary spherocytosis
Dermatomyositis	
Retinal vasculitis (Eale's disease)	

The following observations are offered in support of this classification of retinopathy:

1. Many of the changes described in diabetic retinopathy are known to occur in other retinopathies associated with venular disease. For example, extravascular lesions are observed in sickle cell disease, multiple myeloma, macroglobulinemia, leukemia, and in many forms of anemia (see Chapter III). Microaneurysms are found in sickle cell disease, multiple myeloma, and macroglobulinemia (see Chapter V).

2. The alterations associated with the connective tissue diseases are dominantly arteriolar and may, in part, be the result of the associated hypertension. The extravascular lesions are commonly found in the accelerated form of hypertension as well as in such connective tissue diseases as polyarteritis nodosa, scleroderma, lupus erythematosus, and dermatomyositis (see Chapter III). Microaneurysms may be observed in accelerated hypertension and the vasculitis of Eale's disease (see Chapter V).

When the retinal changes include both arteriolar and venular disease, it may be difficult to assess the relative importance of each. That problem frequently arises when hypertension and diabetes mellitus coexist.

Since many systemic and intraocular diseases adversely affect the retina and optic nerve, the ophthalmoscopic examination may serve as an invaluable source of clinical information. Armed with an understanding of the clinical pathological correlation of lesions of those tissues, the clinician may utilize funduscopy in several ways:

1. The ophthalmoscopic findings may provide the initial objective evidence of either systemic or intraocular disease. The discovery of a broad and deep physiologic cup of the optic disc may arouse suspicion of glaucoma. Related to systemic disease, maturity onset diabetes mellitus may be suspected when either retinal venular tortuosity, microaneurysms, or extravascular lesions are discovered before overt abnormalities of carbohydrate tolerance are observed.

2. Funduscopic changes may provide diagnostic clues. For example, subhyaloid hemorrhage and nuchal rigidity, accompanied by a history of sudden onset of headache, suggest a diagnosis of spontaneous subarachnoid hemorrhage associated with a ruptured aneurysm of the circle of Willis. A well–known example is the association of papilledema and the expanding intracranial lesion. Another is the relationship of such systemic granulomatous diseases as tuberculosis, syphilis, histoplasmosis, toxoplasmosis, and sarcoidosis with chorioretinitis.

3. The development of certain retinal abnormalities may serve as an indicator of progression of the underlying systemic disease. This is best exemplified in the hypertensive state when acceleration of the process is heralded by the development of extravascular lesions, often associated with papilledema.

References

1. Wolff, E.: *Anatomy of the Eye and Orbit, Including the Central Connections, Development, and Comparative Anatomy of the Visual Apparatus*, 5th ed., revised by R. J. Last, Saunders, Philadelphia, 1961.
2. Hogan, M. J. and Zimmerman, L. E. (eds.): *Ophthalmic Pathology. An Atlas and Textbook*, 2nd ed., Saunders, Philadelphia, 1962.
3. Cogan, D. G.: *Neurology of the Visual System*, Charles C Thomas, Springfield, Ill., 1966.
4. Ballantyne, A. J. and Michaelson, I. C.: *Textbook of the Fundus of the Eye*, 2nd ed., Williams & Wilkins, Baltimore, 1970.
5. Wolter, J. R.: *The Cells of Remak and the Astroglia of the Normal Human Retina*, Arch. Ophthalmol., **53:** 832, 1955.
6. VanBuren, J. M.: *The Retinal Ganglion Cell Layer*, Charles C Thomas, Springfield, Ill., 1963.
7. Singh, S. and Dass, R.: *The Central Artery of the Retina. Part II, A Study of Its Distribution and Anastomoses*, Br. J. Ophthalmol., **44:** 280, 1960.
8. Francois, J. and Neetens, A.: *Vascularization of the Optic Pathway. Part I, Lamina Cribrosa and Optic Nerve*, Br. J. Ophthalmol., **38:** 472, 1954.
9. Francois, J. and Neetens, A.: *Central Retinal Artery and Central Optic Nerve Artery*, Br. J. Ophthalmol., **47:** 21, 1963.
10. Fry, W. E.: *Variations in the Intraneural Course of the Central Vein of the Retina*, Arch. Ophthalmol., **4:** 180, 1930.
11. Michaelson, I. C.: *Retinal Circulation in Man and Animals*, Charles C Thomas, Springfield, Ill., 1954.
12. Toussaint, D., Kuwabara, T., and Cogan, D.G.: *Retinal Vascular Patterns. Part II, Human Retinal Vessels Studied in Three Dimensions*, Arch. Ophthalmol., **65:** 575, 1961.
13. Kuwabara, T. and Cogan, D. G.: *Studies of Retinal Vascular Patterns. Part I, Normal Architecture*, Arch. Ophthalmol., **64:** 904, 1960.
14. Ashton, N. and de Oliveira, F.: *Nomenclature of Pericytes. Intramural and Extramural*, Br. J. Ophthalmol., **50:** 119, 1966.
15. Bloodworth, J. M. B., Jr.: *Diabetic Retinopathy*, Diabetes, **11:** 1, 1962.
16. Hogan, M. J. and Feeney, L.: *The Ultrastructure of the Retinal Vessels. Part II, The Small Vessels*, J. Ultrastruct. Res., **9:** 29, 1963.
17. Kuwabara, T. and Cogan, D. G.: *Retinal Vascular Patterns. Part VI, Mural Cells of the Retinal Capillaries*, Arch. Ophthalmol., **69:** 492, 1963.
18. Lerman, S.: *Basic Ophthalmology*, pp. 252–263, McGraw-Hill, New York, 1966.
19. Burditt, A. F. and Caird, F. I.: *Natural History of Lens Opacities in Diabetics*, Br. J. Ophthalmol., **52:** 433, 1968.
20. Paton, D. and Duke, J. R.: *Primary Familial Amyloidosis. Ocular Manifestations with Histopathologic Observations*, Am. J. Ophthalmol., **61:** 736, 1966.
21. Bard, L. A.: *Asteroid Hyalitis. Relationship to Diabetes and Hypercholesterolemia*, Am. J. Ophthalmol., **58:** 239, 1964.
22. Smith, J. L.: *Asteroid Hyalitis and Diabetes Mellitus*, Trans. Am. Acad. Ophthalmol. and Otolaryngol., **69:** 269, 1965.
23. Duke-Elder, W. S.: *Normal and Abnormal Development. Part II, Congenital Deformities*, in Duke-Elder, W. S. (ed.): *System of Ophthalmology*, Vol. III, Mosby, St. Louis, 1963.
24. Novotny, H. R. and Alvis, D. L.: *A Method of Photographing Fluorescence in Circulating Blood in the Human Retina*, Circulation, **24:** 82, 1961.
25. Oosterhuis, J. A. and Lammens, A. J. J.: *Fluorescein Photography of the Ocular Fundus*, Ophthalmologica, **149:** 210, 1965.
26. Hodge, J. V. and Clemett, R. S.: *Improved Method for Fluorescence Angiography of the Retina*, Am. J. Ophthalmol., **61:** 1400, 1966.
27. David, N. J., Norton, E. W. D., Gass, J. D., and Beauchamp, J.: *Fluorescein Angiography in Central Retinal Artery Occlusion*, Arch. Ophthalmol., **77:** 619, 1967.
28. Wolter, J. R. and Liddicoat, D. A.: *Secondary Glaucoma Following Occlusion of the Central Artery of the Retina*, Am. J. Ophthalmol., **46:** 182, 1958.
29. Fisher, C. M.: *Observations of the Fundus Oculi in Transient Monocular Blindness*, Neurology, **9:** 333, 1959.
30. Hollenhorst, R. W.: *Significance of Bright Plaques in the Retinal Arterioles*, JAMA, **178:** 23, 1961.
31. Ashby, M., Oakley, N., Lorentz, I., and Scott, D.: *Recurrent Transient Monocular Blindness*, Br. Med. J., **2:** 894, 1963.
32. Russell, R. W. R.: *Atheromatous Retinal Embolism*, Lancet, **2:** 1354, 1963.
33. Marshall, J. and Meadows, S.: *The Natural History of Amaurosis Fugax*, Brain, **91:** 419, 1968.
34. Swash, M. and Earl, C. J.: *Transient Visual Obscurations in Chronic Rheumatic Heart-Disease*, Lancet, **2:** 232, 1970.
35. Dahrling, B. E.: *The Histopathology of Early Central Retinal Artery Occlusion*,

Arch. Ophthalmol., **73:** 506, 1965.
36. Kroll, A. J.: *Experimental Central Retinal Artery Occlusion,* Arch. Ophthalmol., **79:** 453, 1968.
37. Gunning, A. J., Pickering, G. W., Robb-Smith, A. H. T., and Russell, R. R.: *Mural Thrombosis of the Internal Carotid Artery and Subsequent Embolism,* Q. J. Med., **33:** 155, 1964.
38. Haney, W. P. and Preston, R. E.: *Ocular Complications of Carotid Arteriography in Carotid Occlusive Disease. A Report of Three Cases,* Arch. Ophthalmol., **67:** 127, 1962.
39. McBrien, D. J., Bradley, R. D., and Ashton, N.: *The Nature of Retinal Emboli in Stenosis of the Internal Carotid Artery,* Lancet, **1:** 697, 1963.
40. David, N. J., Klintworth, G. K., Friedberg, S. J., and Dillon, M.: *Fatal Atheromatous Cerebral Embolism Associated with Bright Plaques in the Retinal Arterioles. A Report of a Case,* Neurology, **13:** 708, 1963.
41. Cogan, D. G., Kuwabara, T., and Moser, H.: *Fat Emboli in the Retina Following Angiography,* Arch. Ophthalmol., **71:** 308, 1964.
42. Zimmerman, L. E.: *Embolism of Central Retinal Artery, Secondary to Myocardial Infarction with Mural Thrombosis,* Arch. Ophthalmol., **73:** 822, 1965.
43. Manschot, W. A.: *Embolism of the Central Retinal Artery, Originating from an Endocardial Myxoma,* Am. J. Ophthalmol., **48:** 381, 1959.
44. Holley, K. E., Bahn, R. C., McGoon, D. C., and Mankin, H. T.: *Spontaneous Calcific Embolization Associated with Calcific Aortic Stenosis,* Circulation, **27:** 197, 1963.
45. Holley, K. E., Bahn, R. C., McGoon, D. C., and Mankin, H. T.: *Calcific Embolization Associated with Valvotomy for Calcific Aortic Stenosis,* Circulation, **28:** 175, 1963.
46. Penner, R. and Font, F. L.: *Retinal Embolism from Calcified Vegetations of Aortic Valve. Spontaneous Complication of Rheumatic Heart Disease,* Arch. Ophthalmol., **81:** 565, 1969.
47. Cooke, W. T., Cloake, P. C. P., Govan, A. D. T., and Colbeck, J. C.: *Temporal Arteritis. A Generalized Vascular Disease,* Q. J. Med., **15:** 47, 1946.
48. Manschot, W. A.: *A Fatal Case of Temporal Arteritis with Ocular Symptoms,* Ophthalmologica, **149:** 121, 1965.
49. Evans, H.: *Periarteritis Nodosa with Marked Eosinophilia,* Proc. R. Soc. Med., **37:** 40, 1943.
50. Font, R. L. and Naumann, G.: *Ocular Histopathology in Pulseless Disease,* Arch. Ophthalmol., **82:** 784, 1969.
51. Walsh, F. B., Clark, D. B., Thompson, R. S., and Nicholson, D. H.: *Oral Contraceptives and Neuro-Ophthalmologic Interest,* Arch. Ophthalmol., **74:** 628, 1965.
52. Irey, N. S., Manion, W. C., and Taylor, H. B.: *Vascular Lesions in Women Taking Oral Contraceptives,* Arch. Pathol., **89:** 1, 1970.
53. Ellis, C. J., Hamer, D. B., Hunt, R. W., Lever, A. F., Lever, R. S., Peart, W. S., and Walker, S. M.: *Medical Investigation of Retinal Vascular Occlusion,* Br. Med. J., **2:** 1093, 1964.
54. Baghdassarian, S. A., Crawford, J. B., and Rathbun, J. E., Jr: *Calcific Emboli of the Retinal and Ciliary Arteries,* Am. J. Ophthalmol., **69:** 372, 1970.
55. Fritz, M. H. and Hogan, M. J.: *Fat Embolization Involving the Human Eye,* Am. J. Ophthalmol., **31:** 527, 1948.
56. Kearns, T. P.: *Fat Embolism of the Retina, Demonstrated by a Flat Retinal Preparation,* Am. J. Ophthalmol., **41:** 1, 1956.
57. Cullen, J. F.: *Occlusion of the Central Retinal Artery Following a Closed Head Injury,* Am. J. Ophthalmol., **57:** 670, 1964.
58. Jennings, G. H.: *Arteritis of the Temporal Vessels,* Lancet, **1:** 424, 1938.
59. Johnson, R. H., Harley, R. D., and Horton, B. T.: *Arteritis of the Temporal Vessels Associated with Loss of Vision,* Am. J. Ophthalmol., **26:** 147, 1943.
60. Wagener, H. P.: *Temporal Arteritis and Loss of Vision,* Am. J. Med. Sci., **212:** 225, 1946.
61. Crosby, R. C. and Wadsworth, R. C.: *Temporal Arteritis. Review of the Literature and Report of Five Additional Cases,* Arch. Intern. Med., **81:** 431, 1948.
62. Bruce, G. M.: *Temporal Arteritis as a Cause of Blindness. Review of Literature and Report of a Case,* Trans. Am. Ophthalmol. Soc., **47:** 300, 1949.
63. Smith, C. and Greene, P. B.: *Ocular Complications of Temporal Arteritis,* Am. J. Ophthalmol., **32:** 685, 1949.
64. Parsons-Smith, G.: *Ophthalmic Manifestations of Temporal Arteritis,* Br. J. Ophthalmol., **36:** 615, 1952.
65. Parsons-Smith, G.: *Sudden Blindness in Cranial Arteritis,* Br. J. Ophthalmol., **43:** 204, 1959.
66. Simmons, R. J. and Cogan, D. G.: *Occult Temporal Arteritis,* Arch. Ophthalmol., **68,** 8, 1962.
67. Miller, G. R. and Smith, J. L.: *Ischemic Optic Neuropathy,* Am. J. Ophthalmol., **62:** 103, 1966.
68. Henkind, P., Charles, N. C., and Pear-

son, J.: *Histopathology of Ischemic Optic Neuropathy,* Am. J. Ophthalmol., **69:** 78, 1970.

69. Birkhead, N. C., Wagener, H. P., and Shick, R. M.: *Treatment of Temporal Arteritis with Adrenal Corticosteroids. Results in Fifty-Five Cases in Which Lesion Was Proved at Biopsy,* JAMA, **163:** 821, 1957.
70. Ostler, H. B.: *Pulseless Disease (Takayasu's Disease),* Am. J. Ophthalmol., **43:** 583, 1957.
71. Shimizu, K. and Sano, K.: *Pulseless Disease,* J. Neuropathol. and Clin. Neurol., **1:** 37, 1951.
72. Hedges, T. R.: *The Aortic Arch Syndromes,* Arch. Ophthalmol., **71:** 28, 1964.
73. Dowling, J. A. and Smith, T. R.: *An Ocular Study of Pulseless Disease,* Arch. Ophthalmol., **64:** 236, 1960.
74. Tour, R. L. and Hoyt, W. F.: *The Syndrome of the Aortic Arch. Ocular Manifestations of "Pulseless Disease" and a Report of a Surgically Treated Case,* Am. J. Ophthalmol., **47** (5, pt. 2): 35, 1959.
75. Shimizu, K.: *Takayasu's Disease. A Fluorescein Angiographic Study,* Jap. J. Ophthalmol., **11:** 23, 1967.
76. Welch, R. B. and Goldberg, M. F.: *Sickle-Cell Hemoglobin and Its Relation to Fundus Abnormality,* Arch. Ophthalmol., **75:** 353, 1966.
77. Kabakow, B., Van Weimokly, S. S., and Lyons, H. A.: *Bilateral Central Retinal Artery Occlusion. Occurrence in a Patient with Cortisone-Treated Systemic Lupus Erythematosus, Sickle Cell Trait, and Active Pulmonary Tuberculosis,* Arch. Ophthalmol., **54:** 670, 1955.
78. Ellis, R. A.: *Central Retinal Artery Occlusion Associated with Cryoglobulinemia* Arch. Ophthalmol., **57:** 327, 1957.
79. Salmon, M. L., Winkelman, J. Z., and Gay, A. J.: *Neuro-Ophthalmic Sequelae in Users of Oral Contraceptives,* JAMA, **206:** 85, 1968.
80. Masi, A. T. and Dugdale, M.: *Cerebrovascular Diseases Associated with the Use of Oral Contraceptives. A Review of the English-Language Literature,* Ann. Intern. Med., **72:** 111, 1970.
81. Leishman, R.: *The Eye in General Vascular Disease. Hypertension and Arteriosclerosis,* Br. J. Ophthalmol., **41:** 641, 1957.
82. Wagener, H. P. and Keith, N. M.: *Diffuse Arteriolar Disease with Hypertension and the Associated Retinal Lesions,* Medicine, **18:** 317, 1939.
83. Scheie, H. G.: *Evaluation of Ophthalmoscopic Changes of Hypertension and Arteriolar Sclerosis,* Arch. Ophthalmol., **49:** 117, 1953.
84. Cohen, M.: *Ophthalmoscopic Changes Associated with Hypertensive Vascular Disease as a Guide to Sympathectomy,* Arch. Ophthalmol., **37:** 491, 1947.
85. Duke-Elder, W. S. and Dobree, J. H.: *Diseases of the Retina,* in Duke-Elder, W. S. (ed.): *System of Ophthalmology,* Vol. X, Mosby, St. Louis, 1967.
86. Sieker, H. O. and Hickam, J. B.: *Normal and Impaired Retinal Vascular Reactivity,* Circulation, **7:** 79, 1953.
87. Lockhart, G., van Noorden, G., Duston, H. P., Corcoran, A. C., and Page, I. H.: *The Course of Retinopathy in Treated Malignant Hypertension,* Arch. Intern. Med., **106:** 205, 1960.
88. Kirkendall, W. M. and Armstrong, M. L.: *Effect of Blood Pressure Reduction on Vascular Changes in the Eye,* in Moyer, J. H. (ed.): *Hypertension. The First Hahnemann Symposium on Hypertensive Disease,* p. 472, Saunders, Philadelphia, 1959.
89. Ellis, P. P. and Fonken, H. A.: *Retinopathies of Chronic Glomerulonephritis. A Study of Cases Treated with Renal Transplantation,* Arch. Ophthalmol., **75:** 36, 1966.
90. Stokoe, N. L. and Turner, R. W. D.: *Normal Retinal Vascular Patterns. Arteriovenous Ratio as a Measure of Arterial Calibre,* Br. J. Ophthalmol., **50:** 21, 1966.
91. Friedenwald, H.: *Pathological Changes in the Retinal Blood-Vessels in Arteriosclerosis and Hypertension,* the Doyne Memorial Lecture, Trans. Ophthalmol. Soc. U. K., **50:** 452, 1930.
92. Friedenwald, J. S.: *Disease Processes Versus Disease Pictures in Interpretation of Retinal Vascular Lesions,* Arch. Ophthalmol., **37:** 403, 1947.
93. Seitz, R.: *The Retinal Vessels. Comparative Ophthalmoscopic and Histologic Studies on Healthy and Diseased Eyes,* translated by F. C. Blodi, Mosby, St. Louis, 1964.
94. Keyes, J. E. L. and Goldblatt, H.: *Experimental Hypertension. Part VIII, Vascular Changes in the Eyes,* Arch. Ophthalmol., **20:** 812, 1938.
95. Marshall, R. A.: *A Review of Lesions in the Optic Fundus in Various Diseases of the Blood,* Blood, **14:** 882, 1959.
96. Loewenstein, A., Michaelson, I. C., and Hill, J.: *Retinal Vasculitis of the Young. A Pathological Report,* Trans. Ophthalmol. Soc. U. K., **66:** 211, 1946.
97. King, E. F.: *Ocular Involvement in a Case of Periarteritis Nodosa,* Trans. Ophthalmol. Soc. U. K., **55:** 246, 1935.

98. Wolter, J. R. and Liss, L.: *The Evoluation of Hyaline Corpuscles (Cytoid Bodies) in the Human Optic Nerve,* Am. J. Ophthalmol., **43:** 885, 1957.
99. Wolter, J. R.: *Pathology of a Cotton-Wool Spot,* Am. J. Ophthalmol., **48:** 473, 1959.
100. Friedenwald, J. S.: *A New Approach to Some Problems of Retinal Vascular Disease,* the Jackson Memorial Lecture, Am. J. Ophthalmol., **32:** 487, 1949.
101. Ashton, N.: *Hypertensive Retinopathy,* Lancet, **1:** 866, 1963.
102. Klien, B. A.: *Comments on the Cotton-Wool Lesion of the Retina,* Am. J. Ophthalmol., **59:** 17, 1965.
103. Banker, B. Q., Victor, M., and Chester, E. M.: *Hypertensive Encephalopathy and Retinopathy,* in preparation.
104. Chester, E. M. and Banker, B. Q.: *The Role of Lipid Thrombi in the Pathogenesis of Diabetic Retinopathy,* Arch. Intern. Med., **120:** 397, 1967.
105. Ashton, N. and Henkind, P.: *Experimental Occlusion of Retinal Arterioles (Using Graded Glass Ballotini),* Br. J. Ophthalmol., **49:** 225, 1965.
106. Dollery, C. T., Henkind, P., Patterson, J. W., Ramolho, P. S., and Hill, D. W.: *Focal Retinal Ischaemia. Part I, Ophthalmoscopic and Circulatory Changes in Focal Retinal Ischaemia,* Br. J. Ophthalmol., **50:** 285, 1966.
107. Shakib, M. and Ashton, N.: *Focal Retinal Ischaemia. Part II, Ultrastructural Changes in Focal Retinal Ischaemia,* Br. J. Ophthalmol., **50:** 325, 1966.
108. Margolis, G. and Brown, I. W.: *Hyperbaric Oxygenation. The Eyes as a Limiting Factor,* Science, **151:** 466, 1966.
109. Ashton, N., Pears, M. A., and Pickering, G. W.: *Neuroretinopathy Following Haemorrhage, with a Discussion on the Nature of Cytoid Bodies,* Br. J. Ophthalmol., **45:** 385, 1961.
110. Saltzman, H. A., Hart, L., Sieker, H. O., and Duffy, E. J.: *Retinal Vascular Response to Hyperbaric Oxygenation,* JAMA, **191:** 290, 1965.
111. Toussaint, D., Cogan, D. G., and Kuwabara, T.: *Extravascular Lesions of Diabetic Retinopathy,* Arch. Ophthalmol., **67:** 42, 1962.
112. Kohner, E. M., Dollery, C. T., and Bulpitt, C. J.: *Cotton-Wool Spots in Diabetic Retinopathy,* Diabetes, **18:** 691, 1969.
113. Baehr, G., Klemperer, P., and Schifrin, A.: *A Diffuse Disease of the Peripheral Circulation (Usually Associated with Lupus Erythematosus and Endocarditis),* Trans. Assoc. Am. Physicians, **50:** 139, 1935.
114. Maumenee, A. E.: *Retinal Lesions in Lupus Erythematosus,* Am. J. Ophthalmol., **23:** 971, 1940.
115. Herson, R. N. and Sampson, R.: *Ocular Manifestations of Polyarteritis Nodosa,* Q. J. Med., **18:** 123, 1949.
116. Bruce, G. M.: *Retinitis in Dermatomyositis,* Trans. Am. Ophthalmol. Soc., **36:** 282, 1938.
117. Liebman, S. and Cook, C.: *Retinopathy with Dermatomyositis,* Arch. Ophthalmol., **74:** 704, 1965.
118. Pollack, I. P. and Becker, B.: *Cytoid Bodies of the Retina, in a Patient with Scleroderma,* Am. J. Ophthalmol., **54:** 655, 1962.
119. Allen, R. A. and Straatsma, B. R.: *Ocular Involvement in Leukemia and Allied Disorders,* Arch. Ophthalmol., **66:** 490, 1961.
120. Schwab, P. J., Okun, E., and Fahey, J. L.: *Reversal of Retinopathy in Waldenstrom's Macroglobulinemia by Plasmapheresis. A Report of Two Cases,* Arch. Ophthalmol., **64:** 515, 1960.
121. Coyle, J. T., Frank, P. E., Leonard, A. L., and Weiner, A.: *Macroglobulinemia and Its Effect upon the Eye,* Arch. Ophthalmol., **65:** 75, 1961.
122. Henry, M. D. and Chapman, A. Z.: *Vitreous Hemorrhage and Retinopathy Associated with Sickle-Cell Disease,* Am. J. Ophthalmol., **38:** 204, 1954.
123. Holt, J. M. and Gordon-Smith, E. C.: *Retinal Abnormalities in Diseases of the Blood,* Br. J. Ophthalmol., **53:** 145, 1969.
124. Hollenhorst, R. W.: *Ocular Manifestations of Insufficiency or Thrombosis of the Internal Carotid Artery,* Am. J. Ophthalmol., **47:** 753, 1959.
125. Hollenhorst, R. W.: *The Ocular Manifestations of Internal Carotid Arterial Thrombosis,* Med. Clin. North Am., **44:** 897, 1960.
126. Hodge, J. V. and Dollery, C. T.: *Retinal Soft Exudates. A Clinical Study by Colour and Fluorescence Photography,* Q. J. Med., **33:** 117, 1964.
127. Gass, J. D. M.: *A Fluorescein Angiographic Study of Macular Dysfunction Secondary to Retinal Vascular Disease. Part III, Hypertensive Retinopathy,* Arch. Ophthalmol., **80:** 569, 1968.
128. Cohen, M.: *Chorioretinal Arteriolar Necrosis in Malignant Hypertension,* Arch. Ophthalmol., **23:** 1052, 1940.
129. Friedman, E., Smith, T. R., Kuwabara, T., and Beyer, C. K.: *Choroidal Vascular Patterns in Hypertension,* Arch. Ophthalmol., **71:** 842, 1964.
130. Goldsmith, J.: *Periarteritis Nodosa with Involvement of the Choroidal and Retinal Arteries,* Am. J. Ophthalmol., **29:** 435, 1946.
131. Manschot, W. A.: *Generalized Scleroderma with Ocular Symptoms,* Ophthal-

mologica, **149:** 131, 1965.
132. Rubenstein, R. A., Yanoff, M., and Albert, D. M.: *Thrombocytopenia, Anemia, and Retinal Hemorrhage,* Am. J. Ophthalmol., **65:** 435, 1968.
133. Dollery, C. T. and Oakley, N. M.: *Reversal of Retinal Vascular Changes in Diabetes,* Diabetes, **14:** 121, 1965.
134. King, R. C., Dobree, J. H., Kok, D. A., Foulds, W. S., and Dangerfield, W. G.: *Exudative Diabetic Retinopathy. Spontaneous Changes and Effects of a Corn Oil Diet,* Br. J. Ophthalmol., **47:** 666, 1963.
135. Van Eck, W. F.: *The Effect of Low Fat Diet on the Serum Lipids in Diabetes and Its Significance in Diabetic Retinopathy,* Am. J. Med., **27:** 196, 1959.
136. Duncan, L. J. P., Cullen, J. F., Ireland, J. T., Nolan, J., Clarke, B. F., and Oliver, M. F.: *A Three-Year Trial of Atromid Therapy in Exudative Diabetic Retinopathy,* Diabetes, **17:** 458, 1968.
137. Farkas, T. G., Sylvester, V., Archer, D., and Altona, M.: *The Histochemistry of Drusen,* Am. J. Ophthalmol., **71:** 1206, 1971.
138. Farkas, T. G., Sylvester, V., and Archer, D.: *The Ultrastructure of Drusen,* Am. J. Ophthalmol., **71:** 1196, 1971.
139. Deutman, A. F. and Jansen, L. M. A. A.: *Dominantly Inherited Drusen of Bruch's Membrane,* Br. J. Ophthalmol., **54:** 373, 1970.
140. Goodman, R. M., Smith, E. W., Paton, D., Bergman, R. A., Siegel, C. L., Otteson, O. E., Shelley, W. M., Pusch, A. L., and McKusick, V. A.: *Pseudoxanthoma Elasticum. A Clinical and Histopathological Study,* Medicine, **42:** 297, 1963.
141. Winter, F. C.: *The Lens and Vitreous,* Arch. Ophthalmol., **78:** 229, 1967.
142. Regnault, F. R.: *Vitreous Hemorrhage: An Experimental Study. Part I, A Macroscopic and Isotopic Study of the Evolution of Whole Blood and Hemoglobin,* Arch. Ophthalmol., **83:** 458, 1970.
143. Duke-Elder, W. S.: *Diseases of the Lens and Vitreous. Glaucoma and Hypotony,* in Duke-Elder, W. S. (ed.): *System of Ophthalmology,* Vol. XI, p. 365, Mosby, St. Louis, 1969.
144. Kennedy, J. E. and Wise, G. N.: *Clinicopathological Correlation of Retinal Lesions. Subacute Bacterial Endocarditis,* Arch. Ophthalmol., **74:** 658, 1965.
145. Tarkanian, M. A., Mills, P., and Chester, E. M.: The Roth Spot. Clinical Pathological Correlation (personal observation).
146. Doherty, W. B. and Trubek, M.: *Significant Hemorrhagic Retinal Lesions in Bacterial Endocarditis (Roth's Spots),* JAMA, **97:** 308, 1931.
147. Wong, V. G. and Bodey, G. P.: *Hemorrhagic Retinoschisis Due to Aplastic Anemia,* Arch. Ophthalmol., **80:** 433, 1968.
148. Merin, S. and Freund, M.: *Retinopathy in Severe Anemia,* Am. J. Ophthalmol., **66:** 1102, 1963.
149. Williams, D. K. and Rentiers, P. K.: *Spontaneous Expulsive Choroidal Hemorrhage. A Clinicopathologic Report of Two Cases,* Arch. Ophthalmol., **83:** 191, 1970.
150. Klien, B. A.: *Sidelights on Retinal Venous Occlusion,* Am. J. Ophthalmol., **61:** 25, 1966.
151. Ballantyne, A. J. and Michaelson, I. C. III: *Retina and Optic Nerve. Some Aspects of Disease Affecting the Retinal Veins,* Trans. Ophthalmol. Soc. U. K., **67:** 59, 1947.
152. Becker, B. and Post, L. T., Jr.: *Retinal Vein Occlusion. Clinical and Experimental Observations,* Am. J. Ophthalmol., **34:** 677, 1951.
153. Verhoeff, F. H.: *Obstruction of the Central Retinal Vein,* Arch. Ophthalmol., **36:** 1, 1907.
154. Spalter, H. F.: *Abnormal Serum Proteins and Retinal Vein Thrombosis,* Arch. Ophthalmol., **62:** 868, 1959.
155. Paton, A., Rubinstein, K., and Smith, V. H.: *Arterial Insufficiency in Retinal Venous Occlusion,* Trans. Ophthalmol. Soc. U. K., **84:** 559, 1964.
156. Kearns, T. P. and Hollenhorst, R. W.: *Venous-Stasis Retinopathy of Occlusive Disease of the Carotid Artery,* Proc. Mayo Clin., **38:** 304, 1963.
157. Hayreh, S. S.: *An Experimental Study of the Central Retinal Vein Occlusion* (in Discussion of Reference #155), Trans. Ophthalmol. Soc. U. K., **84:** 586, 1964.
158. Wunsh, S. and Leopold, I. H.: *Ocular Manifestations of Ischemic Disease,* in Sherry, S., Brinkhous, K. M., Genton, E., and Stengle, J. M. (eds.): *Conference on Thrombosis,* Washington, D. C., 1967, pp. 166–169, National Academy of Sciences, 1969.
159. Gass, J. D. M.: *A Fluorescein Angiographic Study of Macular Dysfunction Secondary to Retinal Vascular Disease. Part II, Retinal Vein Obstruction,* Arch. Ophthalmol., **80:** 550, 1968.
160. Hauswirth, L. and Eisenberg, A. A.: *Disseminated Venofibrosis (Phlebosclerosis). Its Clinicopathologic Significance,* Arch. Pathol., **11:** 857, 1931.
161. Agatson, S. A.: *Clinicopathologic Study of Diabetic Retinitis,* Arch. Ophthalmol., **24:** 252, 1940.
162. O'Brien, C. S. and Allen, J. H.: *Unusual Changes in the Retinal Veins in Diabetes,* Arch. Ophthalmol., **24:** 742, 1940.

163. Ballantyne, A. J. and Loewenstein, A.: *The Pathology of Diabetic Retinopathy,* Trans. Ophthalmol. Soc. U. K., **63:** 95, 1943.
164. Wolter, J. R.: *Diabetic Retinopathy,* Am. J. Ophthalmol., **51:** 1123, 1961.
165. Ballantyne, A. J.: *The State of the Retina in Diabetes Mellitus,* Trans. Ophthalmol. Soc. U. K., **66:** 503, 1946.
166. Lundbaek, K.: *Long-Term Diabetes,* p. 118, Munksgaard, Copenhagen; and Lange, Maxwell and Springer Ltd., London and New York, 1953.
167. Burditt, A. F., Caird, F. I., and Draper, G. J.: *The Natural History of Diabetic Retinopathy,* Q. J. Med., **37:** 303, 1968.
168. Kornerup, T.: *Retinopathia Diabetica Proliferans,* Acta Ophthalmol., **36:** 87, 1958.
169. Larsen, H. W.: *Diabetic Retinopathy. An Ophthalmoscopic Study with a Discussion of the Morphologic Changes and the Pathogenetic Factors in This Disease,* Acta Ophthalmol., Suppl.: 60, 1960.
170. Joplin, G. F., Oakley, N. W., Hill, D. W., Kohner, E. M., and Fraser, T. R.: *Diabetic Retinopathy. Part II, Comparison of Disease Remission Induced by Various Degrees of Pituitary Ablation by* Y^{90}, Diabetalogia, **3:** 406, 1967.
171. Ashton, N., Kok, D. A., and Foulds, W. S.: *Ocular Pathology in Macroglobulinaemia,* J. Pathol. Bacteriol., **86:** 453, 1963.
172. Ashton, N.: *Ocular Changes in Multiple Myelomatosis,* Arch. Ophthalmol., **73:** 487, 1965.
173. Sanders, T. E., Podos, S. M., and Rosenbaum, L. J.: *Intraocular Manifestations of Multiple Myeloma,* Arch. Ophthalmol., **77:** 789, 1967.
174. Dollery, C. T., Hodge, J. V., and Engel, M.: *Studies of the Retinal Circulation with Fluorescein,* Br. Med. J., **2:** 1210, 1962.
175. Friedenwald, J. S.: *Diabetic Retinopathy,* Am. J. Ophthalmol., **33:** 1187, 1950.
176. Wagener, H. P.: *Retinal Microaneurysms,* Am. J. Med. Sci., **225:** 205, 1953.
177. Cogan, D. G., Toussaint, D., and Kuwabara, T.: *Retinal Vascular Patterns. Part IV, Diabetic Retinopathy,* Arch. Ophthalmol., **66:** 366, 1961.
178. Yamashita, T. and Rosen, D. A.: *Electron-Microscopic Study of Diabetic Capillary Aneurysm,* Arch. Ophthalmol., **67:** 785, 1962.
179. Bloodworth, J. M. B., Jr.: *Diabetic Microangiopathy,* Diabetes, **12:** 99, 1963.
180. Toussaint, D. and Dustin, P.: *Electron Microscopy of Normal and Diabetic Capillaries,* Arch. Ophthalmol., **70:** 96, 1963.
181. Zacks, S. I., Pegues, J. J., and Elliott, F. A.: *Interstitial Muscle Capillaries in Patients with Diabetes Mellitus. A Light and Electron Microscope Study,* Metabolism, **11:** 381, 1962.
182. Siperstein, M. D., Norton, W., Unger, R. H., and Madison, L. L.: *Muscle Capillary Basement Membrane Width in Normal, Diabetic and Prediabetic Patients,* Trans. Assoc. Am. Physicians, **79:** 330, 1966.
183. Banson, B. B. and Lacey, P. E.: *Diabetic Microangiopathy in Human Toes, with an Emphasis on the Ultrastructural Change in Dermal Capillaries,* Am. J. Pathol., **45:** 41, 1964.
184. Ashton, N.: *Vascular Changes in Diabetes with Particular Reference to the Retinal Vessels,* Br. J. Ophthalmol., **33:** 407, 1949.
185. McCulloch, C. and Pashby, T. J.: *The Significance of Conjunctival Aneurysms in Diabetics,* Br. J. Ophthalmol., **34:** 495, 1950.
186. Funahashi, T. and Fink, A. I.: *The Pathology of the Bulbar Conjunctiva in Diabetes Mellitus. Part I, Microaneurysms,* Am. J. Ophthalmol., **55:** 504, 1963.
187. Tamura, T.: *Electron Microscopical Observation of the Capillaries of the Bulbar Conjunctiva in Diabetic and Non-Diabetic Patients,* Jap. J. Ophthalmol., **11:** 193, 1967.
188. MacKenzie, S.: *A Case of Glycosuric Retinitis, with Comments by E. Nettleship,* Ophthal. Hosp. Rep., **9:** 134, 1877.
189. Ashton, N.: *Diabetic Micro-Angiopathy,* Bibl. Ophthalmol., **52:** 1, 1958; also Adv. Ophthalmol., **8:** 1, 1958.
190. Wolter, J. R.: *Diabetic Capillary Microaneurysms of the Retina,* Arch. Ophthalmol., **65:** 847, 1961.
191. Cogan, D. G.: *Diabetic Retinopathy,* N. Engl. J. Med., **270:** 787, 1964.
192. Pope, C. H., Jr.: *Retinal Capillary Microaneurysms. A Concept of Pathogenesis,* Diabetes, **9:** 9, 1960.
193. Cook, C. A. G.: *Role of Fat Emboli in Diabetic Retinopathy,* Br. J. Ophthalmol., **41:** 741, 1957.
194. Kohner, E. M., Dollery, C. T., Paterson, J. W., and Oakley, N. W.: *Arterial Fluorescein Studies in Diabetic Retinopathy,* Diabetes, **16:** 1, 1967.
195. Edington, G. M. and Sarkies, J. W. R.: *Two Cases of Sickle-Cell Anaemia Associated with Retinal Microaneurysms,* Trans. R. Soc. Trop. Med. Hyg., **46:** 59, 1952.
196. Wexler, D. and Branower, G.: *Retinal Capillary Lesions in Malignant Hypertension,* Arch. Ophthalmol., **44:** 539, 1950.
197. Becker, B.: *Diabetic Retinopathy,* Ann.

Intern. Med., **37:** 273, 1952.
198. Patz, A. and Maumenee, A. E.: *Studies on Diabetic Retinopathy. Part I, Retinopathy in a Dog with Spontaneous Diabetes Mellitus,* Am. J. Ophthalmol., **54:** 532, 1962.
199. Hausler, H. R., Sibay, T. M., and Campbell, J.: *Retinopathy in a Dog Following Diabetes Induced by Growth Hormone,* Diabetes, **13:** 122, 1964.
200. Musacchio, I. T. L., Palermo, N., and Rodriguez, R. R.: *Microaneurysms in the Retina of Diabetic Rats,* Lancet, **1:** 146, 1964.
201. Engerman, R. L. and Bloodworth, J. M. B., Jr.: *Experimental Diabetic Retinopathy in Dogs,* Arch. Ophthalmol., **73:** 205, 1965.
202. Patz, A., Berkow, J. W., Maumenee, A. E., and Cox, J.: *Studies on Diabetic Retinopathy. Part II, Retinopathy and Neuropathy in Spontaneous Canine Diabetes,* Diabetes, **14:** 700, 1965.
203. Mutlu, F. and Leopold, I. H.: *Allergic Response of Retinal Vessel 6 after Intravitreal Foreign Protein,* Arch. Ophthalmol., **72:** 513, 1964.
204. Berken, A.: *Ocular Changes in the Schwartzman Reaction. Their Possible Relationship to Diabetic Retinopathy,* Arch. Ophthalmol., **67:** 505, 1962.
205. Ashton, N.: *Retinal Micro-Aneurysms in the Non-Diabetic Subject,* Br. J. Ophthalmol., **35:** 189, 1951.
206. Snell, A. C.: *Angiomatosis Retinae. A Clinical Report of One Case,* Am. Ophthalmol. Soc., **25:** 216, 1927.
207. Ashton, N.: *Retinal Angiogenesis in the Human Embryo,* Br. Med. Bull., **26:** 103, 1970.
208. Michaelson, I. C. and Campbell, A. C. P.: *Anatomy of Finer Retinal Vessels and Some Observations on Their Significance in Certain Retinal Diseases,* Trans. Ophthalmol. Soc. U. K., **60:** 71, 1940.
209. Michaelson, I. C.: *The Mode of Development of the Vascular System of the Retina, with Some Observations on Its Significance for Certain Retinal Diseases,* Trans. Ophthalmol. Soc. U. K., **68:** 137, 1948.
210. Davis, M. D.: *Vitreous Contraction in Proliferative Diabetic Retinopathy,* Arch. Ophthalmol., **74:** 741, 1965.
211. Madsen, P. H.: *Aneurysms on New-Formed Pre-Papillary and Pre-Retinal Vessels in Proliferative Diabetic Retinopathy,* Br. J. Ophthalmol., **50:** 527, 1966.
212. Wise, G. N.: *Retinal Neovascularization,* Trans. Am. Ophthalmol. Soc., **54:** 729, 1956.
213. Ballantyne, A. J.: *New-Formed Vessels in the Fundus Oculi,* Ophthalmologica, **118:** 611, 1949.
214. Ashton, N.: *Pathological Basis of Retrolental Fibroplasia,* Br. J. Ophthalmol., **38:** 385, 1954.
215. Reese, A. B., Blodi, F. C., and Locke, J. C.: *The Pathology of Early Retrolental Fibroplasia, with an Analysis of the Histologic Findings in the Eyes of Newborn and Stillborn Infants,* Am. J. Ophthalmol., **35:** 1407, 1952.
216. Ashton, N., Ward, B., and Serpell, G.: *Effect of Oxygen on Developing Retinal Vessels with Particular Reference to the Problem of Retrolental Fibroplasia,* Br. J. Ophthalmol., **38:** 397, 1954.
217. Lewis, W. H.: *The Outgrowth of Endothelium and Capillaries in Tissue Culture,* Bull. Johns Hopkins Hosp., **48:** 242, 1931.
218. Clark, E. R. and Clark, E. L.: *Microscopic Observations on the Growth of Blood Capillaries in the Living Mammal,* Am. J. Anat., **64:** 251, 1939.
219. Ashton, N.: *Neovascularization in Ocular Disease,* Trans. Ophthalmol. Soc. U. K., **81:** 145, 1961.
220. Imre, G.: *Studies on the Mechanism of Retinal Neovascularization. Role of Lactic Acid,* Br. J. Ophthalmol., **48:** 75, 1964.
221. Goldberg, M. F.: *Classification and Pathogenesis of Proliferative Sickle Retinopathy,* Am. J. Ophthalmol., **71:** 649, 1971.
222. Andersson, B. and Samuelson, A.: *A Case of Hyperglobulinemia with Pronounced Eye Changes and Acrocyanosis,* Acta Med. Scand., **117:** 248, 1944.
223. Heath, P.: *Retrolental Fibroplasia as a Syndrome. Pathogenesis and Classifications,* Arch. Ophthalmol., **44:** 245, 1950.
224. Ray, B. S., Pazianos, A. G., Greenberg, E., Peretz, W. L., and McLean, J. M.: *Pituitary Ablation for Diabetic Retinopathy. Part I, Results of Hypophystectomy (A Ten-Year Evaluation),* JAMA, **203:** 79, 1968.
225. Ray, B. S., Pazianos, A. G., Greenberg, E., Peretz, W. L., and McLean, J. M.: *Pituitary Ablation for Diabetic Retinopathy. Part II, Results of Yttrium 90 Implantation in the Pituitary Gland,* JAMA, **203:** 85, 1968.
226. Kohner, E. M., Dollery, C. T., Fraser, T. R., and Bulpitt, C. J.: *Effect of Pituitary Ablation on Diabetic Retinopathy Studied by Fluorescence Angiography,* Diabetes, **19:** 703, 1970.
227. Okun, E. and Cibis, P. A.: *The Role of Photocoagulation in the Therapy of Proliferative Diabetic Retinopathy,* Arch. Ophthalmol., **75:** 337, 1966.

228. Meyer-Schwickerath, G.: *Indications and Limitations of Light Coagulation of the Retina,* Trans. Am. Acad. Ophthalmol. and Otolaryngol., **63:** 725, 1959.
229. Wetzig, P. C. and Worlton, J. T.: *Treatment of Diabetic Retinopathy by Light-Coagulation,* Br. J. Ophthalmol., **47:** 539, 1963.
230. Okun, E. and Collins, E. M.: *Histopathology of Experimental Photocoagulation in the Dog Eye. Part I, Graded Lesions, Vitreous Effect and Complications,* Am. J. Ophthalmol., **54:** 3, 1962.
231. Powell, J. O., Bresnick, G. H., Yanoff, M., Frisch, G. D., and Chester, J. E.: *Ocular Effects of Argon Laser Radiation. Part II, Histopathology of Chorioretinal Lesions,* Am. J. Ophthalmol., **71:** 1267, 1971.
232. Dobree, J. H.: *Proliferative Diabetic Retinopathy. Evolution of the Retinal Lesions,* Br. J. Ophthalmol., **48:** 637, 1964.
233. Friedenwald, J. S., Owens, W. C., and Owens, E. U.: *Retrolental Fibroplasia in Premature Infants. Part III, The Pathology of the Disease,* Trans. Am. Ophthalmol. Soc. (1951), **49:** 207, 1952.
234. Hanum, S.: *Diabetic Retinitis. Clinical Studies of 195 Cases of Retinal Changes in Diabetics,* Acta Ophthalmol., Suppl.: 16, 1939.
235. Klien, B. A.: *Retinitis Proliferans. Clinical and Histologic Studies,* Arch. Ophthalmol., **20:** 427, 1938.
236. Tolentino, F. I., Lee, P. F., and Schepens, C. L.: *Biomicroscopic Study of Vitreous Cavity in Diabetic Retinopathy,* Arch. Ophthalmol., **75:** 238, 1966.
237. Root, H. F., Mirsky, S., and Ditzel, J.: *Proliferative Retinopathy in Diabetes Mellitus. Review of Eight Hundred Forty-Seven Cases,* JAMA, **169:** 903, 1959.
238. Beetham, W. P.: *Visual Prognosis of Proliferating Diabetic Retinopathy,* Br. J. Ophthalmol., **47:** 611, 1963.
239. Goldberg, M. F.: *Natural History of Untreated Proliferative Sickle Retinopathy,* Arch. Ophthalmol., **85:** 428, 1971.
240. Goldberg, M. F. and Fine, S. L. (eds.): *Symposium on the Treatment of Diabetic Retinopathy, 1968,* U. S. Public Health Service, Arlington, Va., 1969.
241. Panisset, A., Kohner, E. M., Cheng, H., and Fraser, T. R.: *Diabetic Retinopathy. New Vessels Arising from the Optic Disc. Part II, Response to Pituitary Ablation by Yttrium 90 Implant,* Diabetes, **20:** 824, 1971.
242. Duke-Elder, W. S.: *Textbook of Ophthalmology,* Vol. III, *Diseases of the Inner Eye,* pp. 2890–2926, Mosby, St. Louis, 1940.
243. Becker, B. and Shaffer, R. N.: *Diagnosis and Therapy of the Glaucomas,* pp. 175, 208, Mosby, St. Louis, 1965.
244. Hohl, R. D. and Barnett, D. M.: *Diabetic Hemorrhagic Glaucoma,* Diabetes, **19:** 944, 1970.
245. Walsh, F. B. and Hoyt, W. F.: *Clinical Neuro-Ophthalmology,* 3rd ed., Vol. I, pp. 567–641, Williams & Wilkins, Baltimore, 1969.
246. Miller, S. J. H., Sanders, M. D., and Ffytche, T. J.: *Fluorescein Fundus Photography in the Detection of Early Papilloedema and Its Differentiation from Pseudo-Papilloedema,* Lancet, **2:** 651, 1965.
247. Dollery, C. T., Mailer, C. M., and Hodge, J. V.: *Studies by Fluorescence Photography of Papilloedema in Malignant Hypertension,* J. Neurol. Neurosurg. Psychiatry, **28:** 241, 1965.
248. Reese, A. B.: *Relation of Drusen of the Optic Nerve to Tuberous Sclerosis,* Arch. Ophthalmol., **24:** 187, 1940.
249. Paton, L. and Holmes, G.: *The Pathology of Papilloedema. A Histological Study of Sixty Eyes,* Brain, **33:** 389, 1911.
250. Leinfelder, P. J.: *Pathogenesis of Papilledema,* Am. J. Ophthalmol., **48:** 107, 1959.
251. Cushing, H. and Bordley, J., Jr.: *Observations of Experimentally Induced Choked Disc,* Johns Hopkins Hosp. Bull., **20:** 95, 1909.
252. Hayreh, S. S.: *Pathogenesis of Oedema of the Optic Disc (Papilloedema),* Br. J. Ophthalmol., **48:** 522, 1964.
253. McAlpine, D.: *Papilloedema Caused by a Cervical Cord Tumour,* Lancet, **2:** 614, 1935.
254. Love, J. G., Wagener, H. P., and Woltman, H. W.: *Tumors of the Spinal Cord Associated with Choking of the Optic Disks,* Arch. Neurol. Psychiatry, **66:** 171, 1951.
255. Miller, A., Bader, R. A., and Bader, M. E.: *The Neurologic Syndrome Due to Marked Hypercapnia, with Papilledema,* Am. J. Med., **33:** 309, 1962.
256. McCormack, W. M. and Spalter, H. F.: *Muscular Dystrophy, Alveolar Hypoventilation, and Papilledema,* JAMA, **197:** 957, 1966.
257. Bronsky, D., Kushner, D. S., Dubin, A., and Snapper, I.: *Idiopathic Hypoparathyroidism and Pseudohypoparathyroidism. Reports and Review of the Literature,* Medicine, **37:** 317, 1958.
258. Leinfelder, P. J. and Paul, W. D.: *Papilledema in General Diseases,* Arch. Ophthalmol., **28:** 983, 1942.
259. Stoebner, R., Kiser, R., and Alperin, J. B.: *Iron Deficiency Anemia and Papilledema. Rapid Resolution with Oral Iron Therapy,* Am. J. Dig. Dis., **15:** 919, 1970.

260. Weiman, C. G., McDowell, F. H., and Plum, F.: *Papilledema in Poliomyelitis,* Arch. Neurol. Psychiatry, **66:** 722, 1951.
261. Drew, A. L. and Magee, K. R.: *Papilledema in the Guillain-Barré Syndrome,* Arch. Neurol. Psychiatry, **66:** 744, 1951.
262. Primrose, J.: *Mechanism of Production of Papilloedema,* Br. J. Ophthalmol., **48:** 19, 1964.
263. Zimmerman, L. E.: *Histology and General Pathology of the Optic Nerve,* Trans. Am. Acad. Ophthalmol. and Otolaryngol., **60:** 14, 1956.
264. Ridley, H.: *Ocular Manifestations of Malnutrition in Released Prisoners of War from Thailand,* Br. J. Ophthalmol., **29:** 613, 1945.
265. Spillane, J. D.: *Nutritional Disorders of the Nervous System,* pp. 158–161, Williams & Wilkins, Baltimore, 1947.
266. Denny-Brown, D.: *Neurological Conditions Resulting from Prolonged and Severe Dietary Restriction (Case Reports on Prisoners of War, and General Review),* Medicine, **26:** 41, 1947.
267. Fisher, M.: *Residual Neuropathological Changes in Canadians Held Prisoners of War by the Japanese (Strachan's Disease),* Can. Serv. Med. J., **11:** 157, 1955.
268. King, J. H. and Passmore, J. W.: *Nutritional Amblyopia. A Study of American Prisoners of War in Korea,* Am. J. Ophthalmol., **39** (4, pt. 2): 173, 1955.
269. Carroll, F. D.: *The Etiology and Treatment of Tobacco-Alcohol Amblyopia,* Am. J. Ophthalmol., **27:** 713, 847, 1944.
270. Victor, M., Mancall, E. L., and Dreyfus, P. M.: *Deficiency Amblyopia in the Alcoholic Patient. A Clinicopatholgic Study,* Arch. Ophthalmol., **64:** 1, 1960.
271. Victor, M. and Dreyfus, P. M.: *Tobacco-Alcohol Ambylopia. Further Comments on Its Pathology,* Arch. Ophthalmol., **74:** 649, 1965.
272. Rodger, F. C.: *Experimental Thiamin Deficiency as a Cause of Degeneration in the Visual Pathway of the Rat,* Br. J. Ophthalmol., **37:** 11, 1953.
273. MacDonald, A. E.: *The Pathology of Methyl Alcohol Amblyopia,* XIII Concilium Ophthalmologicum, Amsterdam, **2:** 440, 1929.
274. Gifford, S. R.: *The Relation of the Paranasal Sinuses to Ocular Disorders, Especially to Retrobulbar Neuritis,* Arch. Ophthalmol., **5:** 276, 1931.
275. Berliner, M. L.: *Acute Optic Neuritis in Demyelinating Diseases of the Nervous System,* Arch. Ophthalmol., **13:** 83, 1935.
276. Benedict, W. L.: *Multiple Sclerosis as an Etiologic Factor in Retrobulbar Neuritis,* Arch. Ophthalmol., **28:** 988, 1942.
277. Levine, J.: *Pellagra as a Cause of Optic Neuritis. Report of a Case,* Arch. Ophthalmol., **12:** 902, 1934.
278. Fine, M. and Lachman, G. S.: *Retrobulbar Neuritis in Pellagra,* Am. J. Ophthalmol., **20:** 708, 1937.
279. Carroll, F. D.: *"Alcohol" Amblyopia, Pellagra, and Polyneuritis. Report of Ten Cases,* Arch. Ophthalmol., **16:** 919, 1936.
280. Victor, M.: *Tobacco–Alcohol Amblyopia. A Critique of Current Concepts of This Disorder, with Special Reference to the Role of Nutritional Deficiency in Its Causation,* Arch. Ophthalmol., **70:** 313, 1963.
281. Skillern, P. G. and Lockhart, G.: *Optic Neuritis and Uncontrolled Diabetes Mellitus in 14 Patients,* Ann. Intern. Med.. **51:** 468, 1959.
282. Freund, M., Carmon, A., and Cohen, A. M.: *Papilledema and Papillitis in Diabetes. A Report of Two Cases,* Am. J. Ophthalmol., **60:** 18, 1965.
283. Hedges, T. R., Jr. and Scheie, H. G.: *Visual Field Defects in Exophthalmos Associated with Thyroid Disease,* Arch. Ophthalmol., **54:** 885, 1955.
284. Wegener, H. P.: *Lesions of the Optic Nerve in Exophthalmos of Endocrine Origin,* Am. J. Med. Sci., **232:** 226, 1956.
285. Henderson, J. W.: *Optic Neuropathy of Exophthalmic Goiter (Grave's Disease),* Arch. Ophthalmol., **59:** 471, 1958.
286. Freeman, A. G. and Heaton, J. M.: *The Aetiology of Retrobulbar Neuritis in Addisonian Pernicious Anemia,* Lancet, **1:** 908, 1961.
287. Drance, S. M.: *Quinine Amaurosis,* Br. J. Ophthalmol., **39:** 178, 1955.
288. Turtz, C. A.: *Transient Loss of Vision Following Use of Quinine,* Am. J. Ophthalmol., **44:** 110, 1957.
289. Wallenstein, I. and Snyder, J.: *Neurotoxic Reaction to Chloromycetin,* Ann. Intern. Med., **36:** 1526, 1952.
290. Cole, J. G., Cole, H. G., and Janoff, L. A.: *A Toxic Ocular Manifestation of Chloramphenicol Therapy. Report of a Case of Optic Neuritis,* Am. J. Ophthalmol., **44:** 18, 1957.
291. Lietman, P. S., diSant'Agnese, P. A., and Wong, V.: *Optic Neuritis in Cystic Fibrosis of the Pancreas. Role of Chloramphenicol Therapy,* JAMA, **189:** 924, 1964.
292. Sutton, P. H. and Beattie, P. H.: *Optic Atrophy after Administration of Isoniazid with P.A.S.,* Lancet, **1:** 650, 1955.

293. Keeping, J. A. and Searle, C. W. A.: *Optic Neuritis Following Isoniazid Therapy,* Lancet, **2:** 278, 1955.
294. Kass, I., Mandel, W., Cohen, H., and Dressler, S. H.: *Isoniazid as a Cause of Optic Neuritis and Atrophy,* JAMA, **164:** 1740, 1957.
295. Kestenbaum, A.: *Clinical Methods of Neuro-Ophthalmologic Examination,* 2nd ed., pp. 147–148, Grune & Stratton, New York, 1961.
296. Kant, A.: *The Ophthalmoscopic Evaluation of Optic Atrophy,* Am. J. Ophthalmol., **32:** 1479, 1949.
297. Verhoeff, F. H.: *Microscopic Observations in a Case of Retinitis Pigmentosa,* Arch. Ophthalmol., **5:** 392, 1931.
298. Hagedoorn, A.: *Amaurotic Idiocy and Related Conditions. Pathology of the Retina in Infantile Amaurotic Idiocy,* Am. J. Ophthalmol., **23:** 735, 1940
299. Goldstein, I. and Wexler, D.: *Niemann-Pick's Disease with Cherry-Red Spots in the Macula,* Arch. Ophthalmol., **5:** 704, 1931.
300. Verhoeff, F. H.: *Amaurotic Family Idiocy. Histological Examination of a Case in Which the Eyes Were Removed Immediately after Death,* Arch. Ophthalmol., **38:** 107, 1909.
301. Hancock, W. I. and Coats, G.: *Pathological Examination of the Freshly Fixed Eyes from a Case of Amaurotic Family Idiocy,* Brain, **33:** 514, 1911.
302. MacMillan, J. A.: *Histology of the Retina in a Case of Tay-Sach's Disease,* Am. J. Ophthalmol., **31:** 1567, 1948.
303. Sugar, H. S.: *The Glaucomas,* 2nd ed., p. 147, Hoeber-Harper, New York, 1957.
304. Wolff, E.: *Schnabel's Cavernous Atrophy,* Trans. Ophthalmol. Soc. U.K., **67:** 133, 1947.
305. Hayreh, S. S.: *Blood Supply of the Optic Nerve Head and Its Role in Optic Atrophy, Glaucoma, and Oedema of the Optic Disc,* Br. J. Ophthalmol., **53:** 721, 1969.
306. Hayreh, S. S.: *Pathogenesis of Visual Field Defects. Role of the Ciliary Circulation,* Br. J. Ophthalmol., **54:** 289, 1970.
307. Hayreh, S. S., Revie, I. H. S., and Edwards, J.: *Vasogenic Origin of Visual Field Defects and Optic Nerve Changes in Glaucoma,* Br. J. Ophthalmol., **54:** 461, 1970.
308. Giannini, D.: *Dell' Influenza dei Disturbi di Circolo Sulla Patogenesi delle Alterazioni Funzionali ed Anatomiche del Nervo Ottico e della Retina Negli Avvelenamenti da Chinino,* Ann. Ottal., **62:** 1069, 1934.
309. Francois, J.: *Heredity in Ophthalmology,* pp. 497–518, Mosby, St. Louis, 1961.
310. Schappert-Kimmijser, J., Henkees, H. E., and Van den Bosch, J.: *Amaurosis Congenita (Leber),* Arch. Ophthalmol., **61:** 211, 1959.
311. Kwittken, J. and Barest, H. D.: *The Neuropathology of Hereditary Optic Atrophy (Leber's Disease). The First Complete Anatomic Study,* Am. J. Pathol., **34:** 185, 1958.
312. Scott, J. G.: *Hereditary Optic Atrophy with Dominant Transmission and Early Onset,* Br. J. Ophthalmol., **25:** 461, 1941.
313. Iverson, H. A.: *Hereditary Optic Atrophy,* Arch. Ophthalmol., **59:** 850, 1958.
314. Kjer, P.: *Infantile Optic Atrophy with Dominant Mode of Inheritance. A Clinical and Genetic Study of 19 Danish Families,* Acta Ophthalmol., Suppl.: 54, 1959.
315. Kok-van Alphen, C. C.: *A Family with the Dominant Infantile Form of Optical Atrophy,* Acta Ophthalmol., **38:** 675, 1960.
316. Cushing, H.: *The Chiasmal Syndrome of Primary Optic Atrophy and Bitemporal Field Defects in Adults with a Normal Sella Turcica,* Arch. Ophthalmol., **3:** 505, 704, 1930.
317. Hartmann, E.: *Optochiasmic Arachnoiditis,* Arch. Ophthalmol., **33:** 68, 1945.
318. Kennedy, F.: *Retrobulbar Neuritis as an Exact Diagnostic Sign of Certain Tumors and Abscesses in the Frontal Lobes,* Am. J. Med. Sci., **142:** 355, 1911.
319. Traquair, H. M., Dott, N. M., and Russell, W. R.: *Traumatic Lesions of the Optic Chiasma,* Brain, **58:** 398, 1935.
320. Walsh, F. B. and Ford, F. R.: *Central Scotomas. Their Importance in Topical Diagnosis,* Arch. Ophthalmol., **24:** 500, 1940.
321. Kennedy, F.: *A Further Note on the Diagnostic Value of Retrobulbar Neuritis in Expanding Lesions of the Frontal Lobes, with a Report of This Syndrome in a Case of Aneurysm of the Right Carotid Artery,* JAMA, **67:** 1361, 1916.
322. Yaskin, H. E. and Schlezinger, N. S.: *Foster Kennedy Syndrome with Non-Neoplastic Intracranial Conditions,* Arch. Ophthalmol., **28:** 704, 1942.
323. Cordes, F. C.: *Optic Atrophy in Infancy, Childhood, and Adolescence. A Survey of 81 Cases,* Am. J. Ophthalmol., **35:** 1272, 1952.
324. Craig, W. McK. and Lillie, W. I.: *Chiasmal Syndrome Produced by Chronic Local Arachnoiditis. Report of Eight Cases,* Arch. Ophthalmol., **5:** 558, 1931.

325. Lillie, W. I.: *Perchiasmal Syndrome Produced by Chronic Local Arachnoiditis. Report of Three Cases,* Arch. Ophthalmol., **24:** 940, 1940.
326. Yaskin, H. E. and Alpers, B. J.: *Foster Kennedy Syndrome with Post-Traumatic Arachnoiditis of Optic Chiasm and Base of Frontal Lobes,* Arch. Ophthalmol., **34:** 399, 1945.
327. Holmes, G. and Lister, W. T.: *Disturbances of Vision from Cerebral Lesions, with Special Reference to Cortical Representation of the Macula,* Brain, **39:** 34, 1916.
328. Greear, J. N. and McGavic, J. S.: *Visual Disturbances Associated with Head Injuries,* Arch. Ophthalmol., **36:** 33, 1946.
329. Woods, A. C.: *Optic Neuropathies. A Simplified Classification and Outline for Etiologic Diagnosis,* Am. J. Ophthalmol., **31:** 1053, 1948.
330. Collis, W. J.: *Acute Unilateral Retrobulbar Neuritis,* Arch. Neurol., **13:** 409, 1965.
331. Croll, M.: *The Ocular Manifestations of Multiple Sclerosis,* Am. J. Ophthalmol., **60:** 822, 1965.
332. Hoyt, W. F.: *Charcot-Marie-Tooth Disease with Primary Optic Atrophy. Report of a Case,* Arch Ophthalmol., **64:** 925, 1960.
333. Austin, J. H.: *Metachromatic Form of Diffuse Cerebral Sclerosis. Part I, Diagnosis During Life by Urine Sediment Examination,* Neurology, **7:** 415, 1957.
334. Robb, R. M. and Watters, G. V.: *Ophthalmic Manifestations of Subacute Sclerosing Panencephalitis,* Arch. Ophthalmol., **83:** 426, 1970.
335. Breakey, A. S.: *Ocular Findings in Cerebral Palsy,* Arch. Ophthalmol., **53:** 852, 1955.
336. Pemberton, J. W. and Freeman, J. M.: *Craniosynostosis. A Review of Experience with Forty Patients with Particular Reference to Ocular Aspects and Comments on Operative Indications,* Am. J. Ophthalmol., **54:** 641, 1962.
337. Riser, R. O.: *Marble Bones and Optic Atrophy,* Am. J. Ophthalmol., **24:** 874, 1941.
338. Ellis, P. P. and Jackson, W. E.: *Osteopetrosis. A Clinical Study of Optic-Nerve Involvement,* Am. J. Ophthalmol., **53:** 943, 1962.
339. Adams, R. D. and Sidman, R. L.: *Introduction to Neuropathology,* pp. 283–287, McGraw-Hill, New York, 1968.
340. Fredrickson, D. S. and Trams, E. G.: *Ganglioside Lipidosis. Tay-Sach's Disease,* in Stanbury, J. B., Wyngaarden, J. B., and Fredrickson, D. S. (eds.): *The Metabolic Basis of Inherited Disease,* 2nd ed., p. 523, McGraw-Hill, New York, 1966.
341. Fredrickson, D. S.: *Sphingomyelin Lipidosis. Niemann-Pick Disease,* in Stanbury, J. B., Wyngaarden, J. B., and Fredrickson, D. S. (eds.): *The Metabolic Basis of Inherited Disease,* 2nd ed., p. 586, McGraw-Hill, New York, 1966.
342. Olivarius, B. de F. and Jensen, L.: *Retrobulbar Neuritis and Optic Atrophy in Pernicious Aenmia,* Acta Ophthalmol., **39:** 190, 1961.
343. Waite, J. H. and Beetham, W. P.: *The Visual Mechanism in Diabetes Mellitus. A Comparative Study of 2002 Diabetics and 457 Non-Diabetics for Control,* N. Engl. J. Med., **212:** 367, 1935.
344. Waite, J. H. and Beetham, W. P.: *The Visual Mechanism in Diabetes Mellitus. A Comparative Study of 2002 Diabetics and 457 Non-Diabetics for Control,* N. Engl. J. Med., **212:** 429, 1935.
345. Stansbury, J. R.: *Optic Atrophy in Diabetes Mellitus. A Report of Three Cases in One Family,* Am. J. Ophthalmol., **31:** 1153, 1948.
346. Lyle, T. K.: *The Management of Hormonal Exophthalmos. Ocular Deviation and Defects of Ocular Movement (and Some Cases Showing Visual Field Defects),* Trans. Ophthalmol. Soc. U. K., **80:** 107, 1960.
347. Naffziger, H. C.: *Pathologic Changes in the Orbit in Progressive Exophthalmos with Special Reference to Alterations in the Extraocular Muscles and the Optic Disks,* Arch. Ophthalmol., **9:** 1, 1933.
348. Jackson, E.: *Methyl Alcohol Poisoning* (editorial), Am. J. Ophthalmol., **3:** 150, 1920.
349. Griscom, J. M.: *Hereditary Optic Atrophy,* Am. J. Ophthalmol., **4:** 347, 1921.
350. Woodworth, J. A., Beckett, R. S., and Netsky, M. G.: *A Composite of Hereditary Ataxias. A Familial Disorder with Features of Olivopontocerebellar Atrophy, Leber's Optic Atrophy, and Fredrickson's Ataxia,* Arch. Intern. Med., **104:** 594, 1959.
351. Waardenburg, P. J., Franceschetti, A., and Klein, D.: *Genetics and Ophthalmology,* Vol. II, *Neuro-Ophthalmological Part,* p. 1617, Charles C Thomas, Springfield, Ill.; Royal Van Corcum Publisher Assen, Netherlands; and Blackwell Scientific Publications Ltd., Oxford, 1963.
352. Jefferson, G.: *Compression of the Chiasma, Optic Nerves, and Optic Tracts by Intracranial Aneurysms,* Brain, **60:** 444, 1937.

353. Marthinsen, R.: *The Supraclinoid Carotid Aneurysm,* Acta Ophthalmol., **19:** 141, 1941.
354. Walsh, F. B. and King, A. B.: *Ocular Signs of Intracranial Saccular Aneurysms. Experimental Work on Collateral Circulation Through the Ophthalmic Artery,* Arch. Ophthalmol., **27:** 1, 1942.
355. Adson, A. W.: *Surgical Treatment of Vascular Diseases Altering the Function of the Eyes,* Am. J. Ophthalmol., **25:** 824, 1942.
356. Ley, A.: *Compression of the Optic Nerve by a Fusiform Aneurysm of the Carotid Artery,* J. Neurol. Neurosurg. Psychiatry, **13:** 75, 1950.
357. White, J. C. and Adams, R. D.: *Combined Supra- and Infraclinoid Aneurysms of Internal Carotid Artery. Report of a Case of Unusual Congenital Dilatation of Intracranial Portion of Carotid Artery and Injuries to Visual, Oculomotor, Sensory, and Taste Fibers,* J. Neurosurg., **12:** 450, 1955.
358. Durston, J. H. J. and Parsons-Smith, B. G.: *Blindness Due to Aneurysm of Anterior Communicating Artery, with Recovery Following Carotid Ligation,* Br. J. Ophthalmol., **54:** 170, 1970.
359. Miller, A. J. and Cuttino, J. T.: *On the Mechanism of Production of Massive Preretinal Hemorrhage Following Rupture of a Congenital Medial-Defect Intracranial Aneurysm,* Am. J. Ophthalmol., **31:** 15, 1948.
360. Fahmy, J. A., Knudsen, V., and Andersen, S. R.: *Intraocular Haemorrhage Following Subarachnoid Haemorrhage,* Acta Ophthalmol., **47:** 550, 1959.
361. White, L. E. and Foltz, E. L.: *Optic Atrophy as an Isolated Sign of Unruptured Carotid Aneurysm,* Neurology, **7:** 803, 1957.
362. Chisholm, I. A.: *Optic Neuropathy of Recurrent Blood Loss,* Br. J. Ophthalmol., **53:** 289, 1969.

Index